Mycobacterium bovis Infection in Animals and Humans

Second Edition

Mycobacterium bovis Infection in Animals and Humans
Second Edition

Charles O. Thoen, DVM, Phd

James H. Steele, DVM, MPH

Michael J. Gilsdorf, DVM, MS

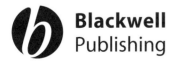
Blackwell Publishing

Charles O. Thoen, DVM, PhD, is Professor in the Department of Veterinary Microbiology and Preventive Medicine, College of Veterinary Medicine, Iowa State University. Dr. Thoen is former Chairman of the Department of Veterinary Microbiology and Preventative Medicine at Iowa State University's College of Veterinary Medicine, Chairman of the International Union against Tuberculosis and Lung Disease Scientific Committee on Tuberculosis in Animals, and former Chairman of the World Health Organization Committee on Animal Tuberculosis.

James H. Steele, DVM, MPH, is Professor Emeritus, Environmental Health, the University of Texas–Houston, School of Public Health, Center for Infectious Diseases, Houston, Texas. Dr. Steele was formerly Chief Veterinary Officer, Assistant Surgeon General, U.S. Public Health Service; Consult to United Nations agencies, World Health Organization, Food and Agriculture Organization, Pan American Health Organization, International Atomic Energy Organization, and World Bank.

Michael J. Gilsdorf is Director at the National Center for Animal Health Programs—Eradication and Surveillance, USDA, APHIS, VS, Riverdale, Maryland.

©2006 Blackwell Publishing

Blackwell Publishing Professional
2121 State Avenue, Ames, Iowa 50014, USA

Orders:	1-800-862-6657
Office:	1-515-292-0140
Fax:	1-515-292-3348
Web site:	www.blackwellprofessional.com

Blackwell Publishing Ltd
9600 Garsington Road, Oxford OX4 2DQ, UK
Tel.: +44 (0)1865 776868

Blackwell Publishing Asia
550 Swanston Street, Carlton, Victoria 3053, Australia
Tel.: +61 (0)3 8359 1011

First edition, 1995 Iowa State University Press
Second edition, 2006

Library of Congress Cataloging-in-Publication Data

Mycobacterium bovis infection in animals and humans / [edited by] Charles O. Thoen, James H. Steele, Michael J. Gilsdorf. - 2nd ed.
    p. cm.
Includes bibliographical references and index.
ISBN-13: 978-0-8138-0919-9 (alk. paper)
ISBN-10: 0-8138-0919-3 (alk. paper)
1. Tuberculosis. 2. Tuberculosis in cattle. 3. *Mycobacterium bovis*. 4. AIDS (Disease)-Complications. I. Thoen, Charles O. II. Steele, James H. III. Gilsdorf, Michael J.

RC311.19.M93 2006
616.9'95—dc22

2005018463

The last digit is the print number: 9 8 7 6 5 4 3 2

Contents

Contributors

David A. Ashford, DVM, MPH, DSc
Lead, Epidemiology, Public Health Emergency Preparedness Team
US Public Health Service
EEHS/NCEH/ATSDR, CDC,
4770 Buford Highway, MS-F16,
Atlanta, GA 30341
DBA4@cdc.gov

Lekan Ayanwale, DVM, MPH, PhD
Associate Professor
Tuskegee University
College of Veterinary Medicine, Nursing and Allied Health
Department of Pathobiology (BIMS)
Computational Epidemiology, Bioinformatics and Risk Analysis
Tuskegee, AL 36088 USA
ayanwal@tuskegee.edu

John Bannantine, PhD
National Animal Disease Center
USDA-ARS
2300 North Dayton Ave.
Ames, IA 50010
jbannant@nadc.ars.usda.gov

Raul G. Barletta, PhD,
Professor
University of Nebraska-Lincoln
Department of Veterinary and Biomedical Sciences
Lincoln, Nebraska 68583-0905
rbarletta@unl.edu

Goran Bölske, DVM, PhD
National Veterinary Institute
SE-75189 Uppsala, Sweden
Goran.bolske@sva.se

Idowu Cadmus, DVM, MVPH
University of Ibadan
Department of Veterinary Public Health and Preventive Medicine
Faculty of Veterinary Medicine
Ibadan, Nigeria
sibcadmus@yahoo.com

Ofelia Chacon, MD, PhD
Research Scientist
University of Nebraska-Lincoln
Department of Veterinary and Biomedical Sciences
Lincoln, Nebraska 68583-0905
ochacon@unlnotes02.unl.edu

Richard Clifton-Hadley, DVM
Statutory and Exotic Bacteria Programme Manager
Veterinary Laboratory Agency (VLA) (Weybridge)
Woodham Lane
New Haw, Addlestone, Surrey, United Kingdom KT15 3NB
r.s.clifton-hadley@vla.defra.gsi.gov.uk

J.D. Collins, MVB, MVM, MS, Dipl. ECVPH, PhD, MRCVS
University College Dublin
Faculty of Veterinary Medicine
Belfield, Dublin 4, Ireland
Dan.Collins@ucd.ie

Debby Cousins, PhD
Department of Agriculture
Animal Health Laboratories
Australian Reference Laboratory for Bovine Tuberculosis
3 Baron-Hay Court
South Perth, Western Australia 6151
dcousins@agric.wa.gov.au

Isabel N. de Kantor, PhD.
WHO, Member Panel of Experts in Tuberculosis
Av. Libertador 7504, 16 A
(1429) Buenos Aires, Argentina
ikantorp@overnet.com.ar

Terry W. Disney, PhD
Risk Analyst
U.S. Department of Agriculture
2150 Centre Ave.
Ft. Collins, CO 80521
terry.w.disney@aphis.usda.gov

Alessandro Dondo, DVM
Chief of Animal Health
Institute of Zooprofilattico Sperimentale del Piemonte
Via Basso 8
Chivasso, Italy
Allessandro.dondo@izsto.it

Eric D. Ebel, DVM, MS
U.S. Department of Agriculture
Animal and Plant Health Inspection Service
Veterinary Services, Animal Health Programs
National Center for Animal Health Programs, Eradication and Surveillance
2150 Centre Ave.
Ft. Collins, CO 80521
eric.D.Ebel@usda.gov

Donald A. Enarson, M.D.
Director of Scientific Committees
International Union Against Tuberculosis and Lung Disease
68 Boulevard Saint-Michel
Paris 75006 France
Denarson@iuatld.org

Ezio Ferroglio, DVM, PhD, Pip. EVPC
Dipartimento Produzioni Animali
Epidemiologia ed Ecologia
Via Leonarda da Vinci
44010095 Grugliasco(TO), Italy
Ezio.ferroglio@unito.it

Patrice A. Frost, DVM
New Iberia Research Center
4401 West Admiral Doyle Drive
New Iberia, LA 70560
Paf1373@louisiana.edu

Michael J. Gilsdorf, DVM, MS
Director of National Animal Health Programs
U.S. Department of Agriculture
Animal and Plant Health Inspection Service
Veterinary Services
Animal Health Programs
National Center for Animal Health Programs, Eradication and Surveillance
4700 River Road
Riverdale, MD 20737
Michael.J.Gilsdorf@aphis.usda.gov

Tony Goodchild, DVM
Epidemiology Workgroup
Centre for Epidemiology and Risk Analysis
Veterinary Laboratory Agency (Weybridge)
Woodham Lane, New Haw, Addlestone, Surrey
United Kingdom KT15 3NB
tony.goodchild@ntworld.com

Mariella Goria, Doctor of Science
Chief of Biotechnology
Institute of Zooprofilattico Sperimentale del Piemonte
Via Sestruere 51/6
10090 Rivoli, Italy
Mariella.goria@izsto.it

N. Beth Harris, PhD
USDA/APHIS/NVSL
Mycobacteria and Brucella Section
1800 Dayton Ave.
Ames, IA 50014
Beth.n.harris@aphis.usda.gov

Lawrence Judge, DVM, PhD
Area Epidemiologist
U.S. Department of Agriculture
Animal and Plant Health Inspection Service
Veterinary Services
3001 Coolidge Road, Suite 325
East Lansing, MI 48823

John B. Kaneene, DVM, PhD
Professor, Director of Population Medicine
Michigan State University
Veterinary Medical Center
East Lansing, MI
kaneene@cvm.msu.edu

Rudovick R. Kazwala, DVM, PhD
Professor
Sokoine University of Agriculture
Morogoro,Tanzania
kazwala@yahoo.com

Maria A. Koller-Jones, DVM
Senior Staff Veterinarian
Animal Health and Production Division
Canadian Food Inspection Agency
59 Camelot Dr.
Ottawa, Ontario, Canada
mkoller@inspection.gc.ca

N. Kriek, DVM, PhD
Dean University of Pretoria
College of Veterinary Medicine
Faculty of Veterinary Science
P/Bag x04
Onderstepoort 0110, Republic of South Africa
nkriek@op.up.ac.za

B. Larsson, DV.M, PhD
Swedish Board of Agriculture
SE-551 82 Jönköping, Sweden
Bengt.larsson@larsson@svj.se

Philip LoBue, MD, FACP, FCCP
Chief, Medical Consultation Team
Centers for Disease Control and Prevention
Division of Tuberculosis Elimination
Field Services and Evaluation Branch
1600 Clifton Road
Atlanta, GA 30333
pgl5@cdc.gov

Cyril Lutze-Wallace
Acting Leader and Research Scientist
Mycobacterial Diseases Center of Expertise
Canadian Food Inspection Agency
Ottawa Laboratory Fallowfield
3851 Fallowfield Rd.
Ottawa, Ontario, Canada
K2H8P9
lwallacecy@insepction.gc.ca

Guiliana Moda, DVM
Head of Animal Health Unit, Region Piemonte
Via Massena
94-10128 Torino, Italy
igieAlle.Settore@regione.piemonte.it

Zhang-Yong Ning, MS
China Agriculture University
College of Veterinary Medicine
Beijing, China
ningzhy@cau.edu.cn

Ivo Pavlik, DVM, MVDr, CSc,
Associate Professor
Veterinary Research Institute
Department of Food and Feed Safety
Mycobacteriology Unit
OIE Reference Laboratory for Paratuberculosis
Hudcova 70,621 32 Brno,The Czech Republic
pavlik@vri.cz

Dirk Pfeiffer, DVM, PhD
Professor
University of London
Royal Veterinary College
Pfeiffer@rvc.ac.uk

P.J. Quinn, MVB, PhD, MRCVS, MVB, MVM, MS, Dipl. ECVPH
University College Dublin
Faculty of Veterinary Medicine
Belfield, Dublin 4, Ireland

Ana Reniero, PhD
PAHO/WHO Temporary Adviser
Capitán Juan de San Martín 1531
(1609) Boulogne, Italy
renieroa@hotmail.com

Viviana Ritacco, MD, PhD
Scientist
CONICET
National Council of Scientific and Technical Research
ANLIS C. Malbran, Mycobacteria Dept.
Av.Vélez Sárfield 563
(1281) Buenos Aires, Argentina
vritacco@anlis.gov.ar

Jan Ake Robertsson, DVM, PhD
Swedish Animal Health Services
SE-18186 Johanneshov, Sweden
Jan.ake.robertsson@svdhv.org

Felix Roth, MA
Swiss Center of Internacional Health
Swiss Tropical Institute
Basel, Switzerland
Felix.roth@unibas.ch

Luigi Ruocco, DVM
Expert of Infectious Diseases in Domestic Animals
Ministry of Health
Via Raffaello swe-Orte-01029, Italy
l.ruocco@sanita.it

Esther Schelling, DVM, PhD
Swiss Tropical Institute
Department of Public Health and Epidemiology
PO Box 4002 Basel, Switzerland
esther.schelling@unibas.ch

María D. Sequeiro, MSc
Assistant Director
National Institute of Respiratory Disease
INER E. Coni
Av. Blas Parera 8260
(3000) Santa Fe, Argentina
msequeira@infovia.com.ar
labconi@infovia.com.ar

James H. Steele, DVM, MPH
Professor Emeritus
The University of Texas
School of Public Health
Health Science Center at Houston
P.O. Box 20186
Houston, Texas 77225
DrJameshsteele@Houston.rr.com

Om Surujballi, PhD
Research Scientist
Mycobacterial Diseases Center of Expertise
Canadian Food Inspection Agency
Ottawa Laboratory Fallowfield
Ottawa, Ontario, Canada
surujballio@inspection.gc.ca

Charles O. Thoen, DVM, PhD,
Professor
Department of Veterinary Microbiology and Preventive Medicine
College of Veterinary Medicine
Iowa State University, Ames, IA
cthoen@iastate.edu

Bruce Thomson, DVM, PhD
U.S. Department of Agriculture
National Veterinary Services Laboratory
Animal Plant Health Inspection Service
Ames, IA
Bruce.V.Thomson@aphis.usda.gov

Pedro Torres, DVM
Chief, TB Control and Eradication Program
National Service of Animal Health
SENASA,
Av. Paseo Colón 367, 4th Floor
(1063)Buenos Aires, Argentina
tuberculosis@senasa.gov.ar

Claude Turcotte, DVM, PhD
Head, Mycobacteriology
Mycobacterial Diseases Center of Expertise
Canadian Food Inspection Agency
Ottawa Laboratory Fallowfield
Ottawa, Ontario, Canada
turcottec@inspection.gc.ca

R. Verma, MSc, MVSc, PhD
Head and I/C Mycobacteria Laboratory
Indian Veterinary Research Institute
Division of Biological Standardization
Izatnagar-243 122 (Uttar Pradesh) India
Rishendra_verma@yahoo.com

P. Vignetta, DVM
Animal Health Unit of Piemonte
Via Asiago 50-10069 Italy
igiealle@regione.piemonte.it

Laurel Voelker, DVM
108-E Northington Pl
Cary NC 27513
laurelvoelker@gmail.com

H. Wahlström, DVM, PhD
National Veterinary Institute
Zoonoses Center
Uppsala, Sweden
Helene.wahlstrom@sva.se

R. Weiss, DVM, PhD
Professor
Justus-Liebeg University, Giessen, Germany
Reinhard.weiss@vetmed.uni-giessen

Gary West, DVM, Dipl. ACZM
Adjunct Assistant Professor and Director of Veterinary Services
Oklahoma State University
College of Veterinary Medicine
The Oklahoma City Zoo
gwest@okczoo.com

Chang D. Wu, PhD
China Agricultural University
College of Veterinary Medicine
Beijing, China
wucd@cau.edu.cn

D. Zhao, PhD
Beijing University
College of Veterinary Medicine CA4
Beijing, China
zhaodm@edu.cn

Jakob Zinsstag DVM, PhD
Assistant Professor
Swiss Tropical Institute
Department of Public Health and Epidemiology
PO Box 4002 Basel, Switzerland
Jacob.zinsstag@unibas.ch

Preface

Considerable progress has been made toward the eradication of tuberculosis caused by *Mycobacterium bovis* from domestic animals. However, sporadic outbreaks continue to occur in many countries in which the disease was nearly eliminated. The importance of *M. bovis* outbreaks in wild and alternate species and the effects these disease outbreaks have on control of tuberculosis in cattle, other domestic farm animals, captive wild animals, and humans is of concern to public health and regulatory officials throughout the world.

Medical professionals and allied health scientists responsible for the development of tuberculosis control programs are confronted with problems related to suppression of host defenses by viral agents such as HIV (human immunodeficiency virus). Because *M. bovis* infections have recently been reported in humans with AIDS in several countries, protocols for therapeutic intervention must be modified. Therefore, it appears imminent that virulence factors be identified so that new approaches may be initiated for management of disease in these patients. A great deal of progress has been made in the last decade in elucidating the genetics of the genus *Mycobacterium*. However, only a limited knowledge of pathogenesis is available. Although research workers have determined the DNA composition of the genome of *M. bovis*, no specific sequence has been identified that codes for virulence.

The importance of various host factors in providing protection against virulent mycobacteria has been investigated in several laboratories; however, definitive information on their importance in host resistance remains unclear. Most recently, studies on the role of nitric oxide indicate that it may contribute to inhibiting the multiplication of tubercle bacilli and participate in the intracellular killing of these organisms. Other reports indicate that cell wall components may be important in entry and survival in the host macrophage. Many individuals are infected with tubercle bacilli, and a percentage develops progressive disease and dies. Therefore, it would be important to identify host factors responsible for resistance to develop interventions that limit the disease process. The development of multiple-drug-resistant (MDR) strains of the *M. tuberculosis* complex and the isolation of MDR strains from animals and humans further emphasizes the need to obtain an improved understanding of the host mechanisms associated with protection.

It is the purpose of the second edition of this text to provide medical professionals, allied health scientists, research workers, diagnosticians, and graduate students with current information on the significance of *M. bovis* in the control and eradication of tuberculosis in animals and humans. The book also includes current updates on the status of *M. bovis* infection in animals and humans in countries in different regions of the world. This information is of value to public health officials, state and federal regulatory veterinarians, practitioners, and producers interested in the importation of animals for herd additions.

Mycobacterium bovis Infection in Animals and Humans
Second Edition

Chapter 1

Introduction

D.A. Enarson, MD

Mycobacterium bovis, in addition to causing disease in animals, is one of three species of the *Mycobacterium tuberculosis* complex that causes tuberculosis in humans. Although its effect on the economy and livelihood of communities through its effects on cattle and other animals is striking and extensively documented, its role in the global epidemic of human tuberculosis is much less well understood and not studied in great detail. Nevertheless, the elimination of tuberculosis from human society will necessitate understanding and controlling this organism.

The extent of bovine tuberculosis in animals has been summarized previously (1,2). Available information shows that only seven countries of Africa report regular control measures for the disease, and of these, three (Algeria, Burkina Faso, and South Africa) note the disease to be enzootic. An additional six (Tunisia, Mali, Ghana, Burundi, Malawi, and Madagascar) are also noted to have enzootic bovine tuberculosis. Five countries of Asia, of which none have enzootic tuberculosis, have organized control measures. Those with reported enzootic disease include Saudi Arabia, Kuwait, Iraq, Afghanistan, Pakistan, Nepal, Laos, Cambodia, Vietnam, Indonesia, and Papua New Guinea. Enzootic locations in the Americas are Guatemala, El Salvador, Dominican Republic, Peru, Bolivia, Chile, and Argentina. Reports from the countries without organized control programs are much less likely to be reliable.

Fanning has further identified countries with a high occurrence of bovine tuberculosis in animals: in Africa, Angola, Cameroon, Central African Republic, Chad, Congo Republic, Mali, Rwanda, Senegal, Sudan, and Zambia; in Europe, Ireland and Spain; in the Americas, Brazil, Nicaragua, and Venezuela.

Very much less is known about the extent of disease in humans caused by *M. bovis*. Kleeberg (3), Fanning and Edwards (4) and Cosivi et al. (1) have summarized the information available. The table summarizes the published materials reporting on cases in the last 40 years that could be comparably assessed. These reports are primarily from countries with mid-to-low levels of human tuberculosis and, in the case of the market economies, that are comprised of either older patients, who were initially infected many years ago, or foreign-born individuals.

Table 1.1. Series of cases of human tuberculosis caused by *Mycobacterium bovis* reported in the past four decades

Location	Period	Reference	Number of Cases	% of Total	% Pulmonary	Bovine Enzootic
Germany	1963–72	26	555		65	low
Canada	1964–70	19	31	0.5	42	low
Canada	1967–76	27	13	0.3	73	low
Australia	1970–94	28	236	1.4	72	low
Germany	1975–80	29	240	4.5	74	low
England	1977–90	30	232	1.2	40	low
Argentina	1977–82	31	54	2.7	82	high
USA	1980–91	32	73	3.0	52	low
Ireland	1982–85	33	9	0.9	89	high
New Zealand	1983–90	34	22	7.2	32	high
Sweden	1983–92	35	96	2.0		low
Ireland	1986–90	36	17	6.4	71	high
Spain	1986–90	37	10	0.9	50	high
Switzerland	1994	38	18	2.6		low

In all instances, *M. bovis* was isolated in a very small proportion (less than 1 in 10) of all cases.

The lack of knowledge of the extent of this organism as a contributor to the global tuberculosis epidemic in humans must be addressed. In the past, mechanisms for systematically collecting such information at a high level of quality were nonexistent. This is no longer the case. A Global Project on Anti-Tuberculosis Drug Resistance Surveillance has been in place for a number of years; it isolates representative samples of patients from all the regions of the world are systematically collected and evaluated. This network can and needs to be used to gather information about the extent of disease due to *M. bovis*.

The understanding of the role of bovine tuberculosis in human disease has changed considerably over time. Koch became increasingly isolated from the mainstream partly because of his belief that the bovine bacillus was of a much-reduced pathogenicity in man (5,6). Investigations in Great Britain in the early twentieth century (7) definitively demonstrated the role of *M. bovis* in the development of human disease. The extent to which human tuberculosis is caused by *M. bovis* has been difficult to determine with accuracy as a result of technical problems in isolating the microorganisms (discussed in other sections of this book). Although newer molecular methods should help to overcome these obstacles, they will do so only if systematically applied.

The role of bovine tuberculosis in the human epidemic of tuberculosis has been noted in the Netherlands (8), where the introduction of pasteurization of milk in 1940 was postulated as the explanation for a sharp acceleration in the decline of tuberculosis in the country. Styblo (9) documented a continuing reduction in the proportion of cases in which *M. bovis* was isolated, from 10% of pulmonary and 17% of extrapulmonary cases in 1933 to 1% and 0%, respectively, in 1950.

The table also summarizes the information available on the sites of the body affected by tuberculosis in the cases reported. In most instances, the majority of the cases are pulmonary (often very similar to the distribution of all forms of tuberculosis). This observation belies a common misconception that cases of tuberculosis caused by *M. bovis* are typically extrapulmonary. This impression arose from observations that, in previous periods, *M. bovis* was particularly frequent in sites thought to represent primary tuberculosis outside the lung. For example, in Great Britain in 1937 (10), proportions were 85% of primary abdominal tuberculosis, 50% of cases of cervical lymphadenitis, 49% of tuberculous lupus, 25% of tuberculous meningitis, and 20% of bone and joint tuberculosis. The contribution of the bovine bacillus to infectious pulmonary cases of tuberculosis was considerably less (0.6% in the south of England, 2.0% in the north of England, and 7.0% in Scotland). The majority of cases among these reports had known occupational exposures to cattle. A recent study from Tanzania (11) showed a similar observation with 29% of isolates from extrapulmonary (primarily cervical and mesenteric lymph nodes) sites yielding *M. bovis.*

One important difference between the diseases caused by the two organisms is the resistance to pyrazinamide in *M. bovis* (12). This may be of consequence because of the important role of pyrazinamide in short-course treatment regimens for the treatment of tuberculosis. However, comparison of treatment outcome in those whose disease is caused by *M. bovis* with those whose disease is caused by the human bacillus has not been reported.

Bovine tuberculosis has been most frequently spread by means of ingesting contaminated milk that had been neither boiled nor pasteurized. The role of ingesting undercooked contaminated meat or offal has never been systematically elucidated, although it has been included as one element in a program to reduce the risk of spread of the disease among hunters (13). Ingestion of contaminated food results in clinical forms of primary disease such as mesenteric and cervical lymphadenitis that are relatively uncommon where milk is boiled and meat is well cooked. A series of studies (14–16) has demonstrated the importance of occupational and recreational exposures to infectious material.

M. bovis is pathogenic for man, but its pathogenicity is less than that of *M. tuberculosis hominis.* It is certainly capable of producing cases of pulmonary tuberculosis that are sputum-smear positive and, therefore, potentially infectious to other humans. Person-to-person spread has been recorded (17–21), but its relative contribution to the overall problem of tuberculosis has not been investigated in detail.

In Denmark (22), a community-based study of the epidemiology of tuberculosis determined that the risk of developing adult pulmonary tuberculosis was inversely proportional to the prevalence of bovine tuberculosis in the area, indicating a relative "protective" effect of infection with *M. bovis* as compared with infection resulting from *M. tuberculosis.* Indeed, the relative risk of development of active tuberculosis, following infection with the bovine bacillus, was estimated to be 7.3 (in the urban area) and 12.5 (in the rural area) less than that following infection with the human bacillus. Similar findings, with an even stronger inverse relationship, have been reported from Sweden (23). The occurrence of bovine tuberculosis in a community is a powerful determinant for the probability of a positive tuberculin reaction, but it has an effect on morbidity subsequent to infection that is much reduced compared with infection with *M. tuberculosis.*

Currently available knowledge is based on old techniques and gives us information that must be extrapolated if we are to understand the pathogenesis of tuberculosis caused by *M. bovis*. Newer molecular techniques are now available and are systematically used to evaluate the pathogenesis and transmission of tuberculosis. They now need to be applied to the study of *M. bovis*.

The control of bovine tuberculosis in man is essentially that of the control of bovine tuberculosis in animals (discussed in another section of this book), coupled with effective treatment of diseased persons. Although less likely to produce disease, *M. bovis* is a contributor to the global tuberculosis epidemic and therefore must be taken into account in the global plan for its containment. This is particularly urgent in the present day, when the convergence of *M. bovis* and the human immunodeficiency virus has the potential (as with every other aspect of the global tuberculosis problem) to exacerbate the situation (24).

References

1. Cosivi, O., J. M. Grange, C. J. Daborn, M. C. Raviglione, T. Fujikura, D. Cousins, R. A. Robinson, H. F. A. K. Huchzermeyer, I. de Kantor, and F.-X. Meslin. 1998. Zoonotic tuberculosis due to *Mycobacterium bovis* in developing countries. *Emerg Infect Dis* 4:59-70.
2. Fanning, E. A. 1998. *Mycobacterium bovis* infection in animals and humans. *In* P. D. O. Davies (ed.), Clinical Tuberculosis. London: Chapman and Hall, 535-552.
3. Kleeberg, H. H. 1984. Human tuberculosis of bovine origin in relation to public health. *Rev Sci Technol Off Int Epiz* 3:11-32.
4. Fanning, A. and Edwards, S. 1991. *Mycobacterium bovis* infection in human beings in contact with elk (*Cervus elaphus*) in Alberta, Canada. *Lancet* 338:1253-55.
5. Gutman, R. B. 1985. The trouble with bovine tuberculosis. *Bull Hist Med* 59:13-29.
6. Collins, C. H. and J. M. Grange. 1983. The bovine tubercle bacillus. *J Appl Bacteriol* 55:13-29.
7. Cobbett, L. 1911. Royal Commission on Tuberculosis. London: Queen's Printer.
8. Ruys, C. A. 1946. Bovine tuberculosis. *Mon Bull Min Health* 5:67-71.
9. Styblo, K., Meijer, J., and I. Sutherland. 1969. The transmission of tubercle bacilli. Its trend in a human population. *Bull Int Union Tuberc* 42:5-104.
10. Griffith, A. S. 1937. Bovine tuberculosis in man. *Vet Rec* 49:529-43.
11. Kazwala, R. R., C. J. Daborn, J. M. Sharp, D. M. Kambarage, S. F. H. Jiwa, and N. A. Mbembati. 2001. Isolation of *Mycobacterium bovis* from human cases of cervical adenitis in Tanzania: a cause for concern? *Int J Tuberc Lung Dis* 5:87-91.
12. Konno, K., F. M. Feldman, and W. McDermott. 1967. Pyrazinamide susceptibility and amidase activity of tubercle bacilli. *Am Rev Respir Dis* 95:461-69.
13. Wilkins, M. J., P. C. Bartlett, B. Frawley, D. J. O'Brien, C. E. Miller, and M. L. Boulton. 2003. *Mycobacterium bovis* (bovine TB) exposure as a recreational risk for hunters: results of a Michigan Hunter Survey, 2001. *Int J Tuberc Lung Dis* 7:1001-1009.
14. Robinson, P., D. Morris, and R. Antic. 1988. *Mycobacterium bovis* as an occupational hazard of abattoir workers. *Aust NZ J Med* 19:701-703.
15. Georghiou, P., A. M. Patel, and A. Konstantinos. 1989. *Mycobacterium bovis* as an occupational hazard in abattoir workers [letter]. *Aust NZ J Med* 19:409-410.

16. de Kantor, I. N. 1992. Bovine tuberculosis: public health importance. *In* Proceedings of the International Conference on Animal Tuberculosis. Cairo: Gen Organ Vet Serv., 212-13.

17. Vaillaud, J. C., J. Viallier, C. Ollagnier, and C. Sarrouy. 1966. Un exemple de contamination interhumaine de la tuberculose pulmonaire a bacilli bovin. *Poumon Coeur* 22:1167-69.

18. Wigle, W. D., M. J. Ashley, E. M. Killough, and M. Cosens. 1972. Bovine tuberculosis in humans in Ontario. *Am Rev Respir Dis* 106:528-34.

19. Collins, C. H., M. D. Yates, and J. M. Grange 1981. A study of bovine strains of *Mycobacterium tuberculosis* isolated from humans in South-East England: 1977-1979. *Tubercle* 62:113-16.

20. Schonfeld, J. K., C. H. Collins, M. D. Yates, and J. M. Grange. 1982. Human-to-human spread of infection by *M. bovis*. *Tubercle* 63:143-44.

21. LoBue, P. A., W. Betancourt, L. Cowan, L. Seli, C. Peter, and K. S. Moser. 2004. Identification of a familial cluster of pulmonary *Mycobacterium bovis* disease. *Int J Tuberc Lung Dis* 8:1142-46.

22. Magnus, K. 1966. Epidemiological basis of tuberculosis eradication. 3. Risk of pulmonary tuberculosis after human and bovine infection. *Bull World Health Org* 35:483-508.

23. Sjogren, I. and I. Sutherland. 1974. Studies of tuberculosis in man in relation to infection in cattle. *Tubercle* 56:113-27.

24. Ayele, W. Y., S. D. Neill, J. Zinsstag, M. G. Weiss, I. Pavlik. 2004. Bovine tuberculosis: an old disease but a new threat to Africa. *Int J Tuberc Lung Dis* 8:924-37.

25. Meissner, G. and K. H. Schroder. 1974. Bovine tuberculosis in man and cattle. *Bull Int Union Tuberc Lung Dis* 49:145-48.

26. Enarson, D. A., M. J. Ashley, S. Grzybowski, E. Ostapkowicz, and E. Dorken. 1980. Non-respiratory tuberculosis in Canada: epidemiologic and bacteriologic features. *Am J Epidemiol* 112:341-51.

27. Cousins, D. V. and D. J. Dawson. 1999. Tuberculosis due to *Mycobacterium bovis* in the Australian population: cases recorded during 1970-1994. *Int J Tuberc Lung Dis* 3:715-21.

28. Krebs, A. and W. Kappler. 1982. Die Bedeutung von *Mycobacterium bovis* in der Tuberduloseepidemiologie. *Zeitschrift Erkrankungen Atmungs Organe* 158:101-109.

29. Grange, J. M. and M. D. Yates. 1994. Zoonotic aspects of *Mycobacterium bovis* infection. *Vet Microbiol* 40:137-51.

30. Dankner, W. M., N. J. Waecker, M. A. Essey, K. Moser, M. Thompson, and C. H. Davis. 1993. *Mycobacterium bovis* infections in San Diego: a clinicoepidemiologic study of 73 patients and a historical review of a forgotten pathogen. Medicine 72:11-37.

31. Collins, C., P. Kelly, C. Byrne, F. Denham, and L. Clancy. 1987. Is bovine, atypical or resistant tuberculosis a problem? *Ir Med J* 80:66-67.

32. Brett, J. L. and M. W. Humble. 1991. Incidence of human tuberculosis caused by *Mycobacterium bovis*. *NZ Med J* 104:13-14.

33. World Health Organization. 1993. Report of WHO meeting on zoonotic tuberculosis. WHO/CDS/VPH/93.130.

34. Cornican, M. G. and J. Flynn. 1992. Tuberculosis in the West of Ireland 1986-1990. *Ir J Med Sci* 161:70-72.

35. Sauret, J., R. Jolis, V. Ausina, E. Castro, and R. Cornudella. 1992. Human tuberculosis due to *Mycobacterium bovis*: report of 10 cases. *Tuber Lung Dis* 73:388-91.

36. Federal Office of Public Health. 1994. La tuberculose en Suisse en 1994. *Bern, Bull* 37:10-11.

Chapter 2
Public Health Significance of *M. bovis*

P. LoBue, MD, FACP, FCCP

Introduction

Tuberculosis control in humans relies on interventions that will both cure patients and interrupt disease transmission. As with other contagious diseases, specific tuberculosis control measures have evolved on the basis of our understanding of the mode of transmission.

When tuberculosis is caused by *Mycobacterium tuberculosis*, transmission with very rare exception occurs from patients with pulmonary tuberculosis to uninfected persons via the airborne route. Therefore, the priority activities for the public health department are to identify patients with active pulmonary tuberculosis, place them in respiratory isolation if contagious, and have the patients complete adequate treatment. In addition, the health department identifies individuals who have been exposed to contagious patients, evaluates those contacts for tuberculosis infection and disease, and places them on treatment for latent infection or disease as needed. Finally, persons in groups known to be at risk of becoming infected with tuberculosis or to progress from infection to disease (e.g., immigrants from high–tuberculosis incidence countries; HIV-infected persons) may be targeted for infection and disease screening.

When tuberculosis in humans is caused by *Mycobacterium bovis,* the goals of the health department are the same: curing patients and interrupting transmission. However, investigative procedures and interventions are more varied because *M. bovis* can be transmitted to humans from a number of mammals, including other humans, and because there are several potential routes of transmission, including gastrointestinal, airborne, and direct inoculation.

Historical Background

Shortly after *M. tuberculosis* and *M. bovis* were discovered to be unique organisms, controversy arose regarding the latter's ability to pose a significant health threat to humans. Robert Koch, for example, did not believe that bovine strains of tuberculosis represented a sufficient danger to humans such that their eradication was necessary (1). Subsequent work by a British Royal Commission and others showed, however, that humans could become infected by drinking contaminated milk, with the resulting disease commonly manifesting as lymphadenitis in children, or via inhalation of droplet nuclei produced by sick cattle, which could result in pulmonary disease (1). In response, *M. bovis* eradication programs were begun in cattle herds, along with widespread pasteurization of dairy products. These measures produced a sharp decline in the incidence of human *M. bovis*. By the 1990s less than 1% of human tuberculosis cases in industrialized countries were caused by this organism (2).

Cow-to-Human Transmission

Although human *M. bovis* disease is rare in technologically advanced nations in general, it appears to be more common in certain geographic regions of the industrialized world. In the United States, for example, the disease is more common in areas along the U.S.-Mexico border such as San Diego, California. Over the last decade, approximately 7% of culture-positive tuberculosis patients in San Diego had disease caused by *M. bovis*. A large majority (90%) of these patients were Hispanic persons born in the United States or Mexico, and most had extrapulmonary disease (3). A study of pediatric tuberculosis in the San Diego region revealed that for many children infected with tuberculosis, the only risk factor was ingestion of unpasteurized dairy products from Mexico (4). These findings have implicated dairy products from Mexican cattle herds as the major source of *M. bovis* infection for patients in San Diego. Ultimately, eradication of human *M. bovis* disease in this setting will require eradication of the organism in the infected dairy herds by culling them. In the short term, more extensive efforts at educating the public about the dangers of consuming raw dairy products may be of value.

In addition to via the consumption of contaminated dairy products, *M. bovis* can be transmitted to humans from cattle via inhalation. Recent reports from the United Kingdom and France have shown that many human cases of *M. bovis* can be attributed to direct contact with cattle. In a description of the molecular epidemiology of *M. bovis* in the United Kingdom, it was reported that 59% of patients worked or lived on a farm (5). In a survey done in France, 13 of 38 patients had an occupational exposure, whereas only three ingested unpasteurized milk (6). Airborne transmission from cattle is also an occupational risk for abattoir workers, as demonstrated by a report from Australia in which five cases of *M. bovis* occurred in a population of 3000 workers during a 2-year period, and for veterinarians and veterinary students (7,8).

In rare cases, humans can become infected with *M. bovis* via direct inoculation (9). Referred to as the Butcher's Wart (analogous to the Prosector's Wart, which is caused by *M. tuberculosis* and is an occupational risk associated with performing autopsies), this skin lesion can occur in persons handling infected meat. It is very rare and generally self-limited.

Because *M. bovis* is either enzootic or found sporadically in much of the developing world, there is clearly a risk for cow-to-human transmission by either ingestion or inhalation (10). As a result of the lack of surveillance data, the actual scope of the problem is unknown, however.

From the public health perspective, eradication programs in cattle and universal pasteurization of milk remain the mainstays of the prevention of a disease in humans that is caused by transmission from cows. These measures should be augmented by public education efforts explaining the dangers of consuming unpasteurized dairy products in areas where *M. bovis* disease in humans is more common.

Other Animal-to-Human Transmission

Spillover of *M. bovis* from cattle to other animal reservoirs represents another possible source of human infection. Cervidae, such as elk and deer, have been confirmed as one such source. During an outbreak of *M. bovis* in domesticated elk in Canada, transmission was documented among persons exposed to live elk and also among those who processed elk carcasses (11). Although most individuals were only found to have latent infection, a veterinary surgeon who examined the index animal case was found to have a positive sputum culture for *M. bovis*. The spread of *M. bovis* to the wild white-tailed deer population of Michigan, where the disease is now endemic, also prompted concerns about possible transmission to humans, and especially hunters. Recent surveillance, however, has not detected any human *M. bovis* cases in Michigan that could be linked to white-tailed deer by either traditional or molecular epidemiologic methods (12). Transmission from more exotic animals has also been reported; in one unusual case, zoo workers were apparently infected by a Southern white rhinoceros (13).

In theory, as with cattle there are three potential routes of transmission from cervidae to humans. Sick deer or elk could transmit *M. bovis* to humans via the airborne route. Direct cutaneous inoculation could result from field dressing an animal or processing a carcass. Finally, there is a theoretical possibility of gastrointestinal transmission through ingestion of undercooked meat, although this has never been documented (12). To prevent disease in humans, education should be provided to persons at risk. The public health message should instruct such individuals to take appropriate precautions such as wearing gloves and cooking meat thoroughly (12).

Human-to-Human Transmission

For *M. tuberculosis*, human-to-human airborne transmission is essentially the only mode of transmission of public health significance, and therefore it has been the primary focus of efforts to control tuberculosis. The potential for human-to-human transmission of *M. bovis* has been recognized for many years, with reports of sporadic, anecdotal examples. However, this route of transmission was felt to be rare and of questionable importance (2,9,14,15).

Several recent lines of evidence indicate that human-to-human transmission of *M. bovis* may be more important than originally believed. During the mid-1990s, multiple nosocomial outbreaks of multidrug-resistant *M. bovis* were documented in Europe (16–19). All of the patients involved were HIV infected; susceptibility of HIV-infected individuals to *M. bovis* has also been documented in other settings (1,3). These findings are of particular concern because of the high rate of HIV infection in places like Africa, where *M. bovis* is enzootic in several countries. In nations with high rates of *M. bovis* infection in cattle and high rates of HIV infection in humans, the potential exists for transmission of *M. bovis* from cattle to immunosuppressed humans, followed by human-to-human spread among immunosuppressed persons (10). Because cultures are not routinely performed in most developing countries with high burdens of tuberculosis, the percentage of cases caused by *M. bovis* in such countries is unknown. Given the high rate of HIV infection in humans and the persistence of *M. bovis* in cattle, it is possible that a substantial fraction of tuberculosis in these countries is of bovine origin.

Although the risk of human-to-human transmission among persons who are not HIV infected is probably substantially less, there is evidence that such transmission occurs. A recent report in which pulmonary *M. bovis* patients were compared with pulmonary *M. tuberculosis* patients showed that these groups of patients were comparably likely to have cavities on chest radiographs and positive sputum smears for acid-fast bacilli (AFB) (20). Both of these characteristics are associated with an increased risk of transmission of tuberculosis in humans. In addition, it was found that contacts exposed to sputum AFB smear–positive patients were equally likely to convert their tuberculin skin test result to positive, regardless of whether the organism infecting the source patient was *M. tuberculosis* or *M. bovis*. This indicates that the contacts had become infected recently, and that it may have been the result of human-to-human transmission. Included in this cohort of patients and contacts were three family members, all of whom had sputum AFB smear–positive pulmonary *M. bovis*, and none of whom was known to be HIV infected. Genotyping revealed the three *M. bovis* isolates to be of one strain, consistent with person-to-person transmission among these individuals (21).

On the basis of these findings, it seems prudent from a public health standpoint to treat pulmonary *M. bovis* patients in the same manner as pulmonary *M. tuberculosis* patients. Respiratory precautions, as determined by local health department policies and procedures, should be instituted for all patients with potentially contagious *M. bovis*. Directly observed therapy is the preferred method of treatment for tuberculosis patients regardless of whether the infecting organism is *M. tuberculosis* or *M. bovis*. Contact investigation should be conducted in the same manner for *M. bovis* and *M. tuberculosis* patients, and priority of the contact investigation should be assigned on the basis of patient characteristics such as sputum AFB smear results or cavity on chest radiograph—not the species of tuberculosis infecting the patient. Finally, it is important that all tuberculosis patients be offered HIV counseling and testing.

Molecular Epidemiology

Over the last decade, genotyping of tuberculosis strains has been shown to be an increasingly valuable tool in tuberculosis control. For disease caused by *M. tuberculosis*, molecular epidemiology has helped to identify unsuspected transmission, determine likely locations of transmission, and measure the extent of transmission (22). Molecular epidemiology serves as a complement to traditional methods of outbreak and contact investigation. Initial studies of the use of molecular epidemiology in examining the transmission of *M. bovis* to humans from other humans and other species indicate that genotyping can play a similar role (5,21).

In one example from the United Kingdom, two siblings were diagnosed with *M. bovis* (23). Both lived on a farm, and neither drank unpasteurized milk. The brother, however, assisted during veterinary examinations of the cattle, and he would become covered with bovine mucus and saliva. The sister had no contact with the cattle. When the brother was diagnosed, he had a positive sputum smear for AFB, and his chest radiograph had a cavity—two characteristics indicative of a high degree of contagiousness. Two years previous to the siblings' diagnosis of *M. bovis* disease, cattle on the farm were found to have *M. bovis* and were slaughtered. Genotyping demonstrated that both siblings' isolates were identical and matched the cattle strain. Thus, molecular epidemiology was able to confirm suspected transmission from cattle to human and subsequent transmission from human to human.

Role of Treatment in Disease Control

For patients with active disease caused by *M. tuberculosis,* treatment serves two public health functions. If patients are contagious, treatment will reduce their disease burden to the point where they are no longer contagious, and eventually to the point where they are cured. If patients are not contagious, treatment will prevent them from becoming contagious. Although controlled clinical trials have not been performed to determine the efficacy of treatment for *M. bovis* in humans, programmatic data indicate that treatment outcomes are similar to those found for treatment of *M. tuberculosis* when standard regimens, based on drug-susceptibility testing, are used (e.g., 9 months of isoniazid and rifampin for *M. bovis* that is susceptible to both drugs) (24).

Treatment of persons with latent tuberculosis infection also plays a role in tuberculosis control. Multiple clinical trials and programmatic reports have repeatedly demonstrated the effectiveness of latent tuberculosis treatment, primarily with isoniazid, in preventing latently infected persons from progressing to active disease (25). Because there is still no diagnostic test that can distinguish *M. tuberculosis* from *M. bovis*, when the infection is latent, there is no method to evaluate the relative efficacy of preventive treatment. Nevertheless, it seems reasonable to treat persons with latent tuberculosis where *M. bovis* is the suspected cause, especially as *M. tuberculosis* infection cannot be excluded as a possibility (11).

Summary

Although disease caused by human *Mycobacterium bovis* is rare in industrialized countries, cases continue to be reported. There are three potential routes of transmission: ingestion of contaminated dairy products (animal-to-human), inhalation of infectious droplet nuclei (animal-to-human or human-to-human), and direct inoculation of the skin (animal-to-human). The different modes of infection require different public health interventions to prevent transmission and additional human cases. Eradication of *M. bovis* in cattle and pasteurization of dairy products are the cornerstones of prevention of human disease. In addition, public education regarding the risks of consumption of unpasteurized dairy products and the precautions that should be taken when field dressing or processing animal carcasses or when cooking meat from animals that are particularly susceptible to the disease (e.g., deer and elk) may be useful in reducing the risks of transmission through ingestion or direct inoculation. Standard public health measures used to manage patients with contagious *M. tuberculosis* should be applied to contagious patients with *M. bovis* to stop airborne person-to-person spread.

Of major concern is the high susceptibility of HIV-infected persons to *M. bovis* infection. Multiple nosocomial outbreaks have already been reported in this population. Perhaps the greatest potential danger is that *M. bovis* could become a sustainable epidemic in areas like Africa, where HIV is rampant and *M. bovis* is enzootic. Even if an epidemic does not become self-sustaining, an increase in human morbidity and mortality, as has occurred with *M. tuberculosis*, is very likely. International efforts to improve *M. bovis* surveillance, provide access to adequate HIV and tuberculosis treatment, and eradicate the disease from animal hosts are needed to avert a resurgence of human *M. bovis* in the developing world.

References

1. Dankner, W. M., N. J. Waecker, M. A. Essey, K. Moser, M. Thompson, and C. E. Davis. 1993. *Mycobacterium bovis* infections in San Diego: a clinicoepidemiologic study of 73 patients and a historical review of a forgotten pathogen. *Medicine* 72:11-37.
2. O'Reilly, L. M. and C. J. Daborn. 1995. The epidemiology of *Mycobacterium bovis* infections in animals and man: a review. *Tuber Lung Dis* 76:1-46.
3. LoBue, P. A., W. Betancourt, C. Peter, and K. Moser. 2003. Epidemiology of *Mycobacterium bovis* disease in San Diego County, 1994-2000. *Int J Tuberculosis Lung Dis* 7:180-85.
4. Besser, R. E., B. Pakiz, J. M. Schulte, S. Alvarado, E. R. Zell, T. A. Kenyon, and I. M. Onorato. 2001. Risk factors for positive Mantoux tuberculin skin tests in children in San Diego, California: evidence for boosting and possible foodborne transmission. *Pediatrics* 108:305-10.
5. Gibson, A. L., G. Hewinson, T. Goodchild, B. Watt, A. Story, J. Inwald, and F. A. Drobniewski. 2004. Molecular epidemiology of disease due to *Mycobacterium bovis* in humans in the United Kingdom. *J Clin Microbiol* 42:431-34.
6. Robert, J., F. Boulahbal, D. Trystram, C. Truffot-Pernot, A.-C. de Benoist, V. Vincent, V. Jarlier, and J. Grosset. 1999. A national survey of human *Mycobacterium bovis* infection in France. *Int J Tuberc Lung Dis* 3:711-14.
7. Robinson, P., D. Morris, and R. Antic. 1988. *Mycobacterium bovis* as an occupational hazard in abattoir workers. *Aust NZ J Med* 18:701-703.
8. Sauret, J., R. Jolis, V. Ausina, E. Castro, and R. Cornudella. 1992. Human tuberculosis due to *Mycobacterium bovis*: report of 10 cases. *Tuber Lung Dis* 73:388-91.

9. Grange, J. M. 2001. *Mycobacterium bovis* infection in human beings. *Tuberculosis* 81:71-77.

10. Cosivi, O., J. M. Grange, C. J. Daborn, M. C. Raviglione, T. Fujikura, D. Cousins, R. A. Robinson, H. F. A. K. Huchzermeyer, I. de Kantor, and F.-X. Meslin. 1998. Zoonotic tuberculosis due to *Mycobacterium bovis* in developing countries. *Emerg Inf Dis* 4:59-70.

11. Fanning, A. and E. Edwards. 1991. *Mycobacterium bovis* infection in human beings in contact with elk (*Cervus elephus*) in Alberta, Canada. *Lancet* 338:1253-55.

12. Wilkins, M. J., P. C. Bartlett, B. Frawley, D. J. O'Brien, C. E. Miller, and M. L. Boulton. 2003. *Mycobacterium bovis* (bovine TB) exposure as a recreational risk for hunters: results of a Michigan Hunter Survey, 2001. *Int J Tuberc Lung Dis* 7:1001-1009.

13. Dalovisio, J. R., M. Stetter, and S. Mikota-Wells. 1992. Rhinoceros' rhinorrhea: cause of an outbreak of infection due to airborne *Mycobacterium bovis* in zookeepers. *Clin Infect Dis* 15:598-600.

14. Kubin, M., Z. Heralt, I. Morongova, R. Ruzhova, and A. Viznerova. 1984. 2 cases of probable interhuman transmission of *Mycobacterium bovis*. *Z Erkr Atmungsorgane* 163:285-91.

15. Schonfeld, J. K. 1982. Human-to-human spread of infection by *M. bovis*. *Tubercle* 63:143-44.

16. Rivero, A., M. Marquez, J. Santos, A. Pinedo, M. A. Sanchez, A. Esteve, S. Samper, C. Martin. 2001. High rate of tuberculosis reinfection during a nosocomial outbreak of multidrug-resistant tuberculosis caused by *Mycobacterium bovis* strain B. *Clin Infect Dis* 32:159-61.

17. Blazquez, J., L. E. E. de Los Monteros, S. Samper, C. Martin, A. Guerrero, J., J. van Embden, F. Baquero, and E. Gomez-Mampaso. 1997. Genetic characterization of multidrug-resistant *Mycobacterium bovis* strains from a hospital outbreak involving human immunodeficiency virus-positive patients. *J Clin Microbiol* 35:1390-93.

18. Samper, S., C. Martin, A. Pinedo, A. Rivero, J. Blazquez, F. Baquero, D. van Soolingen, and J. van Embden. 1997. Transmission between HIV-infected patients of multidrug-resistant tuberculosis caused by *Mycobacterium bovis*. *AIDS* 11:1237-242.

19. Guerrero, A., J. Cobo, J. Fortun, E. Navas, C. Quereda, A. Asensio, J. Canon, J. Blézquez, and E. Gomez-Mampaso. 1997. Nosocomial transmission of *Mycobacterium bovis* resistant to 11 drugs in people with advanced HIV-1 infection. *Lancet* 350:1738-42.

20. LoBue, P. A., J. J. LeClair, and K. S. Moser. 2004. Contact investigation for cases of pulmonary *Mycobacterium bovis*. *Int J Tuberculosis Lung Dis* 8:868-72.

21. LoBue, P. A., W. Betancourt, L. Cowan, L. Seli, C. Peter, and K. Moser. Identification of a familial cluster of pulmonary *Mycobacterium bovis* disease. *Int J Tuberculosis Lung Dis* 8:1142-46.

22. Daley, C. L. and L. M. Kawamura. The role of molecular epidemiology in contact investigations: a US perspective. *Int J Tuberc Lung Dis* 7:S458-S462.

23. Smith, R. M. M., F. Drobniewski, A. Gibson, J. D. E. Montague, M. N. Logan, D. Hunt, G. Hewinson, R. L. Salmon, and B. O'Neill. 2004. *Mycobacterium bovis* infection, United Kingdom. *Emerg Infect Dis* 10:539-41.

24. LoBue, P. A. and K. S. Moser. 2005. Treatment of *Mycobacterium bovis* infected tuberculosis patients, San Diego, California, United States, 1994-2003. *Int J Tuberculosis Lung Dis* 9:333-38.

25. American Thoracic Society and Centers for Disease Control and Prevention. 2000. Targeted tuberculin testing and treatment of latent tuberculosis infection. *MMWR Recomm Rep* 49(RR-6):1-51.

Chapter 3

Human Tuberculosis Caused by *Mycobacterium bovis* in Latin America and the Caribbean

V. Ritacco, MD, PhD, M.D. Sequeira, MSc, and I.N. de Kantor, PhD

At present, in most industrialized countries, human tuberculosis (TB) incidence ranges between 2 and 10/100,000, and TB in cattle has been either controlled or totally eradicated. Milk is pasteurized. Reported bovine TB cases in humans are either persons more than 70 years of age, whose disease is a result of endogenous reactivation of ancient infections, or immigrants from developing countries. A steady relationship between the number of *Mycobacterium bovis* and *Mycobacterium tuberculosis* human TB cases (0.5–1.0%) is observed, mostly because of a constant decrease in the denominator (1–4).

Nowadays, in most Latin American and Caribbean countries, milk is pasteurized, but the quality control of this process is not always complete and reliable, and the coverage is rather low in certain areas, meaning that a part of the population continues consuming unpasteurized milk. In addition, bovine TB infection in cattle continues being prevalent in several countries, and human TB incidence rates are relatively high (30 to >100/100,000). In these conditions, the relationship between *M. bovis*/*M. tuberculosis* human TB cases can be also steadily maintained, but not because of a decrease in the denominator.

Historically, *M. bovis* had been related to extrapulmonary TB in infants and children, because of the consumption of unpasteurized and unboiled milk from TB-infected cattle. With the introduction of habit of boiling milk, and the growing number of milk pasteurization plants all over the world, the digestive route of infection lost its relevance, except in the conditions above described. However, aerogenic infection is still quite frequent among cattle industries and slaughterhouse workers in areas where TB infection in cattle continues to be prevalent (5).

According to data collected in a recent survey (6), at least 7% of the total population in 15 Latin America and Caribbean countries that answered the questionnaire (Mexico, Panama, Costa Rica, Nicaragua, Honduras, Argentina, Chile, Uruguay, Brazil, Paraguay, Peru, Ecuador, Surinam, Cuba, and Jamaica) are in close contact with cattle, including meat processing and veterinary services workers, as well as cattle breeders and farmers. This 7% represents some 21 million people. However, the estimated percentage for these 15 countries would be significantly higher if the peasant population were also considered at risk, as a result of their sporadic or frequent contact with bovines and the habit of drinking raw milk.

In most Latin American and Caribbean countries, the bacteriological diagnosis of pulmonary tuberculosis is usually performed by the Ziehl Neelsen smear examination. This is mainly because of the limited laboratory facilities that exist in these countries. The priority for using culture are, first, patients who are repeatedly smear negative but who are suspected to have TB because of clinical symptoms and thorax radiography; childhood and extrapulmonary TB suspects; those who been associated with HIV; and those who have suffered from suspected failures of treatment and relapses. In addition, culture is used in special surveys, such as those addressed to determine the prevalence of drug resistance in TB.

Information on Human TB Caused By *M. bovis* in Argentina

In Argentina, a study performed in 1982–1984 in 15 provincial laboratories showed that *M. bovis* was the origin of human disease in 0.5% of all TB cases diagnosed by culture, ranging between 2% in Santa Fe and 0.04% in the northwest of the country, where cattle breeding is not frequent (7).

From the late 1970s on, several reference TB laboratories have systematically performed culture and drug susceptibility tests in newly diagnosed patients, using Lowenstein Jensen and Stonebrink media. The use of this last culture media allows us to isolate and to identify *M. bovis* strains.

One of these reference laboratories, the E. Coni Institute, is situated in the Province of Santa Fe, where the main productive activities are cattle breeding, slaughterhouses, dairy industries, and agriculture. In the period 1977–2001, nearly 150,000 persons were investigated for TB. In Table 3.1, the number and percentages of cases with *M. bovis* or *M. avium* complex isolated is presented. The average percentage of cases caused by *M. bovis* versus the total cases caused by any mycobacterial species was 2.3% (97 of 4243 cases; range: 0.0–6.0). There was not any trend in the incidence of *M. bovis*.

Eighty-three percent of patients who had *M. bovis* isolated were men; in 65% of these cases, a direct working relationship with cattle was proved (rural or slaughterhouse workers, veterinary professionals, and other related activities). All cases presented pulmonary localization. No extrapulmonary TB case caused by *M. bovis* was detected during this period. The mean age of *M. bovis* TB patients was 45 years. The youngest patient diagnosed with bovine TB was a 14-year-old girl. In the period 1980–2001, the incidence rate of TB in Santa Fe decreased from 48.1 to 20.3/100,000. Although the total incident cases in the province showed a clear decreasing trend, the number of cases caused by *M. bovis* or MAC (*Mycobacterium avium* complex) did not present any clear trend, either increasing or decreasing.

Table 3.1. Patients with *Mycobacterium spp.* isolations. Number and percentage of *M. bovis* and MAC (*M. avium* Complex) cases, E. Coni Institute, Santa Fe, years 1977–2001; and incidence rates (tuberculosis cases per 100,000 inhabitants) in the Santa Fe Province, Argentina, years 1980–2001.

Year	*M. bovis*	M.A.C. Complex	Total (*)	TB cases/ 100 000
1977	1(0.6)	2 (1.3)	150	—
1978	6 (3.1)	2 (1.1)	189	—
1979	2 (1.0)	2 (1.0)	199	—
1980	2 (1.1)	2 (1.1)	175	48.1
1981	5 (3.2)	2 (1.3)	155	46.4
1982	4 (1.6)	3 (1.2)	246	51.0
1983	7 (2.6)	3 (1.1)	268	46.5
1984	6 (2.7)	2 (0.9)	225	42.2
1985	7 (3.2)	2 (0.9)	216	34.7
1986	7 (3.4)	2 (1.0)	207	33.2
1987	6 (3.5)	4 (2.3)	170	27.3
1988	9 (6.0)	4 (2.7)	149	35.3
1989	4 (2.4)	2 (1.2)	167	31.5
1990	4 (2.3)	3 (1.8)	171	27.2
1991	4 (2.3)	3 (1.7)	174	27.9
1992	2 (1.1)	4 (2.2)	183	30.7
1993	4 (2.4)	5 (2.9)	170	29.1
1994	3 (1.9)	3 (1.9)	161	28.1
1995	4 (2.9)	7 (5.0)	139	26.5
1996	2 (1.5)	4 (3.1)	130	24.7
1997	2 (1.6)	4 (3.1)	128	24.1
1998	2 (1.5)	1 (0.8)	132	22.9
1999	1 (0.7)	4 (3.0)	135	22.0
2000	3 (3.7)	2 (2.5)	81	21.6
2001	0 (0.0)	4 (3.3)	121	20.3
Total	97 (2.3)	76 (1.9)	4 243	—

The percentage of cases caused by MAC in the same period was 1.8% (range: 0.8–5.0). In the case of *M. bovis*, the random variation here found could be related to a rather constant risk of infection (endemic TB in cattle, maintained risk for rural and slaughterhouse workers). The infection risk for MAC seems to be also quite constant, possibly as a result of contact with birds and poultry in a population predominantly residing in small towns with a rural environment (8).

In populations from big cities, two studies were published in the last decade in Argentina. In La Plata, Ferreyra and Poggio (9) found in 1997 that 1.7% of TB cases were caused by *M. bovis*. In Buenos Aires, among 10,000 patients not suspected of being HIV infected who were studied over an 11-year period, 1981–1991, *M. bovis* was the cause of disease in 0.95% of them, and MAC in another 0.32%. Among 240 HIV-positive patients examined in the same laboratory in the period 1985–1991, with mycobacteria isolated by culture, in 0.8% of the patients, the disease was caused by *M. bovis*, and by MAC in another 5.8%. All cases caused by *M. bovis*, either in HIV-infected patients or not, presented pulmonary localization (10).

Bovine TB among Mexican Immigrants, San Diego, California, and Its Possible Relation with TB in Dairy Cattle in Mexico

An interesting piece of information on bovine TB in humans proceeds from San Diego, California, and is directly related to previously mentioned studies concerning rates of TB infection and lesions found predominantly in dairy cattle in Mexico (11–14). In San Diego, 3% of TB cases diagnosed between 1980 and 1991 were caused by *M. bovis*. Of these cases, more than 90% occurred in Hispanic persons, about 25% of patients were children, the main site of disease was extrapulmonary, and 54.3% of the patients were born in Mexico. Of all adults with *M. bovis* disease, 30% tested positive to HIV infection. The authors (16) suggest that the relatively high percentage of extrapulmonary *M. bovis* disease—and particularly abdominal disease, which occurred nine times more frequently in *M. bovis* than in *M. tuberculosis* cases—could be caused by transmission via ingestion of unpasteurized dairy products. As almost all cases were confined to Hispanic persons born in the United States or Mexico, and a large proportion of them were children, it appears that Mexican dairy herds could be the primary source of *M. bovis* in San Diego County. This combination of HIV and contaminated dairy products was considered a very probable origin for the continuing presence of HIV-associated *M. bovis* disease in young adults and children.

References

1. Frieden, T. R., T. K. Sterling, S. S. Munsiff, C. J. Watt, and C. Dye. 2003. Seminar: tuberculosis. *Lancet* 362:887-99.
2. Robert, J., F. Boulhabal, D. Trystam, et al. 1999. A national survey of human *Mycobacterium bovis* infection in France. IJTLD 8:711-14.
3. Cousins, D. V. and D. J. Dawson. 1999. Tuberculosis due to *Mycobacterium bovis* in the Australian population: cases recorded during 1970-1994. *IJTLD* 8:715-21.
4. Grange, J. M. and M. D. Yates. 1994. Zoonotic aspects of *Mycobacterium bovis* infections. *Vet Microbiol* 40:137-53.
5. Myers, J. A. and J. H. Steele. 1969. Bovine tuberculosis control in man and animals. Saint Louis, MO: Warren H. Green.
6. Organización Panamericana de la Salud (OPS/OMS). 2000. Brucelosis y tuberculosis (*Mycobacterium bovis*). Situación de los Programas en las Américas, Publicación PANAFTOSA 4. Centro Panamericano de Fiebre Aftosa, Rio de Janeiro, Enero.
7. Barrera, L. and I. N. Kantor. 1969. Nontuberculous mycobacteria and *Mycobacterium bovis* as a cause of human disease in Argentina. *Trop Geogr Med* 39:222-27.
8. Sequeira, M. D. and O. Latini. 2002. Información sobre tuberculosis bovina en humanos en Argentina. INER E. Coni, Ministerio Salud Pública, Santa Fe, Argentina.
9. Ferreyra, M., and G. Poggio. 1997. Casos de tuberculosis producida por *Mycobacterium bovis* diagnosticados en el Hospital "San Juan de Dios" de la Plata entre los años 1992-1996. Actas del XXVI Congreso Argentino de Tisiología y Neumonología. Santa Fe, Argentina.
10. Di Lonardo, M., N. C. Isola, M. Ambroggi, A. Rybko, and S. Poggi. 1995. Mycobacteria in HIV-infected patients in Buenos Aires. *Tubercle Lung Dis* 76:185-89.

11. Milian, F., L. M. Sanchez, P. Toledo, C. Ramirez, and M. A. Santillan. 2000. Descriptive study of human and bovine tuberculosis in Queretaro, México. *Rev Latinoam Microbiol* 42:13-19.

12. Milian-Suazo, F., M. D. Salman, C. Ramirez, J. B. Payeur, J. C. Rhyan, and M. Santillan. 2000. Identification of tuberculosis in cattle slaughtered in Mexico. *Am J Vet Res* 61:86-9.

13. Brown, W. H. and J. Hernandez de Anda. 1998. Tuberculosis in adult beef cattle of Mexican origin shipped direct-to-slaughter into Texas. *J Am Vet Med Assoc* 212:557-59.

14. Hernandez de Anda, J., T. Renteria Evangelista, G. Lopez Valencia, and M. Montano Hodgers. 1997. An abattoir monitoring system for diagnosis of tuberculosis in cattle in Baja California, Mexico. *J Am Vet Med Assoc* 211:709-11.

15. Brown, W. H., and J. Hernandez de Anda. 1998. Tuberculosis in adult beef cattle of Mexican origin shipped direct-to-slaughter into Texas. *J Am Vet Med Assoc* 212:557-59.

16. Lo Bue, P. A., W. Betacourt, C. Peter, and K. S. Moser. 2003. Epidemiology of *Mycobacterium bovis* disease in San Diego County, 1994-2000. *IJTLD* 7:180-85.

Chapter 4
Pathogenesis of *Mycobacterium bovis*
C.O. Thoen, DVM, PhD, and R.G. Barletta, PhD

Introduction

Mycobacterium bovis, the etiologic agent of bovine tuberculosis, is a slow-growing nonphotochromogenic acid-fast bacillus (1). Bovine tuberculosis can be transmitted from cattle to humans and, thus, is considered a zoonoses. This microorganism is a member of the *Mycobacterium tuberculosis* complex, a designation that, though without taxonomical status, includes important animal and human pathogens. In addition to *M. bovis*, other members of the complex include *M. tuberculosis, Mycobacterium africanum, Mycobacterium canettii*, and *Mycobacterium microti*. Other host-adapted variants of *M. bovis* have been designated *Mycobacterium pinnipedii* (seal-adapted) and *Mycobacterium caprae* (2,3). Interestingly, the antituberculosis vaccine used throughout the world, *Mycobacterium bovis* Bacille Calmette-Güerin (BCG), was attenuated by *in vitro* passage on potato slices. *M. africanum, M. cannettii*, and *M. microti* are human pathogens.

Genomics

This chapter is written at a crucial time when the knowledge of these microorganisms has increased substantially. The new science of genomics has made possible the elucidation of the complete genetic blueprint of *M. bovis* (4) and *M. tuberculosis* (5), which has already provided major insights into evolutionary relationships and virulence factors underlying the molecular basis of disease. Moreover, genetic systems have been developed to create defined mutants and elucidate the function of each gene in the physiopathology of *M. bovis* (6).

A major finding from the genome sequencing project has been that the 65.6% GC *M. bovis* genome (4,345,492 bp for the virulent bovine isolate AF2122/97) is a downsized version of the genome of *M. tuberculosis* (4,411,532 for the human isolate H37Rv), with more than 99.95% identity (Figure 4.1). Moreover, *M. bovis* does not have any new genetic material when compared to *M. tuberculosis*. Thus, DNA deletions in *M. bovis* are the major contributors to these differences, though

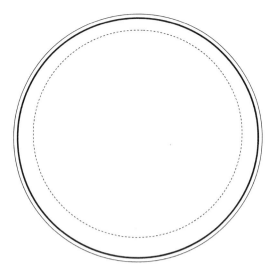

Figure 4.1   Reductive evolution of mycobacterial genomes. Relative sizes of *Mycobacterium tuberculosis* (4,411,532 bp, continuous thin line), *Mycobacterium bovis* (4,345,492 bp, continuous heavy line), and *Mycobacterium leprae* (3,258,203 bp, broken line).

more than 2000 single nucleotide polymorphisms have also been found. It is intriguing how these two microorganisms could have such differences in pathogenicity and host range. However, a comparative genomic analysis indicates that minor genome changes have a profound effect on the phenotype. For example, a point mutation in *M. bovis* is responsible for its resistance to pyrazinamide. The greatest sequence variations have been found in gene coding for cell wall and secreted proteins, such as the PE_PGRS and PPE protein families. Because these proteins may be involved in adhesion functions (7), it is possible that tissue tropism and host range are also affected. Likewise, the TbD 1 locus (present in *M. bovis,* but absent from most *M. tuberculosis* strains) encodes transporter proteins and synthetases involved in lipid trafficking and glycolipid biosynthesis. Other sequence changes involve master regulatory genes controlling the expression of multiple gene families. Likewise, deletions have been found to affect genes involved in transport, cell-surface structures, and intermediary metabolism. Finally, it is important to note that deletions may remove genes that are unnecessary for host adaptation and lead to a different or even wider host range.

Evolutionary Relationships

The analysis of the *M. bovis* genome challenged the natural epidemiological hypothesis that *M. tuberculosis* is a human-adapted variety of *M. bovis* that was acquired from cattle. The irreversible loss of DNA material uncovered by the *M. bovis* genome sequencing project and the systematic analysis of polymorphisms in a large panel of strains indicate quite a different scenario (8,9). This analysis indicates that *Mycobacterium canettii* is likely the ancestral species of the *M. tuberculosis* complex. Successive DNA deletions, starting by the loss of region RD 9 (RD

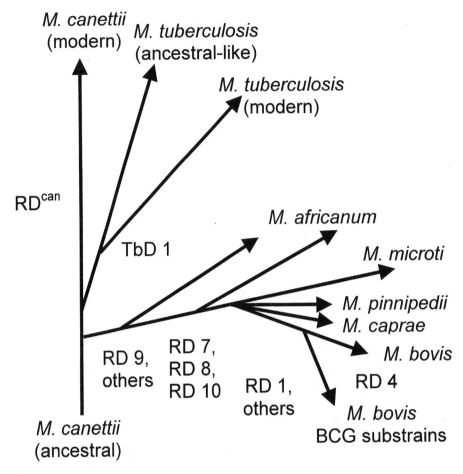

Figure 4.2   Proposed evolution of mycobacterial pathogens from a common ancestral *M. cannetti* strain. During evolution, the ancestral progenitor underwent various deletions (e.g., loss of RD^{can}, RD 9, RD 4, and RD 1), giving origin to the microorganisms of the *Mycobacterium tuberculosis* complex. The scheme is based on Brosch et al. (8), as modified by other studies (5,22,27). Note the two lineages for *M. africanum* with the more ancestral-like lineage originating before the loss of RD 7, RD 8, and RD 10. This scheme is compatible with bovine tuberculosis arising from human tuberculosis.

stands for regions of difference), originated *Mycobacterium africanum, Mycobacterium microti,* and *M. bovis.* Moreover, *M. bovis* BCG experienced further deletions during *in vitro* adaptation, and the loss of region RD1 has been implicated as the mechanism of virulence attenuation. In this view, modern *M. tuberculosis* strains originated later from ancestral *M. canettii* by loss of the TbD 1 locus (Figure 4.2).

Pathogenesis

Aerosol exposure of cattle to *M. bovis* is considered the most frequent route of infection; gross lesions usually involve the lungs and thoracic lymph nodes (10). Cattle exposed by ingestion of food and water contaminated with *M. bovis* often develop primary foci in lymph tissues associated with the intestinal tract. Other mycobacteria including *Mycobacterium* subsp. *avium, Mycobacterium avium* subsp. *paratuberculosis, Mycobacterium intracellulare, Mycobacterium scrofulaceum, Mycobacterium kansassii, Mycobacterium fortuitum,* and *M. tuberculosis* may induce tuberculin skin sensitivity, but they do not produce progressive pulmonary disease in cattle. Experimental investigations in animals comparing intravenous, intratracheal, intraperitoneal injection, as well as oral exposure to *M. bovis*, reveal that the nature and extent of disease varies with the route of exposure and dose of organisms.

Tubercle bacilli were identified more than 100 years ago; however, definitive information on the pathogenesis of *M. bovis* in cattle and other bovidae is not available (1). Aerosol exposure leads to the involvement of the lung and associated lymph nodes. The mucociliary clearance by mucus and epithelial cilia in the upper respiratory passages provides a defense against infection by inhalation of mycobacteria. However, microorganisms on small particles such as dust and water droplets that do not impinge against the mucociliary layer can pass through terminal bronchioles, thus gaining access to alveolar spaces. The estimated size of terminal endings of bronchioles is about 20 μm as compared to 1–4 μm for an acid-fast bacillus. Following aerosol exposure, *M. bovis* is carried to the small air passages, where it is ingested by phagocytes. The phagocytes pass through the lining of the bronchioles, enter the circulation, and are carried to lymph nodes, parenchyma of lungs, or other sites. After ingestion of the bacillus, the mononuclear macrophages attempt to kill the organism; however, virulent tubercle bacilli possess the ability to escape killing. Ingestion of the tubercle bacilli by the phagocytes into phagosomes or intracytoplasmic vacuoles protects the organisms from bactericidal components in serum. Following ingestion into phagocytes, mycobacteria effectively prevent phagolysosome fusion and acidification (11).

Mycobacterial lipids such as lipoarabinomannan (LAM) and phosphatidyl inositol mannoside have been shown to intercalate within endosomal membranes and contribute to the arrest in phagosome maturation (12,13). In addition, mycobacterial proteins of the antigen 85 complex have been shown to localize within cytoplasmic vacuoles free of mycobacteria (14). By this mechanism, mycobacteria survive and multiply within the phagosomes and eventually destroy the phagocytes. *Mycobacterium marinum,* a close relative of *M. tuberculosis and M. bovis*, may lyse the phagosome and enter into the cytoplasm and use actin polymerization to spread from cell to cell (15), a phenomenon that has not been observed with *M. tuberculosis* or *M. bovis*. Nonetheless, phagosomes containing *M. tuberculosis* or *M. bovis* BCG display certain degree of permeability, allowing entrance of cytosol components of up to 70 kDa in size (16). These findings led to the hypothesis that these membrane-permeable phagosomes may allow a bidirectional transfer of mycobacterial products such as peptides, cord factor, or other toxic products from the phagosomes into the cytoplasm. This process may have implications for the role of cytotoxic T cells and class I–mediated antigen presentation in the pathogenesis of mycobacterial infections (16). On the basis of these findings, pathogenic mycobacteria may even gain access to the cytoplasm (17).

Following the stage described above, other phagocytes then enter the area and ingest the increasing numbers of tubercle bacilli. A small cluster of cells referred to as a granuloma develops. Cellular responses attempting to control the disease result in the accumulation of large numbers of phagocytes, and finally the formation of macroscopic lesions, denominated tubercles. After 10–14 days, cell-mediated immunity (CMI) responses develop, and macrophages of the host have an increased capacity to kill the intracellular bacilli. The CMI responses are mediated by T lymphocytes, which release lymphokines (messenger proteins secreted by lymphocytes) that attract, immobilize, and activate additional blood-borne mononuclear cells at the sites where virulent mycobacteria or their products exist. The cellular hypersensitivity that develops contributes to cell death and tissue destruction (caseous necrosis). In some instances, liquefaction and cavity formation occur as a result of enzymatic action on proteins and lipids. Rupture of these cavities into the bronchi allows aerosol spread of bacilli (Figures 4.3). Activated macrophages migrate to blind endings of lymphatic vessels and course to one or more of the thoracic lymph nodes, either bronchial or mediastinal. Lymph nodes are more commonly infected than other tissues because fluids in an animal eventually pass through the nodes, where the meshwork of trabeculae entraps the microorganisms. The enlargement and presence of macrophages in impenetrable passageways between reticular cell fibers of the lymph node provide an environment for mycobacterial growth and development of the granulomatous lesion in the node. On occasion, some phagocytized mycobacteria remain in the lung, and both lung and thoracic nodes are affected. Primary lesions often become localized in a node or nodes and may become large and firm. Fibrous connective tissue development in the dynamics of granuloma formation probably contributes to the localization of lesions.

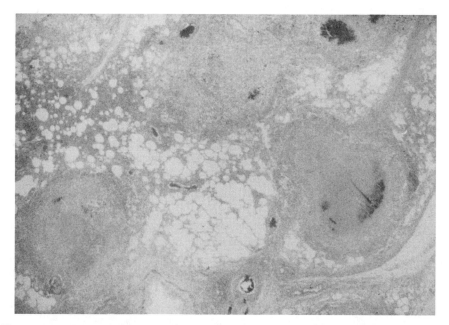

Figure 4.3. Photomicrograph of lung of an elk from which *Mycobacterium bovis* was isolated. Note multiple granulomas, some containing caseation necrosis and mineralization. One granuloma is adjacent to a bronchiole. HE × 63.28.

Granuloma formation is an attempt by the host to localize the disease process and to allow inflammatory and immune mechanisms to destroy bacilli. A few lesions may appear to be regressing while becoming encapsulated by well-organized connective tissue; however, such lesions may contain viable bacilli. Typically, the microscopic appearance of a granuloma (tubercle) is focal and has some caseous necrosis in a central area encircled by a zone of epithelioid cells, lymphocytes, and some granulocytes. Mineralization may be present in necrotic centers; in more advanced lesions, several foci of mineralization may coalesce (Fig. 4.4). Multinucleated giant cells, which contain several nuclei, often in a horseshoe or ring shape near the cytoplasmic border, are often seen in the zone near the necrotic area. An outer boundary of fibrous connective tissue is usually present between the lesions and normal tissue (18). Occasionally, fibrous tissue is not apparent, and the lesion assumes a more diffuse appearance (Fig. 4.5). Lesions caused by *M. bovis* may have few, if any, organisms that can be found by microscopic examination.

Virulence Factors

The development of disease in an animal depends on the ability of *M. bovis* to multiply within phagocytic cells and induce a host response while escaping the host

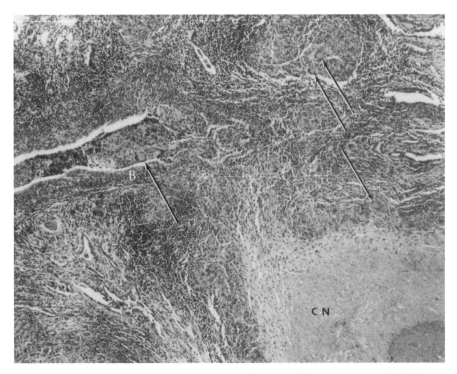

Figure 4.4. Pulmonary tuberculosis in a cow. Section of a mature tubercle in lung with caseous necrosis (*CN*) and slight mineralization present at lower right. Note other lesions of epithelioid cells, some of which have formed multinucleated giant cells (*arrows*). One giant cell is present in debris that occludes a bronchiole. Columnar epithelial cells of the bronchiole are shown at *B. Mycobacterium bovis* was isolated. HE × 65. Photo by E. M. Himes.

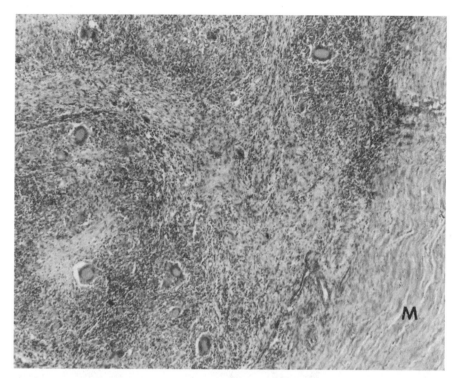

Figure 4.5. Tuberculous metritis in a cow. Diffuse tuberculous granulation tissue of epithelioid cells, lymphocytes, and macrophages are shown at left with lesion adjacent to smooth muscle cells (*M*) of endometrium of the uterus. Numerous multinucleated giant cells are present. HE × 65. Photo by E. M. Himes.

bactericidal action associated with this response. Pathogenicity of mycobacteria is a multifactorial phenomenon requiring the participation and cumulative effects of several components, including complex lipids and proteins in both the cell wall and the cytoplasm of tubercle bacilli (19–21). Moreover, most studies of mycobacterial virulence determinants have been performed with *M. tuberculosis* rather than with *M. bovis*. However, the presence of homologous genes in *M. bovis* and the close relationship between these microorganisms indicate the use of similar virulence determinants and mechanisms of pathogenicity.

Complex lipids, extracted from both virulent and attenuated strains of mycobacteria, have been extensively evaluated by *in vivo* or *in vitro* systems to obtain information on their significance in disease (22–26). The cell wall core of mycobacteria is composed of three covalently attached molecules: peptidoglycan, arabinogalactan, and mycolic acid. Glycolipid complexes present in the cell wall of virulent and attenuated strains of mycobacteria have been extensively examined to obtain information on their significance in granuloma formation. An important property of virulent bovine tubercle bacilli is their ability to form cords when grown in liquid culture medium. These cords are consistently demonstrated in smears. Lipids or lipid complexes present in the cell wall of the virulent tubercle bacilli appear to contribute to the formation of these "ropelike" cords, which represent bacilli aligned in parallel form. Several lipid components have been isolated, chemically characterized, and evaluated in certain *in vivo* and *in vitro* systems to determine their importance in pathogenicity. Cord factor, a glycolipid, extracted with petroleum ether from viable turbercle bacilli, identified as trehalose-6,6′ dimycolate, does not induce tuberculin sensitivity, but it does inhibit the migration of leukocytes and is leukotoxic (27). Moreover, cord factor has been found to induce swelling and disruption of liver mitochondria; the swollen mitochondria have decreased respiratory and phosphorylative activity (28). Also, cord factor was reported to induce disintegration of the rough endoplasmic reticulum and detachment of ribosomes in liver cells (29). Furthermore, gene deletion mutants unable to synthesize cord factor have normal initial replication but fail to persist within and kill infected mice (30), which underlies the importance of this virulence factor.

Improved biochemical techniques for purifying cell wall lipids have permitted the isolation of sulfur-containing glycolipids (sulfolipids, sulfatides) from *M. tuberculosis*. However, sulfated lipids are absent from the envelope of *M. bovis* because the glycolipid sulfotransferase and arylsulphatase genes are disrupted or deleted (4). This difference may also contribute to determine the host range and tissue tropism of *M. bovis*. As described above, LAM, the major mycobacterial glycolipid, may contribute to arrest phagosome maturation. In addition, LAM is a powerful scavenger of oxygen (reactive oxygen intermediates, ROI) and nitrogen (reactive nitrogen intermediates, RNI) reactive intermediates (23,23). Moreover, virulent strains of *M. tuberculosis* and *M. bovis* BCG contain mannosylated LAM. Mannosylated LAM provides another way for mycobacteria to enter phagocytes via mannose receptors, and it serves as a ligand for the interaction with dendritic cells (a major antigen-presenting cell). The macrophage mannose receptor is involved in the presentation of LAM to T cells via CD1 molecules. However, no definitive correlation of mannosylated LAM to mycobacterial virulence has yet been shown (31,32).

Proteins and protein complexes (i.e., lipoproteins) of *M. bovis* and other pathogenic mycobacteria also play an important role in pathogenesis. Of particular interest are the secreted proteins in the antigen 85 complex, as they may play a role in development of CMI and disease in the host (33). Moreover, these proteins have been shown to possess enzymatic activity and catalyze mycolyltransfer reactions involved in the final stages of mycobacterial cell wall assembly (34). Regarding binding activities, fibronectin binds to antigen 85 complex, and the release of large amounts of this antigen could inhibit binding of fibronectin to tubercle bacilli (35). Although little or no evidence exists that fibronectin directly mediates phagocytosis of mycobacteria, there is some evidence that fibronectin enables monocytes to phagocytose C3b-sensitized cells (36). This finding may be of importance, as it has been shown that complement receptors also mediate phagocytosis of *M. tuberculosis* (25,37). Proteins encoded by the *mce* operons seem to play a role in the entry and survival of mycobacteria within phagocytic cells, as well as in the invasion of epithelial cells (38). There are four operons in *M. tuberculosis*, each encoding five to six proteins, whereas the *mce3* operon is absent from *M. bovis* (4,5).

Several stress proteins have been identified as major immunodominant antigens of mycobacteria (39,40). The elevated synthesis of these proteins in response to changes in physiological conditions within the phagosome may protect the mycobacteria from hydrolytic enzymes, ROI (i.e., superoxide anion), and RNI (i.e., nitric oxide—NO). Superoxide dismutases (SODs) are produced and released by several mycobacterial pathogens (41–43). *M. bovis* and *M. tuberculosis* possess a redundant system of two SODs (4,5). The iron–manganese–dependent SOD (Sod A) is secreted and seems the more fundamental enzyme for resistance against reactive oxygen intermediates (42,44). Another membrane-associated copper–zinc–dependent SOD (Sod C) may play an additional role to protect tubercle bacilli against the oxidative burst of activated macrophages (45). In contrast, protection against reactive nitrogen intermediates is provided by two alkyl hydroperoxidases denominated AhpC and AhpD (46,47). In addition, housekeeping functions such as enzymes involved in major metabolic pathways are also important for the virulence of *M. bovis*. For example, it has been shown that *M. tuberculosis* persistence in infected mice and macrophages requires the glyoxylate enzyme isocitrate lyase that is also present in *M. bovis* (48). Furthermore, mutations in many metabolic genes also result in the attenuation of the virulence of tubercle bacilli (49,50).

Effector Mechanisms against Mycobacterial Infections

Discussions will concern primarily CMI against virulent tubercle bacilli or their virulence factors, as these effects are the most relevant to determine protection. However, analysis of serum therapy against human tuberculosis indicates that humoral (antibody) responses against certain antigens (e.g., carbohydrate components or adhesion proteins) also may be protective (51). In this context, a conjugated vaccine of protein-arabinomannan was shown to be protective against tuberculosis in a mice model of infection (52). In contrast, other humoral responses are usually detrimental (e.g., antibodies that alter the surface charge of phagocytic cells enhancing chemotaxis and uptake). Thus, the role of humoral immunity in protection against *M. bovis* is unclear.

The natural and acquired cellular immune response mechanisms of bovines are often successful in limiting proliferation of tubercle bacilli and development of progressive disease. Elimination of *M. bovis* from host tissues depends, in part, on killing the bacillus in mononuclear macrophages that have been activated by lymphokines. Although this mechanism is generally accepted, evidence to support this concept is mostly based on information obtained from studies in small laboratory animals using *M. tuberculosis* or *M. bovis* BCG. Tuberculostatic murine macrophage functions are enhanced following exposure to interferon (IFN) gamma, whereas interleukin 4 and tumor necrosis factor do not increase these activities (53). However, IFN-gamma and tumor necrosis factor act synergistically to induce increased production of NO and RNI in mouse macrophages that are able to inhibit growth and kill intracellular *M. tuberculosis* and *M. bovis* BCG (53,54). Significant studies have been performed on the role of RNI and ROI in mycobactericidal action (47,55). Mouse macrophages release abundant NO production on infection with mycobacteria. This release is mediated by IFN-gamma-inducible nitric oxide synthase (also referred as iNOS or NOS2). Several studies indicated that cultured human macrophages did not produce iNOS upon mycobacterial infections. However, *in vivo* studies have shown significant induction of NO production. Current evidence indicates that human macrophages do possess iNOS activity, but that the levels of NO production are highly dependent on the state of differentiation of the phagocytes and the tissue of origin. For example, alveolar and peritoneal macrophages display significant NO production. In summary, RNI, especially NO, may play the more fundamental role in the control of mycobacterial infections (47,55). This view is supported by the fact that NO has both bactericidal and immunomodulatory effects, in contrast to ROI, which are only bactericidal. Moreover, RNI and ROI may also act synergistically by the formation of the highly bactericidal compound peroxynitrite. In cattle, iNOS activity and NO production have been shown to occur in cultured bovine macrophages in response to mycobacterial infections, but they do not seem to require stimulation with bovine IFN-gamma (56). Thus, iNOS synthesis in cattle seems to differ in its regulation by lymphokines.

Processing of mycobacterial antigens by macrophages and presentation to T lymphocytes also play a key role in the release of the appropriate lymphokines necessary for full activation of the bactericidal mechanisms of phagocytic cells. T lymphocytes can be divided in T-helper (CD4) and T-cytotoxic cells (CD8, CTL). T-helper cells are further subdivided on the basis of their lymphokine profiles (57). Type 1 cells (Th1) produce IFN-gamma and interleukin 2, which stimulate macrophage activation, whereas type 2 cells (Th2) produce interleukin 4, which leads to a humoral response. Th1 and Th2 cells operate in a reciprocal fashion, whereby cellular and humoral immune responses are mutually antagonistic. Thus, Th2 cells are associated with exacerbation and rapid lesion formation in several chronic infectious disease models. Therefore, the existence or absence of an immune response does not predict protection; this is dependent on the balance between the various types of host responses and the virulence of the bacterial strain.

The availability of transgenic "knockout" mice with disruptions in genes critical for immunological functions has provided new tools for delineating the role of the various immune responses in protection from infection. Mice lacking the gene for beta-2 microglobulin are unable to express the major histocompatibility complex class I (MHC class I). MHC class I molecules are required for presenting antigens to CTL; hence, these mice lack the ability to generate CTL. It was assumed that only CD4 T cells capable of making appropriate lymphokines were involved in protection against tuberculosis. However, it has been shown that mice that are unable to generate MHC class I–restricted T cells die extremely rapidly from *M. tuberculosis* infection. Interestingly, these mice can survive *M. bovis* BCG infection, indicating that CTLs are necessary for protection against tuberculosis (58).

Deficiencies of T lymphocyte and macrophage functions have been associated with opportunistic mycobacterial diseases (59,60). These abnormalities may be mediated by increased conversion of arachidonic acid into prostaglandins via the cyclooxygenase pathway. In this context, lymphocyte responses to a purified protein derivative from *M. avium* and *M. intracellulare* improved in cultures containing indomethacin, an inhibitor of cyclooxygenase (61). Activated mononuclear macrophages exhibit marked morphological changes, including increases in the number of mitochondria, spreading ability, and phagocytic and microbicidal activities. Activated alveolar macrophages from rabbits receiving *M. bovis* BCG (heat killed in oil) showed increases in tricarboxylic acid cycle and hexose monophosphate shunt activities in comparison to normal cells.

Macrophage functions such as chemotaxis, phagocytosis, enzyme secretion, and cytotoxicity are also influenced by intracellular nucleotide levels. Studies on the activation of adenylate cyclase in isolated macrophage membranes revealed that guanine-5-monophosphate, present in the macrophage membrane, regulates adenylate cyclase activation (62). Furthermore, certain chemical mediators such as prostaglandins can exert their effect on cyclic adenosine-5-monophosphate production by stimulating membrane-bound adenylate cyclase. Macrophages infected with live *M. bovis* BCG have increased cyclic adenosine-5-monophosphate levels and reduced phagolysosome formation (63).

Concerns when conducting tuberculin skin tests in animals are related most often to the failure of some *M. bovis*–infected animals with advanced lesions to respond to purified protein derivative tuberculin (64). The analytical sensitivity of these tests in detecting tuberculosis varies for animals in a population. In animals with healed lesions, dormant infections, or advanced disease, test responses may be diminished. The problem of nonresponsiveness can be minimized by removing all test-responder animals on the first test. Repeated testing appears to increase the number of *M. bovis*–infected animals failing to respond to *M. bovis* purified protein derivative in populations in which infection persists (10). Changes in responsiveness to tuberculin in skin tests have been attributed in part to lymphokine-induced immunosuppression. *M. bovis* and *M. tuberculosis* are formidable pathogens that appear to require an orchestrated immune response to engender protection. In summary, both CD4-helper T cells producing lymphokines such as IFN-gamma that can activate bactericidal macrophage effector mechanisms and CD8 MHC class I restricted cytotoxic T lymphocytes are necessary. The model would hold that activated macrophages can kill or inhibit the growth of small numbers of invading organisms. However, if mycobacteria escape this immunological surveillance and reach a critical number, an individual macrophage is no longer capable of killing or inhibiting growth of the microorganism and is likely to spread the infection. Thus, only by lysing macrophages overwhelmed by the infection and creating inflammation is it possible to reduce the number of invading bacilli to a level that can be resisted by new infiltrating mononuclear phagocytes. This ultimately raises the question of whether pathogenesis and tissue damage are the price one pays for protection against tuberculosis. However, it is not known whether protective immunity requires a strong delayed-type hypersensitive response (65). In this context, vaccines eliciting strong hypersensitive responses may be less protective than vaccines eliciting weaker responses.

Natural Resistance to Mycobacterial Infections

Some animals and humans display increased natural resistance to mycobacterial infections. The molecular bases of this effect have been extensively investigated, but contradictory results across and within host species have raised substantial controversy. In mice, it seems that the Nramp1 protein plays an important role in resistance (66). This protein is a divalent cation transporter and has affinity for both iron and manganese (67). Definite polymorphisms leading to nonconservative changes in the amino acid sequence of the host Nramp1 protein have been associated with increased natural resistance to mycobacterial infections, with the resistant allele being dominant. More recently, an Nramp1 orthologue (e.g., genes in different species that derive from a common ancestor) has been found in *M. bovis* and *M. tuberculosis* (5). This finding led to the hypothesis that the resistant Nramp1 protein in the host may compete favorably with the mycobacterial counterpart (Mramp) and decrease the availability of iron and manganese for the bacilli (68). However, this hypothesis is difficult to reconcile with the finding that disruption of the bacterial gene in *M. tuberculosis* does not affect virulence in mice (69,70). An Nramp1 orthologue is also present in cattle, but in this case, polymorphisms associated in mice with resistance failed to protect cattle against tuberculosis (71). This indicates that in bovines, Nramp1 polymorphisms cannot account for natural resistance. In humans, some evidence predicts a role of Nramp in resistance (72), but more extensive studies are needed. Moreover, in all animal species, there is a family of Nramp proteins, making it difficult to sort out individual effects (73). Thus, extensive investigations are necessary to reach a more thorough understanding of the resistant phenotype in the various hosts.

References

1. Thoen, C. O. and R. G. Barletta. 2004. Mycobacterium. *In* C. L. Gyles, J. F. Prescott, J. G. Songer, and C. O. Thoen (ed.), Pathogenesis of Bacterial Infections in Animals. Ames, IA: Blackwell Publishing, 69-76.
2. Aranaz, A., D. Cousins, A. Mateos, and L. Dominguez. 2003. Elevation of *Mycobacterium tuberculosis* subsp. caprae Aranaz et al. 1999 to species rank as *Mycobacterium caprae* comb. nov., sp. nov. *Int J Syst Evol Microbiol* 53:1785-9.
3. Cousins, D. V., R. Bastida, A. Cataldi, V. Quse, S. Redrobe, et al. 2003. Tuberculosis in seals caused by a novel member of the *Mycobacterium tuberculosis* complex: *Mycobacterium pinnipedii* sp. nov. *Int J Syst Evol Microbiol* 53:1305-14.
4. Garnier, T., K. Eiglmeier, J. C. Camus, N. Medina, H. Mansoor, et al. 2003. The complete genome sequence of Mycobacterium bovis. *Proc Natl Acad Sci USA* 100:7877-82.
5. Cole, S. T., R. Brosch, J. Parkhill, T. Garnier, C. Churcher, et al. 1998. Deciphering the biology of *Mycobacterium tuberculosis* from the complete genome sequence. *Nature* 393:537-44.
6. Braunstein, M., S. S. Bardarov, and W. R. Jacobs, Jr. 2002. Genetic methods for deciphering virulence determinants of *Mycobacterium tuberculosis*. *Methods Enzymol* 358: 67-99.
7. Brennan, M. J., G. Delogu, Y. Chen, S. Bardarov, J. Kriakov, et al. 2001. Evidence that mycobacterial PE_PGRS proteins are cell surface constituents that influence interactions with other cells. *Infect Immun* 69:7326-33.
8. Brosch, R., S. V. Gordon, M. Marmiesse, P. Brodin, C. Buchrieser, et al. 2002. A new evolutionary scenario for the *Mycobacterium tuberculosis* complex. *Proc Natl Acad Sci USA* 99:3684-9.

9. Fabre, M., J. L. Koeck, P. Le Fleche, F. Simon, V. Herve, et al. 2004. High genetic diversity revealed by variable-number tandem repeat genotyping and analysis of hsp65 gene polymorphism in a large collection of *"Mycobacterium canettii"* strains indicates that the *M. tuberculosis* complex is a recently emerged clone of *"M. canettii". J Clin Microbiol* 42:3248-55.

10. Thoen, C. O. and B. R. Bloom. 1995. Pathogenesis of *Mycobacterium bovis. In* C. O. Thoen and J. H. Steele (ed.), *Mycobacterium bovis* Infection in Animals and Humans. Ames: Iowa State Press, 3-14.

11. Sturgill-Koszycki, S., P. H. Schlesinger, P. Chakraborty, P. L. Haddix, H. L. Collins, et al. 1994. Lack of acidification in *Mycobacterium* phagosomes produced by exclusion of the vesicular proton-ATPase. *Science* 263:678-81.

12. Beatty, W. L., E. R. Rhoades, H. J. Ullrich, D. Chatterjee, J. E. Heuser, and D. G. Russell. 2000. Trafficking and release of mycobacterial lipids from infected macrophages. *Traffic* 1:235-47.

13. Vergne, I., R. A. Fratti, P. J. Hill, J. Chua, J. Belisle, and V. Deretic. 2004. *Mycobacterium tuberculosis* phagosome maturation arrest: mycobacterial phosphatidylinositol analog phosphatidylinositol mannoside stimulates early endosomal fusion. *Mol Biol Cell* 15:751-60.

14. Beatty, W. L. and D. G. Russell. 2000. Identification of mycobacterial surface proteins released into subcellular compartments of infected macrophages. *Infect Immun* 68:6997-7002.

15. Stamm, L. M., J. H. Morisaki, L. Y. Gao, R. L. Jeng, K. L. McDonald, et al. 2003. *Mycobacterium marinum* escapes from phagosomes and is propelled by actin-based motility. *J Exp Med* 198:1361-8.

16. Teitelbaum, R., M. Cammer, M. L. Maitland, N. E. Freitag, J. Condeelis, and B. R. Bloom. 1999. Mycobacterial infection of macrophages results in membrane-permeable phagosomes. *Proc Natl Acad Sci USA* 96:15190-5.

17. McDonough, K. A., Y. Kress, and B. R. Bloom. 1993. Pathogenesis of tuberculosis: interaction of *Mycobacterium tuberculosis* with macrophages. *Infect Immun* 61:2763-73.

18. Thoen, C. O., K. J. Throlson, L. D. Miller, E. M. Himes, and R. L. Morgan. 1988. Pathogenesis of *Mycobacterium bovis* infection in American bison. *Am J Vet Res* 49:1861-5.

19. McNeil, M. R. and P. J. Brennan. 1991. Structure, function and biogenesis of the cell envelope of mycobacteria in relation to bacterial physiology, pathogenesis and drug resistance; some thoughts and possibilities arising from recent structural information. *Res Microbiol* 142:451-63.

20. Shinnick, T. M., M. H. Vodkin, and J. C. Williams. 1988. The Mycobacterium tuberculosis 65-kilodalton antigen is a heat shock protein which corresponds to common antigen and to the *Escherichia coli* GroEL protein. *Infect Immun* 56:446-51.

21. Young, D., R. Lathigra, R. Hendrix, D. Sweetser, and R. A. Young. 1988. Stress proteins are immune targets in leprosy and tuberculosis. *Proc Natl Acad Sci USA* 85:4267-70.

22. Chan, J., X. D. Fan, S. W. Hunter, P. J. Brennan, and B. R. Bloom. 1991. Lipoarabinomannan, a possible virulence factor involved in persistence of *Mycobacterium tuberculosis* within macrophages. *Infect Immun* 59:1755-61.

23. Chan, J., T. Fujiwara, P. Brennan, M. McNeil, S. J. Turco, et al. 1989. Microbial glycolipids: possible virulence factors that scavenge oxygen radicals. *Proc Natl Acad Sci USA* 86:2453-7.

24. Chua, J. and V. Deretic. 2004. *Mycobacterium tuberculosis* reprograms waves of phosphatidylinositol 3-phosphate on phagosomal organelles. *J Biol Chem* 279: 36982-92.

25. Ernst, J. D. 1998. Macrophage receptors for *Mycobacterium tuberculosis. Infect Immun* 66:1277-81

26. Schluger, N. W. and Rom, W. N. 1998. The host immune response to tuberculosis. *Am J Respir Crit Care Med* 157:679-91.

27. Noll, H., H. Bloch, J. Asselineau, and E. Lederer. 1956. The chemical structure of the cord factor of *Mycobacterium tuberculosis. Biochim Biophys Acta* 20:299-309.

28. Kato, M. and K. Fukushi. 1969. Studies of a biochemical lesion in experimental tuberculosis in mice. X. Mitochondrial swelling induced by cord factor *in vivo* and accompanying biochemical change. *Am Rev Respir Dis* 100:42-46.

29. Fukuyama, K., J. Tani, and M. Kato. 1971. Effect of cord factor (mycobacterial toxic glycolipid) on liver microsomes in vivo. *J Biochem (Tokyo)* 69:511-16.

30. Glickman, M. S., J. S. Cox, W. R. Jacobs Jr. 2000. A novel mycolic acid cyclopropane synthetase is required for cording, persistence, and virulence of *Mycobacterium tuberculosis. Mol Cell* 5:717-27.

31. Fenton, M. J., L. W. Riley, and L. S. Schlessinger. 2005. Receptor-mediated recognition of *Mycobacterium tuberculosis. In* S. T. Cole, K. D. Eisenach, D. N. McMurray, and W. R. Jacobs Jr. (ed.). Tuberculosis and the Tubercle Bacillus. Washington, DC: ASM Press, 405-26.

32. Schlesinger, L. S., S. R. Hull, and T. M. Kaufman. 1994. Binding of the terminal mannosyl units of lipoarabinomannan from a virulent strain of *Mycobacterium tuberculosis* to human macrophages. *J Immunol* 152:4070-9.

33. Andersen, P., D. Askgaard, L. Ljungqvist, J. Bennedsen, and I. Heron. 1991. Proteins released from *Mycobacterium tuberculosis* during growth. *Infect Immun* 59:1905-10.

34. Belisle, J. T., V. D. Vissa, T. Sievert, K. Takayama, P. J. Brennan, and G. S. Besra. 1997. Role of the major antigen of *Mycobacterium tuberculosis* in cell wall biogenesis. *Science* 276:1420-2.

35. Abou-Zeid, C., T. L. Ratliff, H. G. Wiker, M. Harboe, J. Bennedsen, and G. A. Rook. 1988. Characterization of fibronectin-binding antigens released by *Mycobacterium tuberculosis* and *Mycobacterium bovis* BCG. *Infect Immun* 56:3046-51.

36. Pommier, C. G., S. Inada, L. F. Fries, T. Takahashi, M. M. Frank, and E. J. Brown. 1983. Plasma fibronectin enhances phagocytosis of opsonized particles by human peripheral blood monocytes. *J Exp Med* 157:1844-54.

37. Schlesinger, L. S., C. G. Bellinger-Kawahara, N. R. Payne, and M. A. Horwitz. 1990. Phagocytosis of *Mycobacterium tuberculosis* is mediated by human monocyte complement receptors and complement component C3. *J Immunol* 144:2771-80.

38. Arruda, S., G. Bomfim, R. Knights, T. Huima-Byron, and L. W. Riley. 1993. Cloning of an *M. tuberculosis* DNA fragment associated with entry and survival inside cells. *Science* 261:1454-7.

39. Mehra, V., J. H. Gong, D. Iyer, Y. Lin, C. T. Boylen, et al. 1996. Immune response to recombinant mycobacterial proteins in patients with tuberculosis infection and disease. *J Infect Dis* 174:431-4.

40. Young, R. A. and T. J. Elliott. 1989. Stress proteins, infection, and immune surveillance. *Cell* 59:5-8.

41. Escuyer, V., N. Haddad, C. Frehel, and P. Berche. 1996. Molecular characterization of a surface-exposed superoxide dismutase of *Mycobacterium avium. Microb Pathog* 20:41-55.

42. Harth, G. and M. A. Horwitz. 1999. Export of recombinant *Mycobacterium tuberculosis* superoxide dismutase is dependent upon both information in the protein and mycobacterial export machinery. A model for studying export of leaderless proteins by pathogenic mycobacteria. *J Biol Chem* 274:4281-92.

43. Liu, X., Z. Feng, N. B. Harris, J. D. Cirillo, H. Bercovier, and R. G. Barletta. 2001. Identification of a secreted superoxide dismutase in *Mycobacterium avium* ssp. paratuberculosis. *FEMS Microbiol Lett* 202:233-8.

44. Edwards, K. M., M. H. Cynamon, R. K. Voladri, C. C. Hager, M. S. DeStefano, et al. 2001. Iron-cofactored superoxide dismutase inhibits host responses to *Mycobacterium tuberculosis*. *Am J Respir Crit Care Med* 164:2213-9.

45. Piddington, D. L., F. C. Fang, T. Laessig, A. M. Cooper, I. M. Orme, and N. A. Buchmeier. 2001. Cu,Zn superoxide dismutase of *Mycobacterium tuberculosis* contributes to survival in activated macrophages that are generating an oxidative burst. *Infect Immun* 69:4980-7.

46. Chen, L., Q. W. Xie, and C. Nathan. 1998. Alkyl hydroperoxide reductase subunit C (AhpC) protects bacterial and human cells against reactive nitrogen intermediates. *Mol Cell* 1:795-805.

47. Nathan, C. and M. U. Shiloh. 2000. Reactive oxygen and nitrogen intermediates in the relationship between mammalian hosts and microbial pathogens. *Proc Natl Acad Sci USA* 97:8841-8.

48. McKinney, J. D., K. Honer zu Bentrup, E. J. Munoz-Elias, A. Miczak, B. Chen, et al. 2000. Persistence of *Mycobacterium tuberculosis* in macrophages and mice requires the glyoxylate shunt enzyme isocitrate lyase. *Nature* 406:735-8.

49. Guleria, I., R. Teitelbaum, R. A. McAdam, G. Kalpana, W. R. Jacobs Jr., and B. R. Bloom. 1996. Auxotrophic vaccines for tuberculosis. *Nat Med* 2:334-7.

50. Hingley-Wilson, S. M., V. K. Sambandamurthy, and W. R. Jacobs Jr. 2003. Survival perspectives from the world's most successful pathogen, *Mycobacterium tuberculosis*. *Nat Immunol* 4:949-55.

51. Glatman-Freedman, A. and A. Casadevall. 1998. Serum therapy for tuberculosis revisited: reappraisal of the role of antibody-mediated immunity against *Mycobacterium tuberculosis*. *Clin Microbiol Rev* 11:514-32.

52. Haile, M., B. Hamasur, T. Jaxmar, D. Gavier-Widen, M. A. Chambers, et al. 2005. Nasal boost with adjuvanted heat-killed BCG or arabinomannan-protein conjugate improves primary BCG-induced protection in C57BL/6 mice. *Tuberculosis (Edinb)* 85:107-14.

53. Chan, J., Y. Xing, R. S. Magliozzo, and B. R. Bloom. 1992. Killing of virulent *Mycobacterium tuberculosis* by reactive nitrogen intermediates produced by activated murine macrophages. *J Exp Med* 175:1111-22.

54. Flesch, I. E. and S. H. Kaufmann. 1991. Mechanisms involved in mycobacterial growth inhibition by gamma interferon-activated bone marrow macrophages: role of reactive nitrogen intermediates. *Infect Immun* 59:3213-8.

55. Chan, E. D., J. Chan, and N. W. Schluger. 2001. What is the role of nitric oxide in murine and human host defense against tuberculosis? Current knowledge. *Am J Respir Cell Mol Biol* 25:606-12.

56. Adler, H., B. Frech, M. Thony, H. Pfister, E. Peterhans, and T. W. Jungi. 1995. Inducible nitric oxide synthase in cattle. Differential cytokine regulation of nitric oxide synthase in bovine and murine macrophages. *J Immunol* 154:4710-8.

57. Salgame, P., J. S. Abrams, C. Clayberger, H. Goldstein, J. Convit, et al. 1991. Differing lymphokine profiles of functional subsets of human CD4 and CD8 T cell clones. *Science* 254:279-82.

58. Flynn, J. L., J. Chan, K. J. Triebold, D. K. Dalton, T. A. Stewart, and B. R. Bloom. 1993. An essential role for interferon gamma in resistance to *Mycobacterium tuberculosis* infection. *J Exp Med* 178:2249-54.

59. Mason 3rd, U. G., L. E. Greenberg, S. S. Yen, and C. H. Kirkpatrick. 1982. Indomethacin-responsive mononuclear cell dysfunction in "atypical" mycobacteriosis. *Cell Immunol* 71:54-65.

60. Uchiyama, N., G. R. Greene, B. J. Warren, P. A. Morozumi, G. S. Spear, and S. P. Galant. 1981. Possible monocyte killing defect in familial atypical mycobacteriosis. *J Pediatr* 98:785-8.

61. K. Kato and K. Yamamoto. 1982. Involvement of prostaglandin E1 in delayed-type hypersensitivity suppression induced with live *Mycobacterium bovis* BCG. *Infect Immun* 36:426-9.

62. M. W. Verghese and R. Snyderman. 1983. Hormonal activation of adenylate cyclase in macrophage membranes is regulated by guanine nucleotides. *J Immunol* 130:869-73.

63. Lowrie, D. B., V. R. Aber, and P. S. Jackett. 1979. Phagosome-lysosome fusion and cyclic adenosine 3':5'-monophosphate in macrophages infected with *Mycobacterium microti, Mycobacterium bovis* BCG or *Mycobacterium lepraemurium. J Gen Microbiol* 110:431-41.

64. Thoen, C. O. 1988. Tuberculosis. *J Am Vet Med Assoc* 193:1045-8.

65. Fine, P. E., J. A. Sterne, J. M. Ponnighaus, and R. J. Rees. 1994. Delayed-type hypersensitivity, mycobacterial vaccines and protective immunity. *Lancet* 344:1245-9.

66. Frehel, C., F. Canonne-Hergaux, P. Gros, and C. De Chastellier. 2002. Effect of Nramp1 on bacterial replication and on maturation of *Mycobacterium avium*-containing phagosomes in bone marrow-derived mouse macrophages. *Cell Microbiol* 4:541-56.

67. Kehres, D. G. and M. E. Maguire. 2003. Emerging themes in manganese transport, biochemistry and pathogenesis in bacteria. *FEMS Microbiol Rev* 27: 263-90.

68. Agranoff, D., I. M. Monahan, J. A. Mangan, P. D. Butcher, and S. Krishna. 1999. *Mycobacterium tuberculosis* expresses a novel pH-dependent divalent cation transporter belonging to the Nramp family. *J Exp Med* 190:717-24.

69. Boechat, N., B. Lagier-Roger, S. Petit, Y. Bordat, J. Rauzier, et al. 2002. Disruption of the gene homologous to mammalian Nramp1 in *Mycobacterium tuberculosis* does not affect virulence in mice. *Infect Immun* 70:4124-31.

70. Domenech, P., A. S. Pym, M. Cellier, C. E. Barry 3rd, and S. T. Cole. 2002. Inactivation of the *Mycobacterium tuberculosis* Nramp orthologue (mntH) does not affect virulence in a mouse model of tuberculosis. *FEMS Microbiol Lett* 207:81-6.

71. Barthel, R., J. A. Piedrahita, D. N. McMurray, J. Payeur, D. Baca, et al. 2000. Pathologic findings and association of *Mycobacterium bovis* infection with the bovine NRAMP1 gene in cattle from herds with naturally occurring tuberculosis. *Am J Vet Res* 61:1140-4.

72. Kim, J. H. , S. Y. Lee, S. H. Lee, C. Sin, J. J. Shim, et al. 2003. NRAMP1 genetic polymorphisms as a risk factor of tuberculous pleurisy. *Int J Tuberc Lung Dis* 7:370-5.

73. Forbes, J. R. and P. Gros. 2001. Divalent-metal transport by NRAMP proteins at the interface of host-pathogen interactions. *Trends Microbiol* 9:397-403.

Chapter 5

Epidemiology of *Mycobacterium bovis*

J.B. Kaneene, DVM, PhD, and D. Pfeiffer, DVM, PhD

Introduction

Bovine tuberculosis (TB) was first recognized in domesticated animals, although its host range is broad and includes most mammalian species. In addition to livestock and wild hoofed mammals, the disease has been reported in elephants, non-human primates, and many other species (1). Apart from the pathogenetic mechanisms, the ability of *Mycobacterium bovis* to infect such a wide variety of species can be attributed to the different routes of transmission by which *M. bovis* can be passed from animal to animal.

Routes of Transmission

There are several routes of transmission for *M. bovis* infection, but the primary routes of infection are via the respiratory and gastrointestinal tracts. Experimental studies involving exposure of animals to *M. bovis* via different routes (intratracheal, oral, intravenous, intraperitoneal) have demonstrated that the nature and extent of tuberculous lesions vary with the route of exposure (2), and the location of tuberculous lesions affects how *M. bovis* is shed from the infected host. These include lesions of the respiratory system, kidneys, mammary glands, and the gastrointestinal system (3,4). Externally draining cutaneous abscesses can also be a source of infection in a wide variety of domestic and wild mammals (4,5).

Inhalation

Respiratory transmission via the inhalation of contaminated aerosols or fomites is the most efficient form of transmission, requiring a low number of organisms as an infective dose (2). Under most circumstances, an infected host generates an aerosol containing *M. bovis* when the animal coughs or sneezes, and the aerosol is inhaled directly by an uninfected host, resulting in infection (2).

Under natural conditions, respiratory transmission has been detected in herding animals, such as domestic and wild bovines, and in captive herds of various cervid species (6). Transmission of *M. bovis* via inhalation is effective in animals that are kept in confinement (7) and in free-ranging wildlife that maintain social or familial groups in underground dens, such as European badgers (*Meles meles*) in the United Kingdom (8) and brushtail possums (*Trichosurus vulpecula*) in New Zealand (9). There have been rare instances in which an indirect aerosol transmission has been documented: pressure-washing facilities at a zoo where a TB-infected rhinoceros was housed may have aerosolized *M. bovis* and resulted in cases of pulmonary TB in primates housed in facilities near the rhinoceros housing (7). Respiratory transmission of *M. bovis* has been detected in wildlife during periods when normal behaviors become altered and result in direct contact between animals, such as white-tailed deer (*Odocoileus virginianus*) behavior in the presence of supplemental winter feeding in Michigan (6,10), or an instance in which a dog acquired TB through inhalation from contact with a tuberculous possum, based on the presence of extensive lesions in the lungs and an absence of lesions elsewhere in the body (11).

Evidence for inhalation transmission is in the location of affected lymph nodes (12). Respiratory transmission has been experimentally demonstrated in a variety of different species, and lymph nodes associated with the respiratory tract, particularly the bronchial and mediastinal, are the most commonly affected by inhaled *M. bovis* (13).

Ingestion

Although respiratory transmission is the most important route of infection in groups of animals that remain in close contact, oral transmission through ingestion of *M. bovis* is another important route. For oral transmission to be accomplished, an uninfected animal has to consume feed or water contaminated with mucous or nasal secretions, feces, or urine that contain the infective organisms, or to receive milk from an infected dam.

Oral transmission of *M. bovis* has been seen in several species through pastures (14) water sources (15), infected animal carcasses (16), and contaminated mucous or abscesses (13). Consumption of infected feeds has also been implicated in interspecies disease transmission in which direct contact between species was not evident (14,17). It has even been suggested that *M. bovis*–infected wild seals in Western Australia contracted the infection from cattle carcasses dumped in the sea by some farmers during the TB eradication process (18).

As in the case of transmission through inhalation, evidence for ingestion transmission is often found through the distribution of tuberculous lesions in naturally infected animals. In these circumstances, the mesenteric lymph nodes are usually affected (3) and have been used to suggest that oral transmission is a more important route of infection in some situations (4).

Transcutaneous

Another less-common form of transmission is through transcutaneous transmission of *M. bovis*. This occurs in humans who handle infected carcasses, where infection had been spread via cuts and abrasions (e.g., butcher's wart in humans) (19).

In animals, transcutaneous transmission is primarily from bites by infected animals. This has been seen in domestic cats (16), ferrets (*Mustela furo*) (16), and European badgers (3).

Vertical

One route of transmission that is less evident in the epidemiology of *M. bovis* is vertical transmission. Vertical transmission has also been identified in some species (12) but has rarely been documented in wildlife under natural conditions. Cases of apparent vertical transmission, or pseudo-vertical transmission, in wildlife can appear through consumption of milk from infected mothers (4), or simply from close contact between mother and offspring (9,13). This form of transmission has been seen in many wildlife species, including badgers (20,21), brushtail possums (9), and white-tailed deer (13).

Issues with Determining Routes of Transmission

Unfortunately, the location of tuberculous lesions is not a conclusive determinant of the route of transmission of the disease (22). Although the lymph nodes of the respiratory and gastrointestinal tracts are commonly affected in naturally transmitted *M. bovis,* lesions in the alimentary canal, such as in retropharyngeal lymph nodes in white-tailed deer (23), can come into contact with the organism through either inhalation or ingestion. Once infection becomes disseminated, or is given at high doses under experimental conditions, severe disease will involve lymph nodes throughout the thorax and abdomen (4). However, some hosts exposed orally to *M. bovis*, such as swine, may only develop lesions in cranial lymph nodes (14,22). Although many of the primary nonaerosol sources of *M. bovis* infection in humans have been removed in industrialized countries, there has been an increase in the number of cases of pulmonary infection with *M. bovis*, which may be caused by several factors: the lung is the usual site of postprimary *M. bovis* infection, regardless of the site of the primary lesion, and cases of pulmonary *M. bovis* infection maybe the result of reactivation of previously quiescent (i.e., nonclinical) primary lesions.

Characteristics of the Epidemiology of *M. bovis*

Given the public health consequences of *M. bovis* infection, the epidemiology of the disease has historically been of great interest. Outbreaks of *M. bovis* infection as well as endemic infection have been reported in animal populations. Outbreaks are characterized by a relatively rapid increase in infection rate over a short period within a population of animals; these outbreaks can occur with the introduction of infected animals to a population (e.g., a cattle herd) that has susceptible animals that have the capacity to spread the disease among their herd mates. However, it is also possible for the infection to spread relatively slowly, depending on the disease progression in infected animals and on the opportunities for contact with other animals within the herd. Endemic mycobacterial infections are characterized by low rates of infection and have also been reported in animal populations. The extent of the disease is not sufficient to affect the survival of the population, but it is sufficient to continue transmission of infection within the populations (24).

The development of molecular techniques for differentiating strains of *M. bovis*, such as DNA fingerprinting (restriction fragment length polymorphism and spoligotyping) has been useful in outbreak investigations in animals and humans to identify potential sources of infection, or relatedness of strains (14,25). Although DNA fingerprinting is a useful tool, the tests must be conducted under carefully controlled conditions to avoid contamination and false-positive findings. More important, results of these tests do not indicate the source and direction of the infection (i.e., results of the test cannot indicate which of two infected populations was the source of infection for the other), but it may be possible to draw causal inferences by taking other epidemiological information into account.

Because of the large number of susceptible species, the differences in pathogenesis, and the variety of possible transmission mechanisms, combined with the lack of effective vaccination and moderately accurate diagnostic methods, bovine TB can be difficult to control. This is particularly the case in epidemiological systems in which wild animal infection reservoirs are present. In such situations, a systems approach, rather than the traditional single-species approach, needs to be applied to disease management to be able to effectively control infection. As part of this approach, epidemiological investigations need to be conducted so that the spillover and key reservoir hosts can be defined. Effective disease management will change a reservoir to a spillover host (1).

M. bovis in Livestock

Bovine TB, as the name implies, was first recognized in domesticated animals. Farmed species that are known to be susceptible to *M. bovis* include cattle (15,26), water buffalo (*Bubalus bubalis*) (27), and other hoof stock (26). There have also been instances in which feral livestock, such as swine, have been infected in the wild (9,22). Of these species, cattle are the most important reservoir for *M. bovis*. The geographic range of *M. bovis* in livestock parallels the distribution of livestock throughout the world. Apart from small-scale studies, little information is available on the *M. bovis* infection rates in livestock in developing countries.

Rates of Disease

United States

Since the inception of national TB control programs in the early 20th century, rates of *M. bovis* infection had dramatically declined to the point at which the disease was eradicated in the majority of the country. Recently, however, there have been outbreaks of *M. bovis* in U.S. cattle herds in four states: Michigan, Texas, New Mexico, and California. Tuberculosis in Michigan has affected a total of 33 beef and dairy cattle operations since 1997, and a wildlife reservoir of *M. bovis* has been presumed to be the source of infection for these cattle (17,28). In Texas, the TB problem is concentrated in the El Paso milkshed area. The states of California and New Mexico have experienced limited outbreaks of TB (affecting two and three dairies, respectively), which have been attributed to cattle imported from areas where *M. bovis* is an ongoing problem. To curtail spread of *M. bovis* throughout the United States, increased surveillance has been implemented at slaughter and in the affected regions in the country. Of 10 newly affected herds in 2003, six were detected through active area test surveillance in Michigan and California (28).

Canada

Since 1993, a total of 12 herds of cattle and farmed bison (*Bison bison*) have been affected by eight separate outbreaks of *M. bovis* infection in five provinces in Canada (28). Recent identification of a wildlife reservoir in Manitoba has implicated wildlife as a possible source of outbreaks in Manitoba (28).

Great Britain

Tuberculosis herd incidence amongst unrestricted herds has increased from 1.3% in 1996 to 3.5% in 2003 (29). One of the reasons for this increase has been the reduction in cattle testing during the foot-and-mouth disease outbreak in 2001. The sources of infection are still debated, despite several scientific reports commissioned by the U.K. government (30). Infection in wild badgers and the movements of infected animals are considered to be important factors, and the relative contribution of these two components is currently being investigated by a large-scale randomized trial (31).

New Zealand

Control programs are in operation to eradicate infection from domestic cattle as well as farmed deer populations. The percentage of infected herds reduced from 3.78% in 1995–1996 to 0.77% in 2003–2004 (32). Infection occurs only in parts of the country where endemic infection is present in wild brushtail possums (9).

Surveillance and Control Programs

Control programs for TB in animals are primarily focused on control of infection with *M. bovis*. These programs can be considered as having four components: prevention, treatment, eradication, and surveillance. Disease prevention primarily focuses on reducing opportunities for animals to be exposed to the pathogen of concern, as well as reducing the likelihood that an exposed animal will become infected after exposure. A final component of any TB control and eradication program is routine surveillance to detect any changes in development of the disease. This includes antemortem testing and slaughter surveillance of livestock and captive animal species.

Antemortem evaluations are a critical component of TB control programs throughout the world. At this time, one of the most reliable and practical methods of diagnosis (albeit tentative) in domestic animals is assessment via the tuberculin skin test. Animals infected with mycobacteria are allergic to the proteins contained in tuberculin and develop characteristic delayed-type hypersensitivity reactions when exposed to those proteins. The deposition of tuberculin intradermally in the deep layers of the skin usually elicits a local reaction characterized by inflammation and swelling in infected animals, whereas such reactions at the injection site fail to develop in uninfected animals. The sensitivity and specificity of the intradermal test depend on the field conditions, prevalence of infection, and other factors, and the test may not be effective or practical for use in all species; however, it has been accepted by the U.S. Department of Agriculture for identification of *M. bovis* in cattle and goats (33).

On cattle farms, the major source of *M. bovis* is infected cattle that either reside on the farm or are introduced to the herd from another facility. In some production systems, as found in the Republic of Ireland, there is also the possibility of contact between animals from neighboring farms. Basic herd hygiene and biosecurity practices (e.g., routine testing for TB and quarantine of imported animals, manure management, and maintenance of feed and water hygiene) have been found to reduce the risks of spread of *M. bovis* on cattle farms (12,17). The Bacille Calmette-Güerin vaccine does not completely prevent infection in cattle or other animals (34); moreover, vaccinated animals yield positive results on the tuberculin skin test, which precludes the use of the vaccine in the United States and other countries with eradication programs. It should be noted that there is considerable interest in the development of new DNA vaccines; however, they have not yet been accepted for use in food producing animals.

In domestic livestock herds, complete depopulation is an effective way of removing *M. bovis* from a livestock operation. The facility can be restocked after a waiting period during which livestock are not allowed onto the depopulated site. Although depopulation is an effective tool for controlling the livestock industry as a whole, the effects can be devastating both financially and emotionally to individual farmers. As an alternative to depopulation of herds in the United States, the U.S. Department of Agriculture allows regulatory agencies to develop herd-specific test and slaughter programs for individual livestock operations (33).

Many countries in Europe and New Zealand conduct control programs that are based on herd testing and removal of test-positive animals. An essential component of these programs is that once at least one animal from a herd tests positive, no movements of animals other than to slaughter are allowed until the herd tests negative (1). Until the discovery of the anti-TB drug isonicotinic acid hydrazide, there was no practical treatment for TB. In Brazil and South Africa, investigators have suggested that it is feasible to treat cattle with isoniazid, and guidelines have been developed for treatment of infective animals with anti-TB drugs, but the treatment of TB in cattle is not permitted in the United States or in many other countries (15).

M. bovis in Free-Ranging Wildlife

Infection with *M. bovis* has been documented in wildlife throughout the world in any area where livestock are raised, and in most situations these cases have been considered to be spillover from infected domestic populations (22,35). Cases have been reported in Europe (8,36), Africa (5), Asia (27), Australia (22) and New Zealand (26), and the Americas (37). Wildlife known to be susceptible to *M. bovis* include cervids and other artiodactylae (6,21,35), insectivora (moles, voles, hedgehogs) (8,24), rodents (24), lagomorphs (26), rhinoceros (5,7), primates (38), and several species of pinnipeds (39). In some species, TB is believed to be spillover through consumption of infected carcasses by carnivores and scavengers under natural conditions (6,8,35).

Although a wide variety of wildlife species are susceptible to *M. bovis*, evidence of infection in a given species is not necessarily proof that the species is a reservoir (40). In many of these situations, when the livestock source of TB is removed from an area, spillover cases in wildlife disappear. This was seen in feral swine on Molokai, Hawaii, where the prevalence of *M. bovis* in swine dropped from 30% in 1980 to 3.2% in 1982, after depopulation of a TB-infected cattle herd in 1981 (41). A wildlife reservoir species may serve as a constant source of infection for another, such as cases of TB in feral red deer contracted from infected brushtail possums in New Zealand (9), and TB infection from white-tailed deer to coyotes in Michigan (6). Often, spillover cases of disease match the spatial distribution of known reservoir species (14).

In recent years, several free-ranging wildlife reservoir hosts have been identified. These species include North American bison (*B. bison*) (37), African buffalo (*Syncerus caffer*) (35), European badgers in United Kingdom (24) and Switzerland (8), brushtail possums in New Zealand (21), white-tailed deer in Michigan (6), and several antelope species in South Africa (35). Studies on these wildlife reservoir hosts for *M. bovis* are providing greater insight into the epidemiology of *M. bovis* in both wildlife and domestic animal populations, which is needed to allow more effective control of the infection in domestic livestock.

Examples of Wildlife Reservoirs—European Badgers in Great Britain

Bovine TB was first identified in badgers in Gloucestershire in 1971, in an area where cattle herds had been experiencing TB outbreaks (42). In this area, as in many parts of the world, wildlife (badgers) and livestock (cattle) have coexisted in the same locations for years, and it has been presumed that cattle served as the primary source of infection for badgers: In the Dorset area, cattle outbreaks preceded infection in badgers, with the first outbreak in cattle recorded in 1970 and the first tuberculous badger found in 1974 (42), and infection levels in badger populations have been highest in the region.

European badgers have been shown to be effective reservoir hosts for *M. bovis*. Badgers are susceptible to *M. bovis*, they can survive for years after infection (24), infected females can reproduce (24), and they may be able to contain the infection for long periods of time until infection is "reactivated" by physical stress (43). Infected badgers can shed *M. bovis* through a variety of routes (e.g., respiratory secretions, urine, feces), and shedding may be intermittent, depending on the host's physical condition (36). Female badgers have been found with mammary lesions, making transmission from mother to offspring through milk possible (20). Although mycobacterial infection can be fatal for an individual badger, TB does not negatively affect the age–sex profile of an infected population (20), indicating that an infected population can continue to reproduce and maintain its numbers.

Badger behavior readily supports transmission of *M. bovis* within social groups. Badgers are animals that live in social groups in underground setts, conditions that put several individuals in close contact in confined spaces, where respiratory transmission of TB is efficient. The use of common "latrine" areas for defecation and urination, which can become heavily contaminated with *M. bovis*, can serve as another source of infection. Finally, aggressive behavior by males can result in transcutaneous transmission of *M. bovis* through bite wounding (3).

Examples of Wildlife Reservoirs—African Buffalo in South Africa

Bovine TB was first reported in Kruger National Park in an impala in 1967 (5), with no other evidence of infection in the area, despite surveys conducted in the 1970s. Later, TB was identified in buffalo in the southern edge of Kruger National Park in 1990, in an area where domestic cattle were known to have outbreaks of TB in the 1960s and early 1980s (5). Tuberculosis was probably passed from domestic cattle to buffalo at these times, as contact between species was suggested by a concurrent outbreak of Corridor Disease (buffalo-associated theileriosis) in the domestic cattle (5). As mentioned above, TB first appeared in southern Kruger National Park in 1967 and has been spreading steadily northward from the southern region to the central and northern regions of the park at a rate of approximately 6 km per year (44).

As in the case of European badgers, buffalo have the qualities necessary for a reservoir host for *M. bovis*. Buffalo are highly susceptible to TB (44), and infection does not appear to affect the fertility or lactation rate of female buffalo, allowing infected cows to reproduce. Natural herding behavior, which keeps animals in close contact, allows easy transmission of TB within free-ranging herds (35).

Examples of Wildlife Reservoirs—White-Tailed Deer in the United States

The presence of a self-sustaining *M. bovis* infection in white-tailed deer in Michigan is unique in the world. The majority of cases of bovine TB in wild deer are sporadic cases in individual animals, often in areas where livestock are known reservoirs of infection. In other areas where free-ranging cervids have had long-standing *M. bovis* infections, these infections have been supported by other wildlife reservoirs, such as bison and captive elk (*Cervus elaphus*) in North America, brushtail possums in New Zealand (16), and European badgers in Great Britain (42).

In white-tailed deer, many diseases can be maintained in nature through winter yarding behavior, in which deer spend large amounts of time together in cedar swamplands, where food and shelter from weather is available, and direct contact between individuals is likely. Behavioral modification can also result in changes that increase the likelihood of the spread of disease in a free-ranging wildlife population, particularly those associated with supplemental feeding. Feeding sites, where large numbers of deer come into very close contact for extended periods, have been suggested as contributing to the spread of TB in Michigan deer (6,10). Unintentional supplemental feeding, as in the utilization of cattle feed, either fed or stored outdoors, by white-tailed deer on Michigan farms, has been implicated as a possible cause of bovine TB for cattle herds (17).

Current control measures in this situation include banning supplemental feeding and baiting to reduce the deer population and to decrease direct contact between deer at feeding or baiting sites (6). This program of reduced deer feeding and intensifying hunting pressure has resulted in a decline in TB levels in the wild deer population since 1998 (45).

Examples of Wildlife Reservoirs—Brushtail Possums in New Zealand

Tuberculosis was first identified in brushtail possums in 1967 and has since then become a major source of infection for cattle and deer in New Zealand (46). The initial source of infection for possums is not clear, but it may be from contact with infected livestock in the past.

Brushtail possums have many of the qualities necessary for an ideal host for *M. bovis*. Possums are highly susceptible to infection, shed *M. bovis* through multiple routes (21), and share dens (9). Respiratory transmission of TB is common (9), and transmission from mother to offspring through direct contact and milk has been seen. High local population densities have been associated with increased prevalence of TB in possums, and levels of TB decreased in areas where population reduction was practiced. Unfortunately, in some instances, culling to reduce populations resulted in dispersing infected animals over greater geographic areas. Edge habitats have been associated with clusters of bovine TB in brushtail possums in New Zealand (21,47).

Tuberculosis levels in possums have shown seasonal variations (20,48). Mating behavior appears to account for some of the seasonal variation (48), as possums gather during mating season (9), and the physical stress of hard winters has been associated with changes in levels of TB in possums (48).

Wildlife Surveillance and Control Programs

Explosive increases in numbers of cases of infection are often easily identified through routine surveillance procedures that detect increases in the prevalence or incidence of infection, or as a result of the identification of sick animals that are not included in surveillance programs. An example of the latter is the detection of *M. bovis* infection in free-ranging white-tailed deer in Michigan that was recognized after a hunter submitted a carcass with suspicious lesions to the state's Department of Natural Resources for investigation (49). However, low rates of infection may be below detectable levels for some surveillance methods; the infection may only be detected when circumstances change to increase the number of cases of disease in the population or when a highly susceptible dead-end host is affected by infection from an endemically infected host species, with dramatic effect. These problems associated with detection of low rates of infection must be taken into consideration when evaluating the effectiveness of any surveillance program. Although it is acknowledged that the Michigan form of TB surveillance in wild white-tailed deer (convenience sample of hunter-harvested heads) will not capture all TB cases, because of reliance on hunter submissions and examination of only heads, rather than complete carcasses (13,23), the system has been able to detect TB at levels less than 1% in the TB-affected area from 1996 to 2000 (45).

In areas where livestock have become infected from wildlife, such as in New Zealand, where wild possums are difficult to track, livestock reinfection can be viewed as an indicator of infection in the local possum population (46). Although the main reservoir of *M. bovis* is cattle, there are several instances in which wildlife reservoirs [including European badgers (8), brushtail possums (46), deer (49), African Cape buffalo (35), and wild boar (14)] have been important sources of infection for cattle. Reservoir animals infected with tubercle bacilli that interact with cattle may be the source of herd infections and significant production losses (17,35).

Depending on the reservoir species involved, eradication of *M. bovis* infection in wildlife can be highly problematic. The size and distribution of wildlife populations is often unknown, the extent of disease in the population can be difficult (if not impossible) to estimate accurately, and aspects of animal behavior associated with the distribution of the disease in the wild may be unclear. The control of TB in cervids and other wild animals is limited to population control, because intradermal skin testing of those animals is not practical. In countries in which *M. bovis* infection has been reported in wildlife with relatively small and stable home ranges (brushtail possums and badgers), a Bacille Calmette-Güerin vaccine has been evaluated as an immunizing agent (34).

Population control is commonly used for disease control in wildlife (40). This is usually accomplished by culling to remove infected animals and to reduce population density, which is effective in handling diseases like TB (45). This is usually exercised through trapping and removal programs (36), by directed hunts to reduce animal numbers (35), or by providing incentives to hunters (i.e., unlimited hunting permits and increased duration of the hunting season) to increase the number of animals removed during the hunting season (6). However, culling large numbers of animals from an area may encourage emigration, and reduction or removal of a species could significantly affect local ecosystem integrity (37). In addition, culling to reduce disease may require levels of killing that result in a critical reduction of genetic diversity in endangered species (35). Culling animals for disease control is often unpopular with the general public, and public sentiment may raise objections to necessary levels of culling (40).

Despite potential problems, however, although it has been demonstrated in test areas in an earlier study that badger population reduction has resulted in decreases in tuberculosis in cattle (24), preliminary results from a large-scale randomized trial in Great Britain showed that localized culling of badger populations around infected herds was associated with in an increase in cattle infection levels. It has been hypothesized that this might have been the result of disturbance of population stability, resulting in increased movements of badgers (31). As part of a review of this trial (31), researchers emphasized that the results should be interpreted very cautiously because of statistical uncertainties as well as the presence of confounding biases.

In addition to population control, wildlife behavior modification has been used as a tool to reduce the spread of the disease in the wildlife population. In the outbreak of *M. bovis* in free-ranging white-tailed deer in Michigan, large-scale winter feeding in one area of the state that had continued for decades had dramatically increased the numbers of deer in the area and created conditions in which large numbers of normally timid animals would congregate around feed piles (10,49). After the discovery of TB in wildlife, bans were placed on feeding and baiting of animals in areas where they may gather during cold weather or under other conditions associated with limited food supply (10). After these measures had been applied over a 6-year period, the apparent prevalence of TB in deer in a 12-county area in Michigan decreased by 50% (6).

M. bovis in Captive Wildlife

The occurrence of *M. bovis* in captive wildlife populations has been well documented, and the epidemiology of the disease in captive populations is very similar to circumstances seen in livestock populations. A wide variety of species have been documented with *M. bovis*, including rhinoceri (5) and primates (38). In addition to zoos, animal parks or "farms" that maintain populations of wildlife have been affected by *M. bovis.* The intradermal tuberculin skin test may not be effective or practical for use in all species, but it has been accepted by the U.S. Department of Agriculture for identification of *M. bovis* in bison and captive cervids (33).

Surveillance and TB control programs for captive wildlife are similar to those exercised for livestock. In the case of some valuable exotic species, animals may receive treatment for the disease, as in the case where elephants have successfully recovered from TB after 6 months of treatment with isonicotinic acid hydrazide along with rifampicin or ethambutol (50).

M. bovis in Humans

Human infection with *M. bovis* is a recognized public health hazard in developing and industrial nations (19). The advent of milk pasteurization and eradication programs has reduced the levels of human bovine TB in industrialized nations, but sporadic cases still occur when individuals come into contact with infected livestock (1), captive wildlife (7), or contaminated animal carcasses (1).

Humans are susceptible to *M. bovis*, and there are numerous instances of human infection resulting from contact with infected animals. Recently, there has been increased interest among public health officials in drug-resistant strains of *Mycobacterium tuberculosis*, *M. bovis*, and *Mycobacterium avium*, because several such strains have been isolated from HIV-infected and nonimmunocompromised humans (1). Infection with *M. bovis* causes pulmonary and extrapulmonary disease

(19). Contact with infected animals is a source of *M. bovis* infection for humans and is a recognized hazard for abattoir workers, veterinarians, and livestock handlers (7).

In the United States and other developed countries, extrapulmonary *M. bovis* infections in humans have been almost eliminated following the introduction of food production procedures such as pasteurization of milk and routine carcass inspection, and many of the primary nonaerosol sources of *M. bovis* infection in humans have been removed in industrialized countries (19). *M. bovis* infection in humans commonly occurs in less-developed countries and in specific demographic groups within developed countries in which consumption of unpasteurized dairy products is practiced. The presence of HIV infection is considered to further complicate the epidemiology in these countries, as infected individuals are more likely to more quickly develop clinical TB (1).

Although there is no active surveillance program specific for *M. bovis* infection for humans in the United States, most of the reported cases appear localized to states with large immigrant populations from countries with recognized *M. bovis* infections in livestock (25). For example, 7% of mycobacterial isolates from 1931 cases of TB in San Diego, California, were identified as *M. bovis*; these infections were associated with ingestion of raw dairy products, 53% of these patients had extrapulmonary disease (25), and 33% of isolates obtained from children were *M. bovis* (25).

Surveillance and Control Programs

Tuberculosis is a reportable disease in the United States, but there is no national active surveillance program for the disease. The existing surveillance program was expanded in 1993 to better monitor and target groups at risk for TB, estimate and follow the extent of drug-resistant TB, and evaluate outcomes of TB cases. When apparent cases are presented to health care workers, an investigation is launched to confirm the diagnosis of TB by clinical case definition (positive tuberculin skin test and signs/symptoms/clinical evidence of TB) with laboratory confirmation (mycobacterial isolation or demonstration of acid-fast bacilli in a clinical specimen). There is no separate surveillance for *M. bovis* in humans in the United States: surveillance is for *M. tuberculosis* complex, which includes *M. bovis*. Cases are identified in the instances in which additional testing is conducted to determine the bacterial species. Following identification of a case of TB, epidemiological investigations are conducted to identify the source of infection, and any other individuals who may have come into contact with the case and may have been exposed to the disease. The Bacille Calmette-Güerin vaccine has been used in humans in some countries in which TB is prevalent in the population.

Conclusions

Bovine TB is a difficult disease to control because of the large number of susceptible species, the variation in pathogenesis, and the limited effectiveness of currently available control methods for wild animals. Effective control requires an understanding of the epidemiology of infection within the ecological system that can include domestic as well as wild animal species. It is also affected by management practices within the livestock production system as well as societal considerations toward the application of control in wild animal reservoir species.

References

1. Pfeiffer, D. U. 2003. Animal tuberculosis. *In* P. D. O. Davies (ed.), Clinical Tuberculosis, 3rd edition. London: Arnold, 449-58.
2. Francis, J. 1971. Susceptibility to tuberculosis and the route of infection. *Aust Vet J* 47:414.
3. Gavier-Widen, D., M. A. Chambers, N. Palmer, D. G. Newell, and R. G. Hewinson. 2001. Pathology of natural *Mycobacterium bovis* infection in European badgers (*Meles meles*) and its relationship with bacterial excretion. *Vet Rec* 148:299-304.
4. Palmer, M. V., W. R. Waters, and D. L. Whipple. 2003. Aerosol exposure of white-tailed deer (*Odocoileus virginianus*) to *Mycobacterium bovis*. *J Wildl Dis* 39:817-23.
5. Bengis, R. G., N. P. J. Kriek, D. F. Keet, J. P. Raath, V. de Vos, and H. F. A. K. Huchzermeyer. 1996. An outbreak of bovine tuberculosis in a free-living African buffalo (*Syncerus caffer*-Sparrman) population in the Kruger National Park: a preliminary report. *Onderstepoort J Vet Res* 63:15-18.
6. Schmitt, S. M., D. J. O'Brien, C. S. Bruning-Fann, and S. D. Fitzgerald. 2002. Bovine tuberculosis in Michigan wildlife and livestock. *Ann N Y Acad Sci* 969:262-68.
7. Stetter, M. D., S. K. Mikota, A. F. Gutter, E. R. Monterroso, J. R. Dalovisio, C. Degraw, and T. Farley. 1995. Epizootic of *Mycobacterium bovis* in a zoologic park. *J Am Vet Med Assoc* 207:1618-21.
8. Delahay, R. J., A. N. S. De Leeuw, A. M. Barlow, R. S. Clifton-Hadley, and C. L. Cheeseman. 2002. The status of *Mycobacterium bovis* infection in UK wild mammals: a review. *Vet J* 164:90-105.
9. Morris, R. S. and D. U. Pfeiffer, 1995. Directions and issues in bovine tuberculosis epidemiology and control in New Zealand. *N Z Vet J* 43:256-65.
10. Miller, R., J. B. Kaneene, S. D. Fitzgerald, and S. M. Schmitt. 2003. Evaluation of the influence of supplemental feeding of white-tailed deer (*Odocoileus virginianus*) on the prevalence of bovine tuberculosis in the Michigan wild deer population. *J Wildl Dis* 39:84-95.
11. Gay, G., H. M. Burbridge, P. Bennett, S. G. Fenwick, C. Dupont, A. Murray, and M. R. Alley. 2000. Pulmonary *Mycobacterium bovis* infection in a dog. *N Z Vet J* 48:78-81.
12. Philips, C. J. C., C. R. W. Foster, P. A. Morris, and R. Teverson. 2003. The transmission of *Mycobacterium bovis* infection to cattle. *Res Vet Sci* 74:1-15.
13. Palmer, M. V., D. L. Whipple, J. B. Payeur, D. P. Alt, K. J. Esch, C. S. Bruning-Fann, and J. B. Kaneene. 2000. Naturally occurring tuberculosis in white-tailed deer. *J Am Vet Med Assoc* 216:1921-24.
14. Serraino, A., G. Marchetti, V. Sanguinetti, M. C. Rossi, R. G. Zanoni, L. Catozzi, A. Bandera, W. Dini, W. Mignone, F. Franzetti, and A. Gori. 1999. Monitoring of transmission of tuberculosis between wild boars and cattle: genotypical analysis of strains by molecular epidemiology. *J Clin Microbiol* 37:2766-71.
15. Anonymous. 1994. Zoonotic tuberculosis (*Mycobacterium bovis*)—memorandum from a WHO meeting (with the participation of FAO). *Bull WHO* 72:851-57.

16. Ragg, J. R., C. G. Mackintosh, and H. Moller. 2000. The scavenging behaviour of ferrets (*Mustela furo*), feral cats (*Felis domesticus*), possums (*Trichosurus vulpecula*), hedgehogs (*Erinaceus europaeus*) and harrier hawks (*Circus approximans*) on pastoral farmland in New Zealand: implications for bovine tuberculosis transmission. *N Z Vet J* 48:166-75.

17. Kaneene, J. B., C. S. Bruning-Fann, L. M. Granger, R. Miller, and B. A. Porter-Spalding. 2002. Environmental and farm management factors associated with tuberculosis on cattle farms in northeastern Michigan. *J Am Vet Med Assoc* 221:837-42.

18. Thompson, P. J., D. V. Cousins, B. L. Gow, D. M. Collins, B. H. Williamson, and H. T. Dagnia. 1993. Seals, seal trainers, and mycobacterial infection. *Am Rev Respir Dis* 147:164-67.

19. Grange, J. M. and M. D. Yates. 1994. Zoonotic aspects of *Mycobacterium bovis* infection. *Vet Microbiol* 40:137-51.

20. Cheeseman, C. L., J. W. Wilesmith, and F. A. Stuart. 1989. Tuberculosis: the disease and its epidemiology in the badger, a review. *Epidemiol Infect* 103:113-25.

21. Jackson, R. 2002. The role of wildlife in *Mycobacterium bovis* infection of livestock in New Zealand. *N Z Vet J* 50:49-52.

22. McInerney, J. P., K. J. Small, and P. Caley. 1995. Prevalence of *Mycobacterium bovis* infection in feral pigs in the Northern Territory. *Aust Vet J* 72:448-51.

23. Fitzgerald, S. D., J. B. Kaneene, K. L. Butler, K. P. Clarke, J. S. Fierke, S. M. Schmitt, C. S. Bruning-Fann, R. R. Mitchell, D. E. Berry, and J. B. Payeur. 2000. Comparison of postmortem techniques for the detection of *Mycobacterium bovis* in white-tailed deer (*Odocoileus virginianus*). *J Vet Diagn Invest* 12:322-27.

24. Clifton-Hadley, R. S. 1996. Badgers, bovine tuberculosis and the age of reason. *Br Vet J* 152:243-46.

25. LoBue, P. A., W. Betacourt, C. Peter, et al. 2003. Epidemiology of *Mycobacterium bovis* disease in San Diego County, 1994-2000. *Int J Tuberc Lung Dis* 7:180-85.

26. Montgomery, R. H. 1999. Mycobacteria in New Zealand. *Surveillance* 26:6-8.

27. Kanameda, M. and Ekgatat, M. 1995. Isolation of *Mycobacterium bovis* from the water buffalo (*Bubalus bubalis*). *Trop Anim Health Prod* 27:227-28.

28. Koller-Jones, M. 2004. Bovine Tuberculosis Eradication in Canada. *Proc 107th Ann Mtg U.S. Animal Health Association.* Chicago, IL, October 14-15, 2003, 580-586. Available at: http://usaha.org/committees/reports/reports03/r03tb.html, accessed 12/21/2004.

29. DEFRA. 2004. The incidence of TB in cattle—Great Britain. Available at: http://statistics.defra.gov.uk/esg/statnot/tbpn.pdf, accessed 01/07/05.

30. Krebs, J., R. Anderson, T. Clutton-Brock, I. Morrison, D. Young, and C. Donnelly. 1997. Bovine tuberculosis in cattle and badgers. Report to The Rt. Hon. Dr. Jack Cunningham, MP. London: Maff Publications.

31. Godfray, H. C. J., R. N. Curnow, C. Dye, D. Pfeiffer, W. J. Sutherland, and M. E. J. Woolhouse. 2004. Independent scientific review of the Randomised Badger Culling Trial and associated epidemiological research. London: Department for Environment, Food and Rural Affairs.

32. AHB. 2004. Progress to official freedom from bovine tuberculosis for New Zealand—December 2004. Technical Report, Animal Health Board, Wellington, New Zealand.

33. U.S. Department of Agriculture. 2005. Bovine tuberculosis eradication: uniform methods and rules, effective January 1, 2005; USDA-APHIS 91-45-011. Available at: http://www.aphis.usda.gov/vs/nahps/tb/tb-umr.pdf, accessed 1/29/2005.

34. Skinner, M. A., D. N. Wedlock, and B. M. Buddle. 2001. Vaccination of animals against *Mycobacterium bovis*. *Rev Sci Tech Off Int Epiz* 20:112-32.

35. Michel, A. L. 2002. Implications of tuberculosis in African wildlife and livestock. *Ann N Y Acad Sci* 969:251-55.
36. Clifton-Hadley, R. S., J. W. Wilesmith, M. S. Richards, P. Upton, and S. Johnston. 1995. The occurrence of *Mycobacterium bovis* infection in and around an area subject to extensive badger (*Meles meles*) control. *Epidemiol Infect* 114:179-93.
37. Nishi, J. S., B. T. Elkin, and T. R. Ellsworth. 2002. The Hook Lake Wood Bison Recovery Project: can a disease-free captive wood bison herd be recovered from a wild population infected with bovine tuberculosis and brucellosis? *Ann NY Acad Sci* 969:229-35.
8. Keet, D. F., N. P. J. Kriek, R. G. Bengis, D. G. Grobler, and A. Michel. 2000. The rise and fall of tuberculosis in a free-ranging Chacma baboon troop in the Kruger National Park. *Onderstepoort J Vet Res* 67:115-22.
39. Tryland, M. 2000. Zoonoses of arctic marine mammals. *Infect Dis Rev* 2:55-64.
40. Artois, M., R. Delahay, V. Guberti, and C. Cheeseman. 2001. Control of infectious diseases of wildlife in Europe. *Vet J* 162:141-52.
41. Essey, M. A., D. E. Stallknecht, E. M. Himes, and S. K. Harris. 1983. Follow-up survey of feral swine for *Mycobacterium bovis* infection on the Hawaiian island of Molokai. *Proc 87th Ann Mtg USAHA* 87:589-595.
42. Wilesmith, J. W., T. W. A. Little, H. V. Thompson, and C. Swan. 1982. Bovine tuberculosis in domestic and wild mammals in an area of Dorset. I. Tuberculosis in cattle. *J Hyg Camb* 89:195-210.
43. Gallagher, J., R. Morris, M. Gavier-Widen, and B. Rule. 1998. Role of infected, non-diseased badgers in the pathogenesis of tuberculosis in the badger. *Vet Rec* 42:710-14.
44. De Vos, V., R. G. Bengis, N. P. J. Kriek, A. Michel, D. F. Keet, J. P. Raath, and H. F. K. Huchzermeyer. 2001. The epidemiology of tuberculosis in free-ranging African buffalo (*Syncerus caffer*) in the Kruger National Park, South Africa. *Onderstepoort J Vet Res* 68:119-30.
45. O'Brien, D. J., S. M. Schmitt, J. S. Fierke, S. A. Hogle, S. R. Winterstein, T. M. Cooley, W. E. Moritz, K. L. Diegel, S. D. Fitzgerald, D. E. Berry, and J. B. Kaneene. 2002. Epidemiology of *Mycobacterium bovis* in free-ranging white-tailed deer, Michigan, USA, 1995-2000. *Prev Vet Med* 54:47-63.
46. Coleman, J. D., M. M. Cooke, R. Jackson, and R. Webster. 1999. Temporal patterns in bovine tuberculosis in a brushtail possum population contiguous with in infected cattle in the Ahaura Valley, Westland. *N Z Vet J* 47:119-24.
47. US Animal Health Association. http://usaha.org/committees/reports/report-tb-2004.pdf, accessed 12/21/2004.
48. Pfeiffer, D. U. and R. S. Morris. 1991. A longitudinal study of bovine tuberculosis in possums and cattle. Symposium on Tuberculosis: Foundation for Continuing Education. *N Z Vet Assoc* 132:17-39.
49. Schmitt, S. M., S. D. Fitzgerald, T. M. Cooley, C. S. Bruning-Fann, L. Sullivan, D. Berry, T. Carlson, R. B. Minnis, J. B. Payeur, and J. Sikarskie. 1997. Bovine tuberculosis in free-ranging white-tailed deer in from Michigan. *J Wildl Dis* 33:749-58.

Chapter 6

Diagnostic Tests for Bovine Tuberculosis

C.O. Thoen, DVM, PhD, and E.D. Ebel, DVM, MS

The intradermal tuberculin test using purified protein derivative (PPD) prepared from the culture filtrate of *Mycobacterium bovis* by precipitation with ammonium sulfate or trichloroacetic acid is widely used to identify tuberculous cattle and other animals in countries throughout the world (1–3). The protein content of the PPD is determined and biologic activity evaluated in sensitized guinea pigs.

The single caudal fold intradermal test, the single cervical intradermal test, and the comparative cervical test are the tuberculin tests used in most bovine tuberculosis control or eradication programs (2,3). In the United States, the caudal fold test is a presumptive test. The injection site is visually observed and palpated at 72 hours following injection of *M. bovis* PPD, and any inflammatory response is classified as suspect. Cattle with suspicious reactions to the caudal fold test are subsequently subjected to a comparative cervical test to determine their relative responsiveness to biologically balanced *M. bovis* and *M. avium ss avium* PPD (4,5).

Cattle infected with *M. bovis* will develop more induration (measured as an increase in skin thickness at the site of injection) in response to the *M. bovis* PPD than to the *M. avium* PPD, except in animals with advanced disease that have become nonresponsive to tuberculin. The increase in skin thickness at each injection site is plotted on a scattergram. The results are classified as negative, suspect, or reactor (positive) (4).

In vitro cell-mediated assays that monitor cell responses to PPD by incorporation of tritiated thymidine or the production of gamma interferon have been developed and evaluated in cattle and other animals in several countries (6,7). In addition, *in vitro* assays have been developed to detect antibodies in *M. bovis*–infected cattle (8,9). The tuberculin skin test, which involves the injection of 0.1 mL PPD intradermally and observation of the injection site at 72 hours in cattle, requires the handling of cattle twice. An *in vitro* blood test would provide a distinct advantage because animals would be restrained only once; this is especially important when working with wild animals (9–11).

The specificity and sensitivity of a diagnostic test should be determined in naturally sensitized *M. bovis*–infected cattle and in cattle in *M. bovis*–free herds in the geographical region under conditions in which the test will be used (2,3,12). This is important because nonspecific sensitization caused by other organisms that share antigenic determinants may vary for different regions and countries (13). For example, it is possible that cattle not infected with *M. bovis* will respond to *M. bovis* because of exposure to other mycobacteria (i.e., *M. avium ss paratuberculosis*)

In vitro Tests

The primary immune response in animals to *M. bovis* infections is cell mediated (14). Because some concerns have been reported concerning the sensitivity and specificity of the tuberculin skin test, considerable research has been conducted to develop *in vitro* correlates of delayed hypersensitivity to monitor cell-mediated responses (6,7). Initial efforts involved the development of lymphocyte blastogenic assays (LBA) using the incorporation of tritiated thymidine following exposure to specific mycobacterial antigen as a measure of cell-mediated responsiveness (6). The stimulation index is determined by comparing the response to specific antigen to nonstimulated controls and is used to determine the status of the animal. Investigations conducted on experimentally infected cattle revealed a good correlation with LBA and skin tests (15). However, the results of LBA and skin test responses in cattle naturally exposed to *M. bovis* varied considerably in different herds within the same geographical region. Systematic studies to determine the conditions of shipment and storage time failed to provide definitive information useful in explaining the variation in findings on LBA. The reproducibility of LBA on the same animals was questioned because results sometimes varied even when conditions for shipment and storage were similar. Therefore, the LBA has not come into widespread use as a stand-alone or supplemental diagnostic test to be used routinely in the diagnosis of bovine tuberculosis.

More recently, a gamma interferon (IFN) assay was described for monitoring cell-mediated responses (6,17). This *in vitro* assay is similar to the LBA in that it requires the collection of blood samples from cattle for antigen stimulation. It differs from the LBA in that IFN produced by the stimulated cells is measured in an ELISA, and no radioactive isotopes are involved in measuring cell stimulation. The IFN assay has been used in detecting tuberculous cattle in several countries, and the results correlate with responses obtained on a tuberculin skin test (7,16–19). This test has been approved as a supplemental test for cattle in the U. S. National Tuberculosis Eradication Program. Nevertheless, a comparison of the sensitivity of the caudal fold test and the IFN assay revealed that the caudal fold test was significantly more sensitive than the IFN for the diagnosis of bovine tuberculosis (19). Maximum overall sensitivity was achieved when results of the caudal fold test and IFN assay were interpreted in parallel. The specificity of the IFN assay has been reported to be 93%; however, the probability that a positive test indicates infection (i.e., the positive predictive value) is reduced when testing cattle in low-prevalence herds. This positive predictive value can only be improved by increasing the specificity of the IFN assay. As with most *in vivo* assays, the success for detecting *M. bovis*–infected animals and minimizing false-positive responses varies with different antigen preparations. *M. bovis* PPD and *M. avium ss avium* PPD are used to stimulate lymphocytes in the plasma sample to produce IFN. The use of proteins secreted by mycobacteria such as ESAT-6 may improve the specificity of the IFN assay (21,22).

Numerous investigations have been conducted to develop antibody-based diagnostic tests (e.g., ELISA) for detecting *M. bovis*–infected cattle and other animals (8–10,23–28). These tests could be used in conjunction with tuberculin skin tests or *in vitro* cell-mediated tests to identify tuberculous animals with advanced disease that fail to elicit a response on intradermal testing with PPD (29). The sensitivity and specificity of serologic tests may be improved by using purified antigens (21). However, it is generally agreed that antibody-based tests are not stand-alone tests, as they fail to detect many *M. bovis*–infected cattle with subclinical disease in a population (3,8). Moreover, nonspecific responses may be observed on these tests because of responses elicited by other mycobacteria or organisms that share antigens with *M. bovis*.

Development of more sensitive and specific serologic tests through continued research could be useful in slaughter surveillance programs and when evaluating progress within individual herds. However, unless sensitivity and specificity are increased dramatically, they would only be considered presumptive tests, and the intradermal and *in vitro* cellular assays would be used in making a final diagnosis.

The use of the intradermal tests, along with herd management, has been successful in eradicating tuberculosis within herds. However, to allay concerns about the specificity of the tuberculin skin tests, *in vitro* cellular assays may improve diagnostic specificity when used in conjunction with the intradermal tests. The *in vitro* tests have the advantage that animals only need to be handled once and the animals can be retested at short time intervals. However, the cost of IFN assay may limit its use.

It is important to emphasize that to confirm a diagnosis of *M. bovis* infection, it is necessary to isolate and identify the acid-fast organism by biochemical tests or molecular techniques (3). A detailed description of the molecular techniques is presented in chapters 7 and 8.

References

1. Haagsma J. A. A. and R. D. Angus. 1995. Tuberculin production. *In* C. O. Thoen and J. H. Steele (eds.), *Mycobacterium bovis* Infection in Animals and Humans. Ames: Iowa State University Press, 73-84.
2. O'Reilly, L. M. 1995. Tuberculin skin tests: sensitivity and specificity. *In* C. O. Thoen and J. H. Steele (eds.), *Mycobacterium bovis* Infection in Animals and Humans. Ames: Iowa State University Press, 85-92.
3. Kaneene, J. B. and C. O. Thoen. 2004. Tuberculosis. *J Am Vet Med Assoc* 224:685-91.
4. Roswurm, J. D. and L. D. Konyha. 1973. The comparative-cervical tuberculin test as an aid to diagnosing bovine tuberculosis. *Proc Annu Meet US Anim Health Assoc* 77:268-389.
5. Duffield, B. J., J. H. Norton, and T. A. Streeten. 1985. Application of the comparative cervical test to the identification of false positive reactions to the bovine tuberculin caudal fold test. *Aust Vet J* 62:424-26.

6. Muscoplat, C. C., C. O. Thoen, A. W. Chen, and D. W. Johnson. (1975). Development of specific *in vitro* lymphocyte responses in cattle infected with *Mycobacterium bovis* and with *Mycobacterium avium. Am J Vet Res* 36:395-98.

7. Wood, P. R., L. A. Corner, J. S. Rothel, J. L. Ripper, T. Fifis, B. S. McCormick, B. Francis, L. Melville, K. Small, K. de Witte, et al. 1992. A field evaluation of serological and cellular diagnostic tests for bovine tuberculosis. *Vet Microbiol* 31:71-79.

8. Thoen, C. O., M. R. Hall, T. A. Petersburg, R. Harrington, and D. E. Pietz. 1975. Application of a modified ELISA for detecting mycobacterial antibodies in sera of cattle from a herd in which *M. bovis* was diagnosed. Proc 87th Annu Meet US Anim Health Assoc, Las Vegas, 603-610.

9. Thoen, C. O., K. Mills, and M. P. Hopkins. 1980. Enzyme-linked protein A: an enzyme-linked immunosorbent assay reagent for detecting antibodies in tuberculous exotic animals. *Am J Vet Res* 40:833-35.

10. Thoen, C. O., K. J. Thorlsen, L. D. Miller, E. M. Himes, and R. L. Morgan. 1988. Pathogenesis of *Mycobacterium bovis* infection in American bison. *Am J Vet Res* 49:1861-65.

11. Thoen, C. O., W. J. Quinn, L. D. Miller, L. L. Stackhouse, B. F. Newcomb, and J. M. Ferrell. 1992. *Mycobacterium bovis* infection in North American elk (*Cervus elaphus*). *J Vet Diagn Invest* 4:423-27.

12. Adams, G. L. 2001. *In vivo* and *in vitro* diagnosis of *Mycobacterium bovis* infection. *Rev Sci Tech Off Int Epiz* 20:1-54.

13. Karlson, A. G. 1962. Nonspecific or cross-sensitivity reactions to tuberculin in cattle. *In* C. A. Brandly and E. L. Jungherr (eds.), Advances in Veterinary Science, Vol. 7. New York: Academic Press, 147-181.

14. Thoen, C. O. and R. G. Barletta. 2004. *Mycobacterium. In* C. L. Gyles, J. F. Prescott, J. G. Songer, and C. O. Thoen (eds.), Pathogenesis of Bacterial Infections in Animals, 3rd ed. Ames, IA: Blackwell Publishing, 69-76.

15. Thoen, C. O., J. L. Jarnagin, C. C. Muscoplat, L. S. Cram, D. W. Johnson, and R. Harrington Jr. 1980. Potential use of lymphocyte blastogenic responses in diagnosis of bovine tuberculosis. *Comp Immunol Microbiol Infect Dis* 3:355-61.

16. Ryan, T. J., G. W. Buddle, and G. W. De Lisle. 2000. An evaluation of the gamma interferon tests for detecting bovine tuberculosis in cattle 8 to 28 days after tuberculin skin testing. *Res Vet Sci* 69:57-61.

17. Wood, P. R., L. A. Corner, J. S. Rothel, C. Badlock, S. L. Jones, D. B. Cousins, B. S. McCormick, B. R. Francis, J. Creeper, and N. E. Tweddle. 1991. Field comparison of the interferon-gamma assay and the intradermal tuberculin test for the diagnosis of bovine tuberculosis. *Aust Vet J* 68:286-90.

18. Gonzalez Llamazares, O. R., C. B. Gutierrez Martin, D. Alvarez Nistal, V. A. de la Puente Redondo, L. Dominguez Rodriquez, and E. F. Rodriguez Ferri. 1999. Field evaluation of the single intradermal cervical tuberculin test and the interferon-gamma assay for detection and eradication of bovine tuberculosis in Spain. *Vet Microbiol* 70:55-66.

19. Whipple, D. L., C. A. Bolin, A. J. Davis, J. L. Jarnagin, D. C. Johnson, R. S. Nabors, J. B. Payeur, D. A. Saari, A. J. Wilson, and M. M. Wolf. 1995. Comparison of the sensitivity of the caudal fold skin test and a commercial gamma-interferon assay for diagnosis of bovine tuberculosis. *Am J Vet Res* 56:415-19.

20. Harboe, M., H. G. Wiker, J. R. Duncan, M. M. Garcia, T. W. Dukes, B. W. Brooks, C. Turcotte, and S. Nagai. 1990. Protein G-based enzyme-linked immunosorbent assay for anti-MPB70 antibodies in bovine tuberculosis. *J Clin Microbiol* 28:913-21.

21. Pollock, J. M. and P. Andersen. 1997. Predominant recognition of the ESAT-6 protein in the first phase of infection with *Mycobacterium bovis* in cattle. *Infect Immun* 65:2587-92.

22. Waters, W. R., B. J. Nonecke, M. V. Palmer, S. Robbe-Austermann, J. Bannantine, J. R. Stabel, D. L. Whipple, J. B. Payeur, D. M. Estes, J. F. Pitzer, and F. C. Minion. 2004. Use of recombinant ESAT-6:CFP-10 fusion protein for differentiation of infections of cattle of *Mycobacterium bovis* and by *M. avium* subsp. *avium* and *M. avium* subsp. *paratuberculosis*. *Clin Diagn Lab Immunol* 11:729-33.

23. Ritacco, V., B. Lopez, L. Barrera, A. Nader, E. Fleiss, and I. N. de Kantor. 1990. Further evaluation of an indirect enzyme-linked immunosorbent assay for the diagnosis of bovine tuberculosis. *Zentralbl Veterinarmed B* 37:19-27.

24. Lilenbaum, W., E. R. Ribeiro, G. N. Souza, E. C. Moreira, L. S. Fonseca, M. A. Ferreira, and J. Schettini. 1999. Evaluation of an ELISA-PPD for the diagnosis of bovine tuberculosis in field trials in Brazil. *Res Vet Sci* 66:191-95.

25. Lightbody, K. A., R. A. Skuce, S. D. Neill, and J. M. Pollock. 1998. Mycobacterial antigen-specific antibody responses in bovine tuberculosis: an ELISA with potential to confirm disease status. *Vet Rec* 142:295-300.

26. Dowling, L. A. and S. M. Schleehauf. 1991. Specified antibody responses to *Mycobacterium bovis* in infected cattle analysed with six mycobacterial antigens in enzyme-linked immunosorbent assays. *Res Vet Sci* 50:157-61.

27. Wood, P. R., L. A. Corner, J. S. Rothel, J. L. Ripper, T. Fifis, B. S. McCormick, B. Francis, L. Melville, K. Small, K. de Witte, et al. 1992. A field evaluation of serological and cellular diagnostic tests for bovine tuberculosis. *Vet Microbiol* 31:71-79.

28. Sugden, E. A., K. Stilwell, E. B. Rohonczy, and P. Marineau. 1997. Competitive and indirect enzyme-linked immunosorbent assays for *Mycobacterium bovis* infections based on MPB70 and lipoarabinomannan antigens. *Can J Vet Res* 61:8-14.

29. Plackett, P., J. Ripper, L. A. Corner, K. Small, K. de Witte, L. Melville, S. Hides, and P. R. Wood. 1989. An ELISA for the detection of anergic tuberculous cattle. *Aust Vet J* 66:15-19.

Chapter 7

Molecular Techniques: Applications in Epidemiologic Studies

N.B. Harris, PhD

Introduction

Mycobacterium bovis continues to be a major pathogen for domestic livestock. Increasingly, contact between production animals and wildlife leads to the establishment of reservoirs of *M. bovis* infections within localized wildlife populations. This in turn facilitates elevated levels of infection in both populations, as well as leads to higher risks of transmission of *M. bovis* between animal species and from animals to humans. Epidemiological identification of reactor and diseased animals is a necessary part of the effective control and eradication of bovine tuberculosis in domestic livestock. By applying molecular techniques together with traditional epidemiology traceback approaches, important insights can be made regarding the sources of infection and the identification of practices or environments that may aid the spread and maintenance of tuberculosis.

The basis of all molecular genotyping techniques relies on the acquisition of genetic mutations over time within specified regions of the bacterial genome, thus creating unique profiles between isolates. Although two bacterial strains of the same species have virtually identical genomes, differences will inevitably occur at a few loci. These differences may be small, such as the alteration of a single nucleotide that may either create or remove a specific restriction enzyme site, or larger changes may occur leading to the replication or deletion of DNA fragments hundreds of base pairs in size. Therefore, epidemiologically related strains will show identical or very similar genetic profiles, whereas unrelated clinical isolates will have divergent patterns.

The specificity and discriminatory power (the ability to differentiate among closely related strains) of any molecular epidemiology technique are dependent on the frequency at which the targeted genetic element is present in the bacterial genome. The higher this frequency, or copy number, the greater the certainty that two identical results from one method represent epidemiologically related strains. When typing methods only detect low copy numbers of a genetic element, no conclusion about clonal identity among bacterial strains can be drawn, and other methods may be needed to verify relationships. Thus, the choice of methods for molecular epidemiology work must be selected with respect to the end goal, be it epidemiological identification of strains involved in a disease outbreak or a more global perspective of biogeographic distribution of isolates from a phylogenetic perspective.

New molecular epidemiological tools beyond the standard fingerprinting reference technique have been described recently for *M. bovis* (1), expanding the repertoire of techniques available for genotyping isolates recovered from disease outbreaks. These new techniques include spacer oligotyping (spoligotyping) and variable number tandem repeat typing. In general, the finding of genetic differences between two strains of *M. bovis* implies that they presumably originate from different sources, which is a fundamental question to be answered during a disease outbreak. Confidence in this assumption can be increased by using more than one typing system to detect genetic differences, as various genetic markers target changes or mutations within different parts of the mycobacterial genome.

IS*6110* Restriction Fragment Length Polymorphism (RFLP)

The insertion sequence IS*6110* is a transposable (mobile) element belonging to the IS*3* family of insertion elements, and it is found only in members of the *Mycobacterium tuberculosis* complex (2). However, the total number of IS*6110* copies found in the genome differs widely between the various *M. tuberculosis* complex species. For example, the *M. tuberculosis* genome may harbor up to 19 copies of IS*6110*, whereas *M. bovis* only contains one to five copies (1). The foundation of any RFLP technique relies on digestion of genomic DNA followed by probing with a specific marker using Southern blotting techniques. Thus, the combination of the restriction enzyme used and the DNA sequence of the probe allows for polymorphisms in the genomic DNA to be visualized. For IS*6110*-RFLP, the variation in the copy number of IS*6110* is a major source of genetic polymorphisms between bacterial isolates. This variation has significantly contributed to IS*6110*-RFLP becoming the standard reference typing technique for *M. tuberculosis* (2). Unfortunately, IS*6110*-RFLP is less useful for differentiating *M. bovis* isolates because strains of *M. bovis* only harbor one to five copies of IS*6110*. Furthermore, this element is routinely present in the same 1.9-kb *Pvu*II fragment of many *M. bovis* strains (1), limiting the differential capacity of this technique. However, utilization of different DNA probes against the same IS*6110* target increases the resolution of this method. For example, Whipple et al. (3) used two different probes against IS*6110* when analyzing 16 *M. bovis* strains from wildlife and domestic cattle. When a fragment internal to IS*6110* was used as a probe, only a single band for each insertion element present in the genomic DNA could be visualized. Reprobing the same strains with a fragment of the inverted repeat region of the insertion element produced two bands per IS*6110* copy, allowing a single-band cluster of isolates to be differentiated into two distinct groups.

Interestingly, the copy number of IS*6110* in clinical strains of *M. bovis* appears to be somewhat correlated with animal species. *M. bovis* isolates recovered from cattle generally carry one copy of IS*6110,* whereas strains harboring multiple copies are more likely to have originated from wildlife or zoo animals (4). However, *M. bovis* strains from Canada appear to be distinct from the usual bovine-origin isolates in that many carry multiple copies of IS*6110* (4).

Polymorphic G/C-Rich Sequence RFLP

The polymorphic G/C-rich sequence (PGRS) loci are microsatellite regions in the mycobacterial genome consisting of multiple short tandem repeat units that are less than 10 bp in length. The DNA residues in these PGRS locales occur within structural genes as repetitive trinucleotide sequences and frequently contain the motif CGG (5). These genes are associated with a unique gene family found only in mycobacteria, in which the encoded proteins contain a signature proline-glutamic acid (PE) amino acid sequence near their amino terminus (6). Although the function of the encoded proteins has yet to be determined, current hypotheses suggest they may be cell surface constituents, presumably involved in antigenic variation designed to evade host immune responses (6). These PE–PGRS genes are randomly dispersed throughout the genome in all *M. tuberculosis* complex bacteria (6), as well as several other mycobacterial species, including *Mycobacterium gastri, Mycobacterium gordonae, Mycobacterium kansasii, Mycobacterium szulgai, Mycobacterium malmoense,* and *Mycobacterium phlei* (7). Thus, by combining multiple genetic targets with coverage throughout the entire genome, these PE–PGRS regions provide greater sensitivity for epidemiological studies and molecular fingerprinting of clinical *M. bovis* isolates than does IS*6110*-RFLP (4,7). However, because of the complexity of the fingerprint pattern obtained with PGRS-RFLP and the poor resolution of bands below approximately 1.5–2 kb in size, most studies limit the analysis of PGRS-RFLP patterns to fragments above this range (4).

Figure 7.1 illustrates typical PGRS-RFLP fingerprints obtained from *M. bovis, M. tuberculosis*, and *M. kansasii*. Isolates of *M. bovis* cultured from a single dairy herd in California demonstrate identical banding patterns (Fig. 7.1, lanes designated CA) and can be distinguished from other *M. bovis* isolates recovered from cattle in Colorado, Wisconsin, Missouri, and Kansas (lanes CO, WI, MO, and KS), as well as from *M. tuberculosis* (M. tb.). The *M. kansasii* PGRS-RFLP pattern shown in lane "M. kansasii" demonstrates that this technique can be applied to other mycobacterial species beyond those in the *M. tuberculosis* complex.

Spoligotyping

Another region of the *M. tuberculosis* complex chromosome that has been exploited recently for molecular epidemiology studies is the direct repeat (DR) locus. This single locus is composed of a series of 43 identical DR sequences. Each DR is 36 bp long, interspersed by spacer sequences varying in length from 35 to 41 bp (8). The DR region is also a preferred "hot spot" for IS*6110* insertions. For *M. bovis* strains carrying only one copy of this transposable element, IS*6110* is inserted into the DR located between spacer sequences 24 and 25 (Fig. 7.2) (8). As a conse-

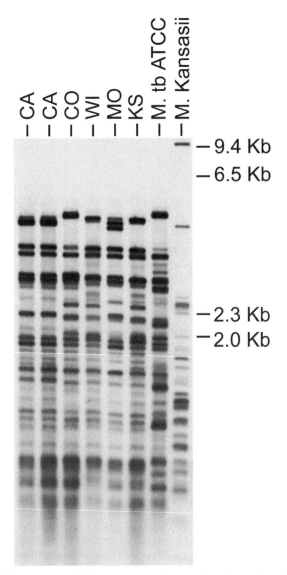

Figure 7.1. RFLP patterns of *Mycobacterium bovis, Mycobacterium tuberculosis*, and *Mycobacterium kansasii* DNA digested with *Alu*I and probed with a 33-bp probe against the PGRS regions. Lanes CA, CO, WI, MO, and KS contain DNA from *M. bovis*. Lanes labeled CA, field isolates recovered from cattle in California; lane CO, bovine isolate from Colorado; lane WI, bovine isolate from Wisconsin; lane MO, bovine isolate from Missouri; lane KS, bovine isolate from Kansas; lane M. tb ATCC, *M. tuberculosis* ATCC strain 14323; lane *M. kansasii, M. kansasii* field isolate from Minnesota. Numbers at right indicate sizes of standard DNA fragments in kilobase pairs.

quence, *M. bovis* genotypic variations in the DR region can be directly correlated with polymorphisms in IS*6110* RFLP types (9).

This DR region is the basis of a novel mycobacterial strain-typing technique called "reverse line blot hybridization," or spoligotyping (defined earlier). In spoligotyping, polymerase chain reaction (PCR) products are amplified using

Direct repeat locus

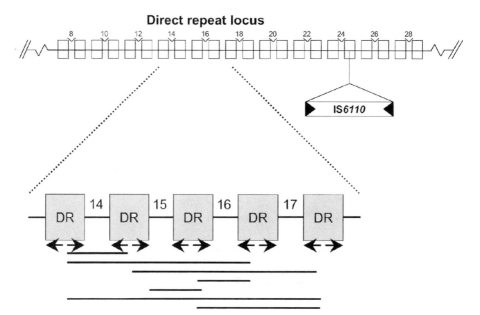

Figure 7.2. Schematic diagram of a segment of the direct-repeat locus in the mycobacterial genome. The direct-repeat sequences are depicted as rectangles, interspersed by variable length spacer regions, labeled 8–28. The site of integration of the IS*6110* insertion element within the DR region is also indicated. The in vitro amplification of the DR region by PCR is represented by the expanded diagram, which illustrates a series of five direct repeats containing spacer regions 14–17. Spoligotyping primers directed against terminal sequences of the DR region are shown as outward-facing arrows, whereas the variable-length polymerase chain reaction products generated from these primers are indicated as solid lines below the diagram.

primers specific for the DR sequences. Thus, products of multiple sizes are generated, representing all the spacer sequences present in an isolate's genome (Fig. 7.2). Using a specialized dot-blot apparatus, this product mixture is then hybridized against a membrane to which the 43 individual spacer sequences have been covalently linked, generating a specific pattern (spoligotype) of positive and negative hybridization signals (Fig. 7.3) (8). Each spacer is then assigned the value of 0 (negative hybridization signal) or 1 (positive signal). The 43 spacers are then divided into a set of 14 triplets with one extra, and each set is then converted to a 15-digit octal code (Fig. 7.3) (10). Differences between spoligotype patterns are mainly the result of deletions of spacer sequence regions (11). Interestingly, the absence of spacers 3, 9, 16, and 39–43 is a characteristic of all *M. bovis* strains (8,9) and is thought to be a result of the deletion of this region by homologous recombination instead of genetic divergence from the *M. tuberculosis* spacer sequence (12).

Spoligotyping has the advantage of being significantly less technically demanding than RFLP fingerprinting, with a much shorter turnaround time. In addition, the degree of differentiation achieved by spoligotyping is higher than that of IS*6110*-RFLP for *M. bovis* (8). One of the major drawbacks to spoligotyping is that it can only identify polymorphisms within the DR cluster, whereas RFLP typing can detect genetic differences arising from multiple loci. Despite this limitation, spo-

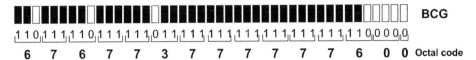

1 1 0	1 1 1	1 1 0	1 1 1	1 1 1	0 1 1	1 1 1	1 1 1	1 1 1	1 1 1	1 1 1	1 1 1	1 1 0	0 0 0	0 0
6	7	6	7	7	3	7	7	7	7	7	7	6	0	0	Octal code

Figure 7.3. Diagram demonstrating the hybridization pattern (spoligotype) and octal code derivation for *M. bovis* BCG. Positive hybridization signals are represented by solid black rectangles, and negative signals are indicated by empty rectangles. The numbers directly below the rectangles are the assigned value of 0 or 1, for negative and positive hybridization signals, respectively. The octal code is derived from these values by first allocating the individual signals into 14 sets of triplets plus one additional singlet. Within each triplet, the first position is arbitrarily assigned the value of 4, the second position is assigned the value of 2, and the third position is assigned the value of 1. These values are then summed for each positive signal within the triplet to arrive at a single digit. The 15 individual digits then form the unique octal code for an isolate.

ligotyping is capable of providing satisfactory sensitivity for routine molecular epidemiologic analyses at both regional and global levels (9).

Figure 7.4 shows *M. bovis* and *M. tuberculosis* spoligotype patterns obtained from infected wildlife, domestic livestock, and exotic animal species. Indicative of all *M. bovis* strains, the field isolates represented in this illustration lack spacers 3, 9, 16, and 39–43. Furthermore, identical spoligotype patterns from *M. bovis* field strains obtained from both wildlife and cattle indicate a potential epidemiological link between these two animal populations.

Variable-Number Tandem Repeat Typing

A more recent PCR-based typing method for the *M. tuberculosis* complex was first described by Frothingham and Meeker-O'Connell (13). This method is based on

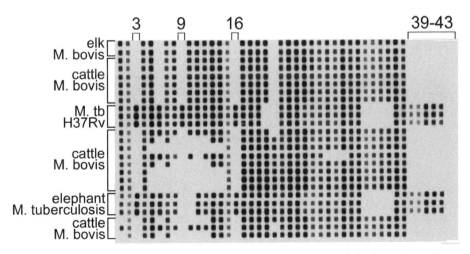

Figure 7.4. Spoligotype patterns of *M. bovis* and *M. tuberculosis* isolates from elk, cattle, and elephants. Spacers 3, 9, 16, and 39–43, characteristically absent from *M. bovis*, are indicated at the top of the figure. Bacterial species designation and animal species of origin are listed at the left. M. tb H37Rv, *M. tuberculosis* strain H37Rv. Photo courtesy of D. Whipple, USDA-ARS.

the variable-number tandem repeats of mycobacterial interspersed repetitive units (MIRU-VNTR). In mycobacteria, isolates are typed by determining the number of copies of specific repeat units at various MIRU-VNTR loci scattered throughout the genome. These short-sequence repeat units are 52–77 nucleotides in length, thus classifying these loci as minisatellite regions. In MIRU-VNTR genotyping, the number of repeat units within a specific locus is determined by PCR amplification of the entire locus, followed by gel electrophoresis, where the number of repeats is determined by the size of the PCR amplicon. The MIRU minisatellite regions have been classified into three major types: type 1, which consists of 77 nucleotide repeat units, type 2, which has a 24-bp gap in the 3′ portion of the type 1 sequence, and type 3, which has a 15-bp gap in the 5′ portion of the type 1 sequence. Mixed type 2 and type 3 MIRUs have also been discovered, which contain gaps in both the 3′ and 5′ regions (14).

Bacteria belonging to the *M. tuberculosis* complex contain 41 different MIRUs randomly located throughout their genomes (Fig. 7.5) (14,15). Within the genome, these MIRUs generally contain an open reading frame that overlaps the termination and initiation codons of their flanking genes. However, some are also found entirely within predicted coding regions (14–16). The purpose of these minisatellite regions in the bacterial chromosome is uncertain, but some evidence indicates that similar to the PE–PGRS genes, they may code repeating amino acid motifs, thus providing another source of antigenic variation (16). Alternatively, these

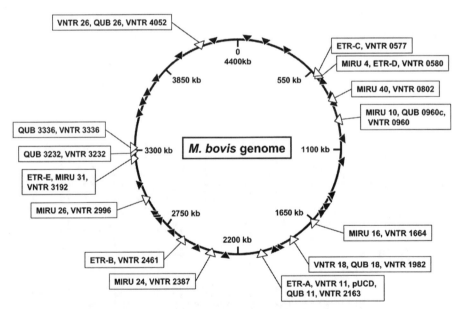

Figure 7.5. Graphic representation of the 41 mycobacterial interspersed repetitive units (MIRU) loci on the *M. bovis* chromosome. Positions along the *M. bovis* chromosome are given in kilobase pairs inside the open circle. The approximate locations of known VNTR-MIRUs are indicated as triangles. Filled triangles represent MIRUs that are invariant among *M. bovis* strains, and the open triangles indicate MIRUs with moderate to high allelic diversity. Published names and aliases of these loci are provided in the accompanying text box.

MIRU-VNTR regions may function in transcriptional or translational regulation (13,17).

Several early studies identified small sets of these MIRU loci that had sufficient allelic variation to differentiate nonrelated bacterial strains, demonstrating the utility of these genetic markers for molecular epidemiology studies. In a landmark study by Frothingham and Meeker-O'Connell, a systematic analysis of the *M. tuberculosis* type strain H37Rv identified 11 tandem repeat loci (13). These 11 loci were PCR amplified and could be reproducibly found in all strains of *M. tuberculosis, M. bovis, M. bovis* BCG, and *Mycobacterium africanum* tested. Only five of these loci (designated ETR-A, ETR-B, ETR-C, ETR-D, and ETR-E) were suitable for epidemiological studies, as the remainder did not demonstrate sufficient allelic diversity to allow discrimination between nonrelated strains (13). Subsequent analyses of both the *M. tuberculosis* and *M. bovis* genomes have identified other novel randomly dispersed loci containing MIRUs suitable for strain discrimination as well (Fig. 7.5) (14,18). Interestingly, one locus from the *M. tuberculosis* genome, MIRU 21, is absent from all *M. bovis* strains tested to date (14). One of the drawbacks of these studies is the lack of uniformity in nomenclature between the various MIRU loci. Thus, careful analysis of the literature is necessary to accurately interpret data regarding specific minisatellite regions and their potential utility in epidemiology studies. To this end, a standardized system of nomenclature has been proposed that uses the first four digits of the exact position of the MIRU with reference to the *M. tuberculosis* H37Rv chromosome (Fig. 7.5) (15).

A recent comprehensive analysis of all published VNTR-MIRUs compared the ability of 30 minisatellite sets to differentiate strains of *M. bovis* and found that individual loci differed significantly in their discriminatory capacity (15). Of the 30 loci evaluated, 12 had no allelic diversity among the 47 different *M. bovis* isolates, and an additional five had diversity indices of < 0.2. However, some of the loci with low discriminatory power in this study demonstrated significantly higher diversity in a different study (18). It is possible that these differences may be attributed in part to the phylogenetic relationship of the bacterial strains used. The study by Roring et al. (17) used field isolates from Northern Ireland and the Republic of Ireland, which may be an overrepresentation of phylogenetically similar strains, whereas the previous research focused on more genetically and geographically diverse groups of isolates. Thus, it appears that the degree of discrimination provided by VNTR typing is dependent on both the individual VNTR loci used and on the test panel of bacterial isolates chosen for analysis. As a consequence, certain MIRU-VNTR markers may be useful for larger population-based studies, whereas others may be more appropriate for outbreak analyses.

References

1. van Soolingen, D., P. W. Hermans, P. E. de Haas, D. R. Soll, and J. D. van Embden. 1991. Occurrence and stability of insertion sequences in *Mycobacterium tuberculosis* complex strains: evaluation of an insertion sequence-dependent DNA polymorphism as a tool in the epidemiology of tuberculosis. *J Clin Microbiol* 29:2578-86.

2. Cave, M. D., K. D. Eisenach, P. F. McDermott, J. H. Bates, and J. T. Crawford. 1991. IS*6110*: conservation of sequence in the *Mycobacterium tuberculosis* complex and its utilization in DNA fingerprinting. *Mol Cell Probes* 5:73-80.

3. Whipple, D. L., P. R. Clarke, J. L. Jarnagin, and J. B. Payeur. 1997. Restriction fragment length polymorphism analysis of *Mycobacterium bovis* isolates from captive and free-ranging animals. *J Vet Diagnostic Investig* 9:381-86.

4. Cousins, D. et al. 1998. Evaluation of four DNA typing techniques in epidemiological investigations of bovine tuberculosis. *J Clin Microbiol* 36:168-78.

5. Otsuka, Y. et al. 2004. Characterization of a trinucleotide repeat sequence (CGG)5 and potential use in restriction fragment length polymorphism typing of *Mycobacterium tuberculosis*. *J Clin Microbiol* 42:3538-48.

6. Brennan, M. J. and G. Delogu. 2002. The PE multigene family: a "molecular mantra" for mycobacteria. *Trends Microbiol.* 10:246-49.

7. Ross, B. C., K. Raios, K. Jackson, and B. Dwyer. 1992. Molecular cloning of a highly repeated DNA element from *Mycobacterium tuberculosis* and its use as an epidemiological tool. *J Clin Microbiol* 30:942-46.

8. Kamerbeek, J., et al. 1997. Simultaneous detection and strain differentiation of *Mycobacterium tuberculosis* for diagnosis and epidemiology. *J Clin Microbiol* 35:907-14.

9. Costello, E., et al. 1999. Study of restriction fragment length polymorphism analysis and spoligotyping for epidemiological investigation of *Mycobacterium bovis* infection. *J Clin Microbiol* 37:3217-22.

10. Dale, J. W. et al. 2001. Spacer oligonucleotide typing of bacteria of the *Mycobacterium tuberculosis* complex: recommendations for standardised nomenclature. *Int J Tubercle Lung Dis* 5:216-19.

11. Fang, Z., N. Morrison, B. Watt, C. Doig, and K. J. Forbes. 1998. IS*6110* transposition and evolutionary scenario of the direct repeat locus in a group of closely related *Mycobacterium tuberculosis* strains. *J Bacteriol* 180:2102-9.

12. Caimi, K., et al. 2001. Sequence analysis of the direct repeat region in *Mycobacterium bovis*. *J Clin Microbiol* 39:1067-72.

13. Frothingham, R. and W. A. Meeker-O'Connell. 1998. Genetic diversity in the *Mycobacterium tuberculosis* complex based on variable numbers of tandem DNA repeats. *Microbiol* 144:1189-96.

14. Supply, P., et al. 2000. Variable human minisatellite-like regions in the *Mycobacterium tuberculosis* genome. *Mol Microbiol* 36:762-71.

15. Roring, S., et al. 2002. Development of variable-number tandem repeat typing of *Mycobacterium bovis*: comparison of results with those obtained by using existing exact tandem repeats and spoligotyping. *J Clin Microbiol* 40:2126-33.

16. Skuce, R. A., et al. 2002. Discrimination of *Mycobacterium tuberculosis* complex bacteria using novel VNTR-PCR targets. *Microbiology* 148:519-28.

17. Roring, S., A. N. Scott, R. Glyn Hewinson, S. D. Neill, and R. A. Skuce. 2004. Evaluation of variable number tandem repeat (VNTR) loci in molecular typing of *Mycobacterium bovis* isolates from Ireland. *Vet Microbiol* 101:65-73.

18. Sola, C., et al. 2003. Genotyping of the *Mycobacterium tuberculosis* complex using MIRUs: association with VNTR and spoligotyping for molecular epidemiology and evolutionary genetics. *Infect Genet Evol* 3:125-33.

Chapter 8

Polymerase Chain Reaction Detection of *Mycobacterium tuberculosis* Complex in Formalin-Fixed Tissues

B. Thomson, DVM, PhD

Polymerase chain reaction (PCR) testing of formalin-fixed tissues is a relatively new and rapid method to diagnose tuberculosis in cattle and other species (1). PCR testing on formalin-fixed tissue has the advantage of being rapid like histopathology, as well as being able to identify whether the bacteria are within the *Mycobacterium tuberculosis* complex, which includes *Mycobacterium bovis*. The test uses formalin-fixed, paraffin-embedded tissue blocks that are used in microscopic slide preparation, which allows retrospective investigations of cases in which only archived paraffin blocks are available because fresh tissue samples were never collected or no longer exist.

Before the development of this test, the primary laboratory methods of bovine tuberculosis diagnosis were histopathology and bacterial culture. Cattle suspected of having tuberculosis, based on the detection of macroscopic tissue granulomas, positive skin test results, or other reasons, are commonly killed, and their tissues are sampled for histopathology and bacterial culture. Histopathology samples are used to confirm the presence or absence of granulomatous lesions with acid-fast bacilli. These lesions would strongly support the diagnosis of a mycobacterial infection, whereas other diagnoses, such as fungal lymphadenitis, effectively rule out the diagnosis of tuberculosis. The testing can be completed rapidly within 24 hours but has the disadvantage of not being definitive for the specific type of mycobacteria present when acid-fast bacteria are identified. In contrast to histopathology, bacterial culture of fresh tissue samples has the advantage of giving a specific genus and species diagnosis, but the significant disadvantage of taking 4–8 weeks to complete the testing.

The Procedure and Interpretation of Positive Results

After acid-fast bacteria have been identified by histopathology, sections from those same paraffin tissue blocks can then be used for PCR testing. This procedure increases the sensitivity of testing by ensuring that there will be bacterial DNA within the sample that is being tested by PCR. The DNA is extracted from the sample, and then PCR is used to amplify any target bacterial DNA within the sample, using highly specific primers, polymerases, and other reagents. Primers are oligonucleotide sequences that bind to complementary bacterial DNA. The primers used in our laboratory, which bind to a fragment of the insertion sequence *6110* (IS*6110*), have been widely used in veterinary and human medicine for the identification of *M. tuberculosis* complex bacteria (1,2). *M. bovis* is a member of the *M. tuberculosis* complex, along with *M. tuberculosis*, *Mycobacterium africanum*, *Mycobacterium canettii*, *Mycobacterium microti*, *Mycobacterium caprae*, and *Mycobacterium pinnipedii* (3). Methods other than PCR for IS*6110* are required to differentiate between the seven species of mycobacteria within the *M. tuberculosis* complex, but the species of the animal diagnosed with tuberculosis and the geographic location of the animal frequently give a strong indication of which member of *M. tuberculosis* complex is involved. *M. bovis* is the primary cause of tuberculosis in cattle and frequently infects many other species, including man. *M. microti* primarily infects voles, *M. caprae* has been identified primarily in goats from Spain, *M. pinnipedii* has been found primarily in seals, and all three infrequently infect other species of animals (3). *M. tuberculosis*, *M. africanum*, and *M. canettii* are all human pathogens; in addition, *M. tuberculosis* occasionally infects a wide variety of animal species (3).

The strains of *M. bovis* commonly found in cattle typically contain a single copy of IS*6110* (4). Because the primers we use amplify a relatively short sequence of DNA (123 base pairs), they are well suited for use on formalin-fixed DNA (Fig. 8.1) (1). Short sequences of DNA are less prone to damage by formalin fixation than are longer sequences, which frequently are damaged by formalin fixation (5). In addition, PCR using primers for other common ruminant mycobacteria, such as *M. avium* or *M. avium paratuberculosis*, can be run concurrently to increase the likelihood of identifying the unknown acid-fast bacteria detected by histopathology.

PCR Performance Compared to Traditional Bacterial Culture

PCR on formalin-fixed tissues has proven to be both complementary and confirmatory to bacterial culture in several studies (5–7). In the majority of cases of bovine tuberculosis, histopathology, PCR testing of fixed tissue, and bacterial culture results are all in agreement (5,6). Miller et al. detected IS*6110* by PCR in 65 of 70 animals that had both microscopic lesions with acid-fast bacteria in formalin-fixed tissue and *M. bovis* cultured from fresh tissues (1). In an additional 133 cases with microscopic lesions typical of *M. bovis* containing acid-fast bacteria, 92% were positive for *M. tuberculosis* complex by PCR and 89% were positive for *M. bovis* by bacterial culture (6). However, 11 of the cases were positive by PCR testing and culture negative, whereas 10 cases had *M. bovis* cultured but were negative by PCR (6). Similar conflicting results were further investigated in another study (7). Seventy bovine cases that had histological lesions of *M. bovis* with acid-fast bacteria but negative culture results were tested by PCR (7). A PCR product,

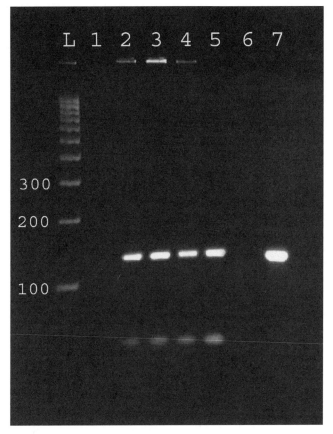

Figure 8.1.   Electrophoresis gel from polymerase chain reaction using primers that amplify a 123–base pair fragment of IS*6110*. Lanes 1 and 6 contain negative controls. Lanes 2–5 are samples from cattle naturally infected with *M. bovis*. Lane 7 contains the positive control sample, and L is the molecular weight ladder in 100–base pair increments.

confirmed to be the IS*6110* sequence by Southern blotting, was detected in 35 of the 70 cases (7). Within human granulomatous lesions in which tuberculosis was previously diagnosed or suspected, PCR testing also detected IS*6110* in tissues that were culture negative (8).

The differing results from PCR and from culture in some animals are not unexpected for a variety of reasons. *M. bovis* infections frequently have very low numbers of bacteria and the bacteria are not evenly distributed throughout the body or even within a single lymph node. When tissue samples are collected and subdivided, with one subsample placed in formalin for PCR and the other subsample used for culture, it is possible that only one of the subsamples will contain bacteria. Of course, PCR detects bacterial DNA, whereas culture detects live bacteria, so the causes of a false negative for PCR are different than the causes of a false negative for bacterial culture.

Potential Causes of False-Negative Results

There are several potential causes of false-negative results in PCR testing. Prolonged formalin fixation progressively increases DNA degradation and eventually leads to false-negative PCR results (5). Decalcifying solutions, which are used commonly to facilitate slide preparation of tissue blocks that contain mineralized granulomas, also decrease the sensitivity of PCR (1). The type of tissue fixation solution used is also important. Ten percent neutral buffered formalin is a commonly used tissue fixative that preserves DNA relatively well, whereas tissues fixed in unbuffered formalin, paraformaldehyde, and Bouin's solution are less useful for PCR (5,9). When using 10% neutral buffered formalin, the best DNA preservation is obtained by placing tissue into formalin as soon as possible after collection, keeping the tissue sample size small and no thicker than 0.5–1 cm, using a ratio of one part tissue to greater than 20 parts formalin, and fixing the tissue for only 3–6 hours at 4°C (5). In diagnostic veterinary medicine, it is frequently impossible to meet these guidelines because samples are collected in the field and then must be shipped to the laboratory. However, by following the basic concept of rapid tissue fixation over a short duration, quality PCR testing results can be obtained despite difficult field conditions.

False-negative bacterial culture results are created by a variety of conditions, such as growth of tissue contaminants during shipping of an improperly preserved tissue sample, and furthermore, the preservation methods themselves can result in decreased numbers of viable mycobacteria (10). Sodium tetraborate, a commonly used transportation medium used when chilling or freezing of tissue during transportation is impractical, results in an 80% loss in viability in *M. bovis* after only 72 hours of storage (10). Understanding the causes of false negatives can help the submitting veterinarian to properly collect samples for testing and to interpret conflicting culture and PCR results. In all cases, a negative test result simply means that the test did not detect the agent in that sample and does not prove that the animal is not infected with *M. bovis*.

False-positive results caused by contamination are possible with both culture and PCR but can be prevented by strict adherence to good laboratory practices and the use of known negative control samples.

An Alternate PCR Method

Other PCR-based methods are also possible for the diagnosis of *M. bovis* in formalin-fixed tissue. One method is to first use PCR to amplify a portion of the 16S rRNA that is common to all prokaryotes (11). The specific mycobacteria in the sample are identified by comparing the genetic sequence of the amplified PCR product to known sequences of many different mycobacterial species (11,12). The advantage of this method is that many different mycobacteria can potentially be identified from a single PCR reaction (11,12). A slight disadvantage of the procedure is that it is necessary to amplify longer strands of DNA, which are more susceptible to formalin degradation, to obtain enough sequence to identify the mycobacteria.

Acknowledgments

I thank Dr. J. M. Miller, Dr. A. Jenny, and my other colleagues, whose original works and guidance have provided me the basis for this chapter.

References

1. Miller, J., A. Jenny, J. Rhyan, D. Saari, and D. Suarez. 1997. Detection of *Mycobacterium bovis* in formalin-fixed, paraffin-embedded tissues of cattle and elk by PCR amplification of an IS*6110* sequence specific for *Mycobacterium tuberculosis* complex organisms. *J Vet Diagnostic Investig* 9:244-49.
2. Eisenach, K. D., M. D. Cave, J. H. Bates, and J. T. Crawford. 1990. Polymerase chain reaction amplification of a repetitive DNA sequence specific for *Mycobacterium tuberculosis. J Infect Dis* 161:977-81.
3. Cousins, D. V., R. Bastida, A. Cataldi, V. Quse, S. Redrobe, S. Dow, P. Duignan, A. Murray, C. Dupont, N. Ahmed, D. M. Collins, W.R. Butler, D. Dawson, D. Rodriguez, J. Loureiro, M. I. Romano, A. Alito, M. Zumarraga, and A. Bernardelli. 2003. Tuberculosis in seals caused by a novel member of the *Mycobacterium tuberculosis* complex: *Mycobacterium pinnipedii* sp. nov. *Int J Syst Evol Microbiol* 53:1305-14.
4. Collins, D. M., S. K. Erasmuson, D. M. Stephens, G. F. Yates, and G. W. DeLisle. 1993. DNA fingerprinting of *Mycobacterium bovis* strains by restriction fragment analysis and hybridization with insertion elements IS*1081* and IS*6110. J Clin Microbiol* 31:1143-47.
5. Srinivasan, M., D. Sedmak, and S. Jewell. 2002. Effect of fixatives and tissue processing on the content and integrity of nucleic acids. *Am J Pathol* 161:1961-71.
6. Miller, J., A. Jenny, and J. Payeur. 2001. Report of the Committee on Tuberculosis: update on PCR on fixed tissues. Proceedings of the One Hundred and Fifth Annual Meeting of the United States Animal Health Association 105, 501-503.
7. Miller, J. M., A. L. Jenny, and J. B. Payeur. 2002. Polymerase chain reaction detection of *Mycobacterium tuberculosis* complex and *Mycobacterium avium* organisms in formalin-fixed tissues from culture-negative ruminants. *Vet Microbiol* 87:15-23.
8. Salian, N. V., J. A. Rish, K. D. Eisenach, M. D. Cave, and J. H. Bates. 1998. Polymerase chain reaction to detect *Mycobacterium tuberculosis* in histologic specimens. *Am J Respir Crit Care Med* 158:1150-55.
9. Greer, C. E., S. L. Peterson, N. B. Kiviat, and M. M. Manos. 1991. PCR amplification from paraffin-embedded tissues. *Am J Clin Pathol* 95:117-24.
10. Corner, L. A. 1994. Post mortem diagnosis of *Mycobacterium bovis* infection in cattle. *Vet Microbiol* 40(1-2):53-63.
11. Hughes, M. S., R. A. Skuce, L. A. Beck, and S. D. Neill. 1993. Identification of Mycobacteria from animals by restriction enzyme analysis and direct DNA cycle sequencing of polymerase chain reaction-amplified 16S rRNA gene sequences. *J Clin Microbiol* 31:3216-22.
12. Appleyard, G. D. and E. G. Clark. 2002. Histologic and genotypic characterization of a novel *Mycobacterium* species found in three cats. *J Clin Microbiol* 40:2425-30.

Chapter 9
Economics of Bovine Tuberculosis

*J. Zinsstag, DVM, PhD, E. Schelling, DVM, PhD,
F. Roth, MA, and R. Kazwala, DVM, PhD*

Introduction

Economics is concerned with how resources are made accessible, allocated, and consumed. The unit of analysis can be the global economy, a particular region, a country, a zone of a country, specific markets, a household, or the individual. Economic analyses are designed to help identify means to maximize welfare with given existing resources. The outcome of most economic analysis of different interventions is to identify the most efficient way of using available resources (i.e., how to get the most benefit for a given budget, or the least costly way to achieve a stated level of benefits) (1,2). The general methods of animal health economics are well established and are not the subject of this chapter, which is the specific economic issues concerning bovine tuberculosis (TB) and its control.

At the end of the 19th century, when control efforts against bovine TB were initiated (Bang in 1884), they were often matched with the control of brucellosis and other zoonoses. These activities occupied a substantial part of the human resources and institutional capacity of the veterinary sector in the 20th century. Compared to its massive logistic, organizational, and financial implications, however, it is surprising to see how few economic and financial analyses of bovine TB control actually exist, especially in countries that have put enormous effort into bovine TB control and that are today declared free of this disease. At the beginning of the 21st century, economic aspects of zoonoses control in general, and specifically of bovine TB, rapidly gained interest in view of continuing and new challenges, including, first, that wildlife reservoirs with bovine TB persist in many countries and slow down substantial and costly efforts of control; second, the World Trade Organization, in its attempt to reduce trade barriers, seeks to standardize sanitary measures to avoid their use for protectionist purposes (3). However, globalized trade and progressively integrated markets with reduced border control increase the risk of the introduction of animal diseases.

Third, the rapidly growing demand for milk and meat in urban centers in developing countries leads to the intensification of livestock production systems, which increases the risk of *M. bovis* transmission to animals and humans. Fourth, zoonoses have been largely eliminated in industrial countries—very important financial and organizational efforts, expended toward animal reservoirs, are not possible in developing countries. An important part of animal disease control programs successes were the result of the compensation of farmers for culled livestock. However, most developing countries would not be able to conduct control schemes based on compensation of livestock owners for culled livestock. Zoonoses, and in particular bovine TB, are considered diseases of poverty (4). In many developing countries, large rural populations—and especially women—are not only at higher risk for zoonotic diseases because of their close interaction with livestock but are also more vulnerable to poverty resulting from the loss of livestock productivity, poor institutional frameworks, and the absence of systematic disease control.

Fourth and fifth, at present, many postcommunist transition countries potentially face a sharp increase of zoonotic disease occurrences resulting from both the breakdown of governmental disease surveillance and their still-weak private health services (5).

The above-stated challenges clearly show that bovine TB is not only a livestock issue but affects public health, wildlife, international trade, tourism, and many other areas of public and private interest. They call for a rethinking of control efforts and their economic consequences. An economic assessment attempting to consider the societal effect of bovine TB must somehow address all of these issues. First of all, the cost of the damage of disease, control, and treatment, both to animals (livestock and wildlife) and humans, needs to be assessed. The latter also involves nonmonetary issues, such as the often-controversial valuing of life years and quality of life. Second, the cost of disease has to be brought into relation to benefits of interventions, again in monetary and nonmonetary terms, to estimate the profitability and cost-effectiveness of disease control. Most important, consideration must be made for the incidence and prevalence of disease, and hence its economic effect changes in a nonlinear way during an intervention.

A disease such as bovine TB affects the individual animal or human not only at the private household's level but also, as a contagious disease, on the level of the whole livestock industry and the public health sector, as well as the national economy. Bovine TB also affects international trade, as many countries ban the import of livestock from countries where it is endemic. Effects may occur also within wildlife ecosystems, with unknown indirect consequences for the whole ecosystem and for economic activities (tourism, agriculture). Current successful intervention schemes based on farmer compensation have to be rethought for their use in developing countries. Hence, an in-depth economic analysis of the profitability of interventions is needed before their recommendation to potential users. This appears to be a fairly complex challenge that only can be sketched in the following pages.

This chapter first presents an overview of the existing productivity and economic analyses and their approaches toward the effects of bovine TB. The second part briefly outlines methods in public health to assess the burden of disease in humans. On the basis of these considerations, an outline is included for a dynamic transsectoral estimation of the burden and cost of disease for bovine TB from a societal perspective. This framework will then be expanded to include the profitability and cost-effectiveness analysis of culling and potential new vaccination interventions, with an outlook on perspectives for bovine TB control in developing countries.

Review of Existing Production and Economic Assessments of the Effects of Bovine TB

Effects on Cattle Productivity

One of the earliest reports on the effects of bovine TB on livestock production was by Meisinger (6), who conducted a cohort study on 8000 cows over 5 years and an abattoir survey in a collectivist production system (Landwirtschaftliche Produktions Genossenschaft) in the former German Democratic Republic. The main productivity losses in cattle are reduced milk and meat production and increased reproduction efforts. Milk productivity, given total livestock contamination, was 10% ± 2.5% lower compared to that of noninfected cows (7). Losses in meat production are divided into losses in beef processing caused by emergency/illness slaughter and losses in processing caused by normal slaughter and reduction of increment meat production. In totally TB infected livestock, 4% (±2%) of the meat production is lost because of emergency and illness slaughter. The losses are mainly in cattle and cows over 18 months of age, and no differences of growth could be found in young animals in fattening schemes.

Overall, bovine TB was found to decrease meat production by 6%–12% (±2.5%), depending on the percentage of cows (30%–70%) in a herd in which more than 80% of all animals or more than 95% of cows are afflicted with the disease (6). Canadian workers (8) assumed a loss of 10% of milk production and one fewer calf in infected cows. They included also a replacement loss of 15% for infected animals. Losses in beef were estimated at 1/5 calf loss and 1/5 replacement loss per year attributed to each infected beef cow. Morris estimates the total losses to 3%–4% of the total cattle and milk output [cited in ref. (9)], but this estimate is not related to a prevalence. Bernues et al. (10) assumed losses in meat production at 10% in calves born from infected cows. Milk losses were assumed at 12% of the total yield, and losses caused by sterility at 5% in infected animals, referring to Denes (11).

Economic Assessments

Existing economic assessments are mainly documents relating to the cost of control efforts and of the disease. Analyses of the profitability of control efforts (benefit/cost) are very rare. Schlegel (12) presents comprehensive data for the cost of controlling bovine TB between 1966 and 1979 in Lower Saxony (Germany), which can be related to herd-level incidence. A benefit/cost analysis of the Canadian TB control program used a stochastic simulation model adapted from the U.S. Animal and Plant Health Inspection Services, known as "Stratified Triple Binomial Herd-to-Herd Disease Population Model in Cost-Benefit Analysis" (8). This comprehensive assessment considers the very complex process of TB transmission between farms, but the authors state that it was most difficult to find documented data on the numerous parameters. The Canadian study resulted in an extraordinary high benefit/cost ratio of 33/1 for the effect of a herd depopulation program compared to that of a "no program" scenario. According to Frye (13), a benefit/cost analysis of *M. bovis* eradication in the United States showed an actual cost of $538 million between 1917 and 1992; current programs cost approximately $3.5–4 million per year. By reducing the number of cattle lost from 100,000 to less than 30 per year, the program saves $150 million per year in replacement costs alone. As a consequence of such efforts, farmers have benefited by eliminating the indirect cost of losses in milk and meat production, stock replacement, and decontamination procedures.

In the Republic of Ireland, the costs of an eradication program of bovine TB, which was inaugurated in 1954, was conveniently rounded to £1 billion by the year 1988 (9). The present value of the benefit exceeded the present value of the costs by 85%, and the rate of return of the scheme was 15.5% and also included the benefits from preserving international market access. In contrast, in the United Kingdom, Power and Watts (14) obtained negative results in the economic evaluation of TB control campaigns, including the control of badgers. In Spain, the payback of an eradication program in two districts of the Huesca Province was infinite (i.e., the accumulated benefits obtained never exceeded the costs) (10). However, none of these analyses included the cost to human health.

In May 2004, we sent out a short questionnaire on the availability of economic analyses on bovine TB to almost 100 national veterinary services based on an OIE (Office International des Epizooties) address list. The received answers and an additional Internet search (October 2004) are summarized in Table 9.1. The table

Table 9.1.   Nonexhaustive list of existing economic studies on bovine tuberculosis

Country	Analysis of Cost of Control	Analysis of Profitability of Control
Andorra	None	None
Australia	Turner (2003) (25)	
Austria	None	None
Canada		Management Consulting Services (1979) (8)
Croatia	None	None
Czech Republic	Pavlas (1999) (26)	
Eritrea	None	None
Germany	Schlegel (1980) (11)	None
Greece	http://www.minagric.gr/greek/data/bov_tuber.doc	
Ireland		Sheehy and Christiansen (1991) (9)
Luxembourg	Internal document	
New Zealand	Animal Health Board (2001) (18)	Animal Health Board (2001) (18)
Portugal	Internal document	
Spain		Bernues et al. (1997) (14)
Slovenia	Internal document	
Switzerland	None	none
Tanzania	Ongoing (Cleaveland and Kazwala)	
United Kingdom	http://www.defra.gov.uk/animalh/tb/stats/stats1.htm	Power and Watts (1987) (13)
United States of America	Frye (1994) (12), Nelson (1999) (27), Meyer (2003) (28)	

shows that in most responding countries, the costs of control programs are assessed. However, analyses of their profitability are lacking, with a few exceptions. We conclude that the profitability of existing bovine TB control programs is highly variable and difficult to compare because of the different epidemiological situations, livestock systems, natural reservoirs, time horizons, and analytical methods. No commonly agreed framework of analysis exists to date.

The Burden of Bovine TB

Within human health, the Disability Adjusted Life Year (DALY) is an instrument developed to determine the relative burden of disease in different settings and at different stages of economic and public health development. As well as being used for ranking of the overall burden of an individual disease, the DALY is also an outcome measure, particularly useful in cost-effectiveness analysis in the frame of economic evaluations. DALYs are composed of years of life lost and years of life lost because of disability (15). Although the number of years of life lost can be estimated by relating the age at death to the life expectancy, the years of life lost because of disability include an estimation of the duration of disease and the severity of disability. There is a lot of controversy in the defining and weighting of disability. For many diseases, discrepancies exist between observed and perceived symptoms that are determined by the sociocultural background and many other factors such as the general health status of the population. Another indicator accounting for perceived preferences and weights of disability is the Quality Adjusted Life Year. For most zoonoses, estimations of DALY do not exist and are currently being developed; for example, for brucellosis (5). For TB, detailed DALY estimates are available and are useful to assess the burden of bovine TB, as in general the clinical outcome in humans is the same as for TB caused by *M. tuberculosis* (16). TB is ranking among the top 10 in the burden-of-disease table because 90% of the DALYs lost are because of premature death (Christopher Dye, World Health Organization, personal communication).

A preliminary estimate of a DALY score for *M. bovis* in the Arusha Region of Tanzania was calculated on the basis of the proportion of culture-positive cases of extrapulmonary TB caused by *M. bovis* (10%), as well as the proportion of extrapulmonary TB cases in Tanzania (20%–30% of cases). The DALY calculation was based on the age-specific incidence of extrapulmonary TB cases resulting from *M. bovis* infection and incorporates both premature death and morbidity/disability. Mortality data were obtained from trace-back of cases. The severity of disease was assessed both from clinical signs reported at the hospital and from duration of disease determined during trace-back studies. Weighting for the disability component for *M. bovis* was given as 0.15 (on a scale of 0–1 in increasing severity) and with guidance from weightings given to other conditions in the Global Burden of Disease study. The overall DALY burden for *M. bovis* in Tanzania was estimated as equivalent to approximately 1.3% of the total burden of TB in the country (Table 9.2). In this preliminary calculation, all extrapulmonary TB cases not caused by *M. bovis* and all pulmonary cases were combined, which resulted in a DALY score of 730,891 for other forms of TB. In the light of results showing a high prevalence of

Table 9.2. Estimates of the DALY burden for tuberculosis infection caused by *Mycobacterium tuberculosis* (anthroponotic transmission) and *Mycobacterium bovis* (zoonotic transmission) in Tanzania in 2000

Age Group, years	*M. tuberculosis* and Atypical Mycobacteria	*M. bovis*
0–4	77,332	547
5–14	154,383	3247
15–44	421,652	5244
45–59	61,066	459
60+	16,458	242
All ages	730,891	9739

atypical *Mycobacteria* in cases of extrapulmonary TB, further refinement of this calculation is needed and a new calculation carried out specifically for TB caused by atypical *Mycobacteria*.

Transsectoral (Public Health, Agriculture, Environment) Economic Analysis of Bovine TB Control

It is widely recognized that many zoonoses can only be eliminated if the disease is controlled in the animal reservoir. However, from a public health sector perspective, the cost-effectiveness of control interventions must be demonstrated. A recent economic analysis of a livestock brucellosis mass vaccination campaign to reduce human brucellosis has shown that for the public health sector, this intervention is not profitable. However, if the benefits for the livestock sector are added and the costs of the intervention are shared between the public health and the agricultural sector proportionally to their benefits, the control of brucellosis is profitable for both sectors (5). For bovine TB, comparable assessments do not exist, and a full societal analysis implies sectors other than health and agriculture (see following).

The transmission of bovine TB changes in a nonlinear way during a control scheme, and consequently, the effects on productivity and public health cannot be assessed by linear extrapolation. Transmission models can provide frameworks to simulate the nonlinear decrease of disease prevalence and the disease transmission with and without control interventions (17). For bovine TB, the transmission to humans must also be included, as was done for brucellosis control (5). In Figure 9.1, we propose a transsectoral framework for the transmission simulation of bovine TB among wildlife, cattle, and humans. The compartmental backbone is flexible and can be adapted to a specific epidemiological situation such as multiple wildlife reservoirs. The black arrows indicate flows of newly infected, infectious, and recovered wildlife, and livestock and human populations between compartments. For example, susceptible cattle become latently infected. Eventually they become infectious as the disease progresses. Infectious livestock (cattle, small ruminants, and camels) may cause human infection (grey arrow), but they also cause infection of wildlife. For every compartment, differential equations can be formulated, and if field data are available, parameters can be estimated for every

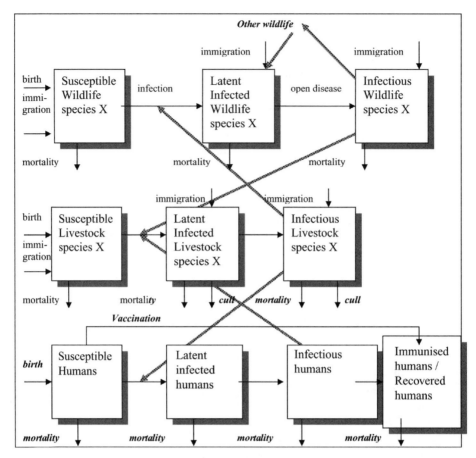

Figure 9.1. Flow chart of transmission of bovine tuberculosis as a backbone to a dynamic transsectoral economic assessment.

flow. If parameter estimates for demographic (birth, death rates) and transmission (contact rates) are available, the transmission of bovine TB can be simulated. Different interventions (test and slaughter, vaccination) can be specified and their effect simulated and possibly validated with field data. The bovine TB control strategy of New Zealand (18) gives particular emphasis to environmental and biodiversity issues in their economic analysis but conclude that "in the absence of an agreed set of values for risk probabilities, costs and benefits all of which are speculative, it is not possible to derive the optimal programme."

As the example from New Zealand shows, in most situations, sufficient data to validate all compartments in Figure 9.1 are not available. A balance has to be found between aspirations to consider complexity and the availability of data to validate a transmission model.

In Figure 9.2, a simplified framework for a model of animal-to-human bovine TB transmission is presented. We consider transmission between cattle (and no other livestock species) and from cattle to humans. Thereby we do not consider aerial and milk transmission separately but aim at estimating one single cattle-to-

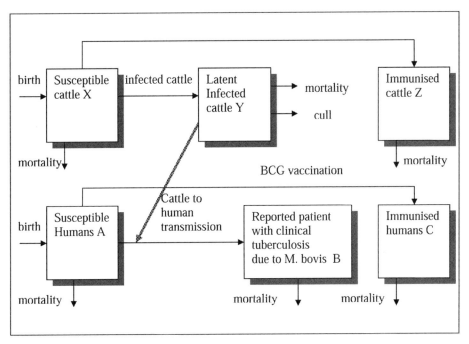

Figure 9.2. Simplified model of transmission of bovine tuberculosis between cattle and humans

human contact rate. Bovine TB affects fertility, growth, and milk production in livestock. The incidence is the product of the number of susceptible animals, the number of infectious animals (via aerosol and milk), and a contact rate, which we intend to estimate. The number of actually infectious animals is breed- and probably prevalence-dependent and can only be estimated by establishing the proportion of tuberculin-positive animals who show lung and udder localizations (78%–85% of all tuberculin-positive animals have gross visible lesions; Almaty Turgenbaev, personal communication). This proportion should be increased by an estimate of the proportion of animals with gross visible lesions that are nonreactors. We tentatively estimate this latter proportion at 3%–6% from observations by Meisinger (7). This proportion can be used to simplify our model considerably. In most cases, only data on the proportion of tuberculin-positive animals will be available. Thus, we use (instead of "infectious" and "recovered" compartments) only one "latent infected" compartment, which contains the number of tuberculin-positive animals. In Equation 9.1, the incidence in cattle is then expressed as the product of γ (proportion of infectious among the latent infected), β (contact rate), the number of susceptible cattle (X), and the number of latent infected (tuberculin-positive) cattle (Y).

$$\text{Incidence}_{cattle} = \gamma\beta XY \qquad\qquad 9.1$$

Compartments and Flows between Compartments

The compartment of susceptible humans A (Figure 9.2) represents the whole population of the area of assessment (district, province) because precise estimates of the population at risk (in general, all ages are at risk if milk is not strictly pasteurized) are often not available. Human TB patients are reported in general, and those affected with *M. bovis* are often not assessed or underestimated.

The description of flows (Figure 9.2) is expressed [see Eqs. (2–7)] as follows: The flow into the susceptible cattle compartment is a result of calf birth. Loss of immunity and immigration/emigration (purchase/sale) are not considered in this outline but can be added easily. Cattle birth (unit: cattle/year) = $\alpha(X + Y)$, where α = birth rate of cattle, multiplied by the sum of $(X + Y)$. Flows out of compartment X are mortality of susceptible cattle, infected cattle, and vaccinated cattle (Bacille Calmette-Güerin and new candidates): Mortality (unit: cattle/year) of susceptible cattle = $-(\mu X)$, where μ is the mortality rate of cattle. Infected cattle (= incidence in cattle; unit: cattle/year) = $-\gamma\beta XY$ in analogy to Equation 9.1 (see above).

$$\frac{dX}{dt} = \alpha(X+Y) - \mu X - \gamma\beta XY \qquad 9.2$$

Flows going into the compartment of latent infected cattle Y are as described above. Flows out of compartment Y are mortality of latent infected cattle and culling of skin test–positive animals. Loss of positive skin-test reactivity is not considered at this stage. Mortality (unit: cattle/year) of latent infected animals = $(\mu_l Y)$, where μ_l is the specific mortality rate of latent infected animals. Culling (test and slaughter; unit: cattle/year) of skin test-positive animals = φY, where φ is the proportion of tested and slaughtered cattle Y.

$$\frac{dY}{dt} = \gamma\beta XY - \mu_l Y - \varphi Y \qquad 9.3$$

Flows into compartment A (susceptible humans) are human births. Human birth (unit: humans/year) = $\alpha_h(A + B + C)$, where α_h = human birth rate multiplied by the sum of all human compartments. Flows out of A are infected humans, mortality, and Bacille Calmette-Güerin vaccination of susceptible humans. Infected humans (unit: humans/year) (cattle-to-human transmission) = $(\gamma\beta_h AY)$, where β_h is the cattle–human contact rate. Mortality (unit: humans/year) of susceptible humans is $\mu_h A$, where μ_h is the mortality rate of humans multiplied with compartment A. Changes of compartment A are expressed in Eq. (9.4) dA/dt. Flows into compartment B are infected humans (as above), which takes a positive sign for this compartment. Flows out of B are mortality. We do not consider recovery. Mortality (unit: humans/year) of annually reported cases = $\mu_h B$ in analogy for compartment A (Equation 9.5). Finally, flows into compartment C are immunized humans, which would be to a limited extent protected from *M. bovis* infections. Immunized humans = λA where λ is the proportion of protected susceptibles (A) (Equation 9.6). The chronic nature of clinical TB development can be considered using delayed time step functions.

$$\frac{dA}{dt} = \alpha_h(A + B + C) - \gamma\beta_h AY - \mu_h A \qquad 9.4$$

$$\frac{dB}{dt} = \gamma\beta_h AY - \mu_h B \qquad\qquad 9.5$$

$$\frac{dC}{dt} = \lambda A - \mu_h C \qquad\qquad 9.6$$

Estimates of the transmission parameters obtained by fitting such a model, possibly over 5–10 years, can be used to simulate different scenarios both with and without interventions. Outcomes of the simulations are prevalences in cattle and humans, which are changing over time. They can be used as inputs into the economic assessment by linking them to human health costs and livestock productivity (5). For example, milk production in tuberculin-positive animals is reduced by 10% (6). Comparable links between productivity and disease occurrence can also be established for other productivity parameters (10) and used as input parameters of livestock production simulation (e.g., Livestock Development Planning System, Food and Agriculture Organization or the United Nations).

During control interventions the costs of control include administrative costs such as salaries and fees paid to veterinarians, hired labor, administrators, and field workers; compensation costs; and field material. The economic analysis of an intervention to control bovine TB should include the effect on human health costs and income loss, the coping costs, and the effect on livestock production. Benefits in monetary terms can then be computed for three different sectors:

1. For the agricultural sector: the benefit resulting from the avoided losses in animals and animal products:
   a. Avoided on-farm losses, which include milk losses, calf losses, meat losses (condemnations), herd restriction (reduced herd size), and replacement losses (difference between salvage value and purchase price of replacement)
   b. Avoided costs and losses in processing reactors: losses incurred through processing reactors ordered to be slaughtered including costs of removal of a reactor such as disinfection of the barn, movement of tuberculin reactors to approved slaughter facility, and destruction of affected carcasses and condemned organs
   c. Other avoided costs (e.g., material used, travel, rent)
   d. Avoided administrative costs: salaries and fees paid to veterinarians and field material to deal with ill animals
2. For the public health sector: the benefit resulting from the avoided costs to the public health sector, such as drug expenses, medical costs, or hospital costs.
3. For private households with patients suffering from bovine tuberculosis: the benefit resulting from avoided out-of-pocket payment for treatment, income loss (opportunity costs), and coping costs (e.g., hiring extra labor capacity).

The sum of the benefits in all three mentioned sectors will be considered as a benefit for the society as a whole and represents monetary valuation of bovine TB control. The methodology avoids double counting of common costs between the public health sector and the payments made by patients for treatment. For every sector, the present monetary value of the intervention can then be computed. A specific feature of zoonoses is that improvements in public health are obtained through interventions in the livestock sector. Hence, it is obvious that the public sector should somehow contribute to the costs of the intervention. Economic methods for the sharing of cost between different sectors are existent, and an example is given by reference (5), in which basic elements of the technique for joint cost allocation in multipurpose projects are applied and adapted. All costs are regarded as joint costs and are allocated proportionally to the benefit. By sharing the costs of the intervention between sectors that benefited from the intervention, the public health sector does not bear the whole cost, and interventions against zoonoses may become cost-effective for human health. Cost-effectiveness to the public health sector is expressed as financial cost per averted DALY.

Using the above approach, the nonlinear change of disease occurrence, in the course of different interventions, can be considered and compared directly. This provides results based on a transmission process that can be validated. If data are available, economic assessments can be expanded to include other sectors, as outlined in Figure 9.1. In addition, benefits derived from retaining access to premium markets that would be lost or curtailed in the absence of the scheme should be added as appropriate. Benefits from access to export markets contributed significantly to the profitability of the Irish control scheme (9).

Developing World Perspectives—Sub-Saharan Africa and Outlook to Financing

The livestock industry in most of Sub-Saharan Africa is significantly underproductive in comparison to that in South Africa, Asia, and Europe. Despite a large herd size, comparable to that of Europe and larger than that of the United States, returns are very low (19). There are many facets to this underperformance, but it is mainly a result of livestock diseases causing relatively low outputs. Economic returns from cattle in Africa are rather low and do not provide impetus to control major diseases, which hampers trade with developed countries. In addition, most developed countries impose strict regulations on imported livestock and products to prevent the introduction of disease from foreign countries.

As an OIE List B disease, bovine TB is one of the significant diseases that affects the international trade of animals and animal products between countries. List B diseases are transmissible diseases that are considered to be of socioeconomic or public health importance within countries. According to OIE bovine TB records within the last 5 years (1998–2003), 31 of 50 African countries have reported the occurrence of TB in their respective countries (20). Control measures have been put in place in 35 of the 50 African countries reporting to OIE.

Despite these control measures, not a single country has been able to eliminate or effectively control bovine TB. There is also a general scarcity of data from individual countries as a result of a lack of a coordinated African, regional, or subregional effort in TB surveillance. It is obvious that some countries are not reporting bovine TB for political, social, and economic motives. For these reasons, the lack of control in the majority of African countries is not surprising. In South Africa, whose performance in livestock productivity is comparable to that of most developed countries, bovine TB has been strongly reduced in the livestock population. However, it remains in the wildlife, particularly in Kruger National Park's buffalo population. The ensuing efforts to attain this success emanated from efforts carried out in the early 20th century, when mandatory tuberculin testing was enforced. Test-and-slaughter approaches (stamping out) have been successful in Europe (except Britain and Ireland), Australia, Canada, and the United States. The major obstacles have been the involvement of wildlife and, up until now, difficulties in realizing the economic benefits of control strategies. Benefit cost analyses fail to produce favorable results and in some cases give negative benefits, making the diseases hard to control with current strategies. In Africa, wildlife involvement in the spread of bovine TB has been documented; however, it is not clear how much wildlife transmission contributes to the occurrence of bovine TB in domesticated animals, and therefore its economical effect on the control of bovine TB in livestock.

The effect of bovine TB on human populations in Africa has not been assessed, bearing in mind that routes of transmission for both pulmonary and extra pulmonary TB exist. In some communities, close housing with cattle is not uncommon for social and security reasons. Aerosol transmission from animals may occur as a result of close contact to infected cattle. Eating habits also exacerbate the transmission of bovine TB (e.g., by consuming raw and undercooked meat and drinking unpasteurized milk).

Bovine TB was completely eliminated in many U.S. herds, at a cost of $450 million over 50 years, using a "test-and-slaughter" program combined with surveillance at slaughter. In Africa, and particularly in Sub-Saharan Africa, such resources are not available. It should be noted that as much as 90% of the human population in Africa live in countries where cattle and dairy cows undergo no or only partial disease controls. In many areas, pasteurization of locally produced milk is not feasible, and 13%–90% of milk is consumed fresh (unboiled) or soured. Cattle testing and meat inspection surveillance are often not conducted because of lack of trained personnel, lack of resources, or fear of economic loss. Unlike the United States, where less than 5% of the population has regular, direct exposure to cattle, more than half of the population in Africa has close contact with potentially infected animals and, therefore, is at risk of acquiring *M. bovis*.

Data from the World Health Organization shows that at present, more than 95% of the estimated 8 million new TB cases occurring each year are in the developing world, where more than 80% of cases occur among people between the ages of 15 and 59 years. It is estimated that there are about 2 million adult deaths annually from TB in developing countries, which accounts for a quarter of all avoidable adult deaths, and in Sub-Saharan Africa, TB is a leading cause of mortality. Data from Tanzania show that up to 20% of all human cases of TB are of extrapulmonary form, and among the culture-positive cases of extrapulmonary-positive TB, 10% were caused by *M. bovis*. If such figures are extrapolated to the African continent data, the magnitude of the involvement of *M. bovis* in total TB cases should not be underestimated, particularly now with the HIV/AIDS coinfection with TB cases approaching more than 31% (21).

The economic situation in most of the developing countries may not be able to maintain the approaches presently used by developed countries. The major factors limiting control of bovine TB in developing countries are as follows:

- Economic constraints
- Absence of culture and strain characterization
- Lack of resources for compensation of culled animals and vaccination, opposed by financial constraints and controversial effectiveness of Bacille Calmette-Güerin
- Inadequate reporting systems, collaboration, and communication between public health and veterinary services
- Low food safety standards in informal dairy systems
- Low public awareness of risk factors
- Absence of national control programs
- Lack of government commitment
- Use of modern methods limited by resources

It is imperative that alternative cheaper control approaches are developed and tested for their profitability and cost-effectiveness to reduce the incidence of bovine TB in both animals and humans. Such approaches may include strengthening public education, raising awareness, correction of misperceptions on risk factors, and correction of unfavorable customs and beliefs. Milk sold by small-scale holders and informal channels should be pasteurized. Grazing management should be changed to avoid contact with wildlife. Intermixing between herds at common watering points and markets should be reduced. If possible, larger herds should be managed as smaller and separate units. Finally, effects of new and existing vaccines in high-risk livestock and wildlife should be assessed.

These approaches, however, involve promoting research and training on risk factors, feasibility and effectiveness of control measures, distribution of strains and patterns of spread, and transmissions and new diagnostic methods.

There is sufficient evidence that the control and elimination of bovine TB is possible. Economic analyses help identify the most cost-effective strategies in a particular context. However, if seen from a global perspective, the shortfalls of current control efforts in developing countries should be of interest for all countries. In a globalized world, with falling trade barriers, endemic diseases in one part of the world will always threaten the spread of disease to disease-free zones. The most recent examples are the foot-and-mouth disease epidemic in the United Kingdom and the risk of the spread of avian influenza and SARS. Many developing countries, however, will not be able by their own means to invest in control and elimination programs for decades.

For human health, the report on macroeconomics and health to the World Health Organization (22) advocates subsidized funding by the international community of minimal health care in the poorest countries. First efforts for this have been made by creating the Global Fund to control malaria, HIV/AIDS, and TB, which provides substantial means to countries in need for the control of these priority diseases (23). Analogously, international organizations such as OIE, Food and Agriculture Organization or the United Nations, and the World Health Organization should enhance their leading role in the development of plans for international financing of animal disease control. This financing also should be expanded to zoonotic diseases as a poverty-reduction strategy (4). A past successful example of international animal disease control is the Pan African Rinderpest Campaign, within the Global Rinderpest Eradication Programme, which is currently expanded to other infectious diseases by the Pan African Programme for the Control of Epizootics (24). Finally, the control of bovine TB should also be seen in a broader disease control perspective, as in many countries the control of bovine TB was linked to brucellosis and other disease control measures. Thereby, the cost of control could be reduced even further.

Acknowledgment

We acknowledge the following persons for providing information on economic assessments of bovine TB in their countries:

Andorra: Frances Alay, Chief of Veterinary Services, Department of Agriculture
Australia: Animal Health Australia
Austria: Dr. Renate Krassnig, Bundesministerium für Gesundheit und Frauen, Vienna
Canada: Dr. Maria Koller-Jones, Senior Staff Veterinarian, Canadian Food Inspection Agency
Croatia: Dr. Mate Brstilo, Ministry of Agriculture, Zagreb
Eritrea: Dr. Tesfaalem Teklghiorghis, Central Veterinary Laboratory, Asmara
Germany: Dr. Bätza, Federal Ministry of Consumer Protection, Food and Agriculture, Berlin
Ireland: ERAD Division, Department of Agriculture and Food, Kildare
Luxembourg: Dr. Arthur Besch, Veterinary Services
New Zealand: P. G. Livingstone, Animal Health Board, Wellington
Portugal: Dr. Agrela Pinheiro, Director General de Veterinaria, Lisbon
Slovenia: Simona Salamon, MAFF, Veterinary Administration of the Republic of Slovenia
Switzerland: Dr. Hansueli Ochs, Federal Veterinary Office, BVET, Bern
Tanzania: Prof. R. Kazwala, Sokoine University, Morogoro
United Kingdom: Chief Veterinary Officer, Dr. Debby Reynolds.

References

1. Dijkuizen, A. A. and R. S. Morris. 1997. Animal Health Economics, Principles and Applications. Post Graduate Foundation, University of Sydney, Australia, 306.
2. Perry, B. D., T. F. Randolph, J. J. McDermott, K. R. Sones, and P. K. Thornton. 2003. Investing in Animal Health Research to Alleviate Poverty, International Livestock Research Institute, Nairobi, Kenya.

3. Leslie, J. and M. Upton. 1999. The economic implications of greater global trade in livestock and livestock products, the economics of animal disease control. *Rev Sci Tech Off Int Epizoo* 18:440-58.

4. Coleman, P. G. 2003. Zoonotic diseases and their impact on the poor. *In* B. D. Perry, T. F. Randolph, J. J. McDermott, K. R. Sones, and P. K. Thornton (eds.), Investing in Animal Health Research to Alleviate Poverty. Nairobi: International Livestock Research Institute.

5. Roth F., Zinsstag J., et al. 2003. Human health benefits from livestock vaccination for brucellosis: economic analysis in Mongolia. *Bull World Health Org* 81:867-76.

6. Meisinger, G. 1969. Untersuchungen über die ökonomischen Auswirkungen der Rindertuberkulosetilgung auf die Produktivität der Rinderbestände, 1. Mitteilung: Auswirkung auf die Milchproduktion, Münchener Tierrztliche Wochenschrift, 806-809.

7. Meisinger, G. 1970. Untersuchungen über die ökonomischen Auswirkungen der Rindertuberkulosetilgung auf die Produktivität der Rinderbestände. 2. Mitteilung: Auswirkung auf die Fleischproduktion. Münchener Tierrztliche Wochenschrift 25: 7-13.

8. Management Consulting Services. 1979. Evaluation of alternative tuberculosis programs by benefit/cost analysis, (Project 78028). Canada Department of Agriculture, Ottawa, Vols. 2 and 2

9. Sheehy, S. J. and K. H. Christiansen. 1991. Cost/benefit analysis of Irish bovine tuberculosis eradication scheme. Dublin: University College Dublin, 79.

10. Bernues, A., E. Manrique, and M. T. Maza. 1997. Economic evaluation of bovine brucellosis and tuberculosis eradication programmes in a mountain area of Spain. *Prev Vet Med* 30:137-49.

11. Denes, B. 1986. Some economic aspects of the bovine tuberculosis eradication in Hungary. *Tech Ser OIE* 3:207-11.

12. Schlegel, H. L. 1980. Die Entwicklung der wichtigsten Tierseuchen in Niedersachsen und die Kosten ihrer Bekämpfung in den Jahren 1966-1976. Deutsche Tierrztliche Wochenschrift 87:163-67.

13. Frye, G. 1994. Bovine tuberculosis eradication, *In* C. O. Thoen and J. H. Steele (eds.), *Mycobacterium bovis* Infection in Humans and Animals. Ames: Iowa State University Press.

14. Power, A. P. and B. G. A. Watts. 1987. The badger control policy: an economic assessment. London: Ministry of Agriculture, Fisheries, and Food, 41.

15. Murray, C. J. L. and A. D. Lopez (eds.). 1994. Global comparative assessments in the health sector, disease burden, expenditures and interventions packages. Geneva: World Health Organization, 196.

16. Cosivi, O., et al. 1998. Zoonotic tuberculosis due to *Mycobacterium bovis* in developing countries. *Emerging Infect Dis* 4:59-70.

17. Perry, B. (ed.). 2003. The economics of animal disease control. *Rev Sci Tech Office Int Epizoo* 18:295-561.

18. Animal Health Board. 2001. Bovine tuberculosis pest management strategy 2001-2013. Wellington: Animal Health Board.

19. Agricultural Bulletin Board on Data Collection. Dissemination and Quality of Statistics. Available at: http://faostat.fao.org/abcdq/about.htm.

20. HANDISTATUS II. Available at: http://www.oie.int/hs2/report.asp.

21. Corbett E. L., C. J. Watt, N. Walker, D. Maher, B. G. Williams, M. Raviglione C., and C. Dye. 2003. The growing burden of tuberculosis: global trends and interactions with the HIV epidemic. *Arch Int Med* 163:1009-21.

22. Commission on Macroeconomics and Health. Available at: http://www.cmhealth.org.
23. The Global Fund to Fight AIDS, Tuberculosis, and Malaria. Available at: http://www.theglobalfund.org.
24. Pan African Programme for the Control of Epizootics. Available at: http://www.fao.org/ag/AGA/AGAH/EMPRES/grep/pace.htm.
25. Turner, A. 2003. Tuberculosis freedom assurance program, Final report 1998-2002. Animal Health Australia, 59.
26. Pavlas, M. 1999. The 30th anniversary of eradication of bovine tuberculosis in cattle in Czechoslovakia. *Acta Vet Brno* 68:155-62.
27. Nelson, A. M. 1999. The cost of disease eradication, smallpox and bovine tuberculosis. *Ann N Y Acad Sci* 894:83-91.
28. Meyer R. M. 2003. Current status of bovine tuberculosis eradication program in the United States. Available at: http://www.animalagriculture.org/proceedings/2003%20Proc/Meyer.htm.

Chapter 10

A Tuberculosis Outbreak in Farmed Deer in Sweden and Its Economic Consequences

*G. Bölske, DVM, PhD, H. Wahlström, DVM, PhD,
B. Larsson, DVM, PhD, and J.Å. Robertsson, DVM, PhD*

History of Bovine Tuberculosis in Cattle in Sweden

Tuberculosis caused by *Mycobacterium bovis* (BTB) was probably imported to Sweden with infected breeding cattle in the middle of the 19th century and then, from breeding centers, spread all over the country (1). At that time, the dairy industry was developing rapidly, and at the end of the 19th century, it became common to return unpasteurized skim milk to farms for the feeding of calves. This resulted in an increased spread of BTB among cattle, and in the 1930s, about 30% of the slaughtered adult cattle had TB lesions. This route of infection was arrested in 1925, when pasteurization of milk used for feeding livestock became compulsory.

Control for BTB was initiated in the early 20th century. In 1930–1940, control was intensified, and in 1958 Sweden was one of the first countries in the world to be declared free from BTB (2). After 1958, sporadic cases have occurred in cattle, the most recent in 1978. The compulsory tuberculin testing of all cattle was abolished in 1970, and national BTB control is now based on meat inspection (3). In Swedish wildlife, only two cases of TB have been reported, both in free-living moose (*Alces alces*) in the 1940s. In humans, fewer than 10 cases of *M. bovis* are notified annually in Sweden. Most of those infected are elderly people, infected in their youth before BTB was eradicated in Sweden, or immigrants from areas where BTB is still common.

Legislation

BTB in animals has been notifiable under the Swedish legislation for epizootic diseases since 1958. If *M. bovis* is confirmed in a herd, the whole herd is depopulated and a 1-year standstill is implemented on the deer enclosures. Farmers are compensated for any loss resulting from actions taken by the Swedish Board of Agriculture. Before 1999, the compensation rate for animal value, cleaning and disinfection, and production losses was 100%. After 1999, the compensation rate for production losses was reduced to 50%.

TB in Farmed Deer

In 1991, BTB was diagnosed for the first time in farmed fallow deer (*Dama dama*) in Sweden (4,5). A total of 13 BTB-infected deer farms have been identified, the latest being in 1997 (as of February 2005). All identified infected deer were fallow deer. A consignment of fallow deer imported in 1987 was identified as the source of infection. This tracing to a common source of infection was supported by results from restriction fragment analysis (4) and restriction fragment length polymorphism. This *M. bovis* strain produced seven bands in the restriction fragment length polymorphism, considerably more than the typical one to two bands for *M. bovis* (6).

TB Control Program for Deer Farms

As all imported deer could not be traced, a voluntary control program, based on tuberculin testing, was implemented in July 1994, and in June 2003 the control program became compulsory. In brief, a herd obtains BTB-free status (A status) after three consecutive whole-herd tuberculin tests of all deer older than 1 year, with negative results. Furthermore, all deer that are killed or die as a result of other reasons shall be meat inspected/necropsied. Only herds with A status may trade in live deer, and to maintain the A status, all female deer in the herd have to be tested after 2 years and then every third year without positive findings. BTB-free status can also be obtained by slaughter and meat inspection of the whole herd and repopulation with deer from BTB-free herds. Herds that do not continue to tuberculin test are downgraded to BTB-free herds with B status, which prohibits trade in live deer.

Since the program's inception, it has become evident that on certain large extensive deer farms, it is difficult to muster all animals in the herd. Therefore, if there is no indication that the flock includes imported deer, the farmer may apply for an alternative control for BTB, based on slaughter and meat inspection. These herds can be declared BTB-free when at least 20% of the herd (equally distributed over sex and age classes) has been slaughtered annually for at least 15 years and the carcasses submitted for meat inspection without any findings of BTB (7).

Meat inspection became compulsory for farmed deer in 1990 and was extended to include free-living red deer (*Cervus elaphus*) and fallow deer in 1994.

The BTB control program is administered by a veterinary company providing official health control programs (Swedish Animal Health Service) in accordance with regulations issued by the Veterinary Authority (Swedish Board of Agriculture).

Deer Farming in Sweden

Fallow deer is the deer species most commonly farmed in Sweden. To a lesser extent, red deer, indigenous to Sweden, are also farmed. The interest in deer keeping increased in the 1990s when government subsidies to promote alternative use of

farmland made deer farming more profitable. Most deer are kept for venison production, and velvetting is prohibited. A few producers sell live deer, and in certain
large herds (game parks), deer are kept for shooting purposes. Deer farming in
Sweden is an extensive production. Farmed deer are not allowed to be kept on areas
smaller than 5 metric hectares. Furthermore, the size of the deer herd is required to
be adjusted to the size and biotope of the deer enclosure, so that supplementary
feeding is not needed during the plant-growing period.

At present (February 2005), there are approximately 20,000 farmed deer, of
which approximately 80% are fallow deer and 20% red deer distributed between
370 herds. In addition, there are 239 empty, depopulated farms, bringing the total
number of registered deer farms to 609. In all, 515 (85%) herds have obtained
BTB-free status, and about 40 of these continue to test to maintain their A status.

Costs for eradicating BTB

The total cost for elimination of BTB in the 13 BTB-infected herds was 15,000,000
SEK (2,146,000 USD). The cost per herd varied between 61,000 and 7,000,000
SEK. These figures include the costs for initial investigations to identify the infected herds. In some herds, this could include building handling facilities to make it
possible to tuberculin-test deer. The figures also include production losses for the
farmer during depopulation, standstill period, and repopulation of the herd, as well
as costs for cleaning and disinfection. Direct costs for the farmer caused by the disease per se, such as rejection of carcasses at meat inspection or deer dying from
TB, are not included.

Costs for trace-back and trace-forward investigations, as well as costs for the
investigation of other suspected BTB infections in farmed deer for the 7 years from
1998 to 2004, were about 1,500,000 SEK (214,600 USD). Corresponding figures
for 1991–1997 are not available. However, as all 13 BTB infected herds were
detected between 1991 and 1997, it is probable that this figure is much higher than
for the figure for 1998–2004.

Costs for the Control Program

Government subsidies to the control program, from its inception in July 1994 to
December 2004, have been 31,000,000 SEK (4,435,000 USD). This covers the
administrative costs and approximately 50% of the costs for TB testing or total
slaughter and meat inspection of the herd. The remaining costs have been covered
by the farmers themselves. Costs for necropsies are covered by other governmental funding for necropsies in food-producing animals.

Total Governmental Cost for Eradication and Control
Program

The total cost for the eradication of BTB in farmed deer until December 2004 is
not possible to calculate, as the total costs for 1991–1997 cannot be retrieved. It

can, however, be concluded that the total costs exceed 47,500,000 SEK (6,795,000 USD). Furthermore, this figure does not include costs for the government staff members who administrated the control and eradication of BTB, nor does it include costs for legal service.

As BTB infection in farmed deer has not spread to cattle, Sweden's official BTB-free status has not been affected, and there have been no additional costs for routine tuberculin testing in cattle.

Additional Costs for the Deer Farmers

As mentioned earlier, approximately 50% of the costs of the TB control in deer herds are paid by the farmers. However, in herds in which deer are tuberculin tested, owners also have to build handling facilities for deer. Furthermore, in herds in which all deer are slaughtered and meat inspected within the program, there probably are production losses during the first years of the repopulation of the herd. It can also be assumed that production losses have occurred for certain farmers as a result of the restriction of live animal movement from 1994, when only BTB-free herds with A status were allowed to sell live deer. The market for live-animal sale initially came to a standstill but has subsequently increased as the control program has progressed. At present, this has probably led to an increased income for herds with A status. Although there are no official statistics, it is judged that export of deer never has been a major issue. Therefore, losses, if any, resulting from decreased export are probably negligible.

Benefits of the Program

Apart from the major benefit of obtaining BTB-free status in all farmed deer herds, there are also some additional benefits. The implementation of the control program has increased the government's control of farmed deer herds, which is of benefit from a disease-control point of view. Furthermore, it has been reported that in herds with handling facilities for deer, the owners have more control over the production, to optimize it, and to thereby increase their economic return from deer farming.

References

1. Björkman, G. 1982. Bekómpandet av nötkreaturstuberkulosen i Sverige [The eradication of bovine tuberculosis in Sweden]. *Svensk Vet* 34:59-64. (English abstract in 17th International Symposium on the History of Veterinary Medicine, June 5–8, 1981, Helsinki, World Association for the History of Veterinary Medicine.)
2. Myers, J. A., and J. H. Steele. 1969. Bovine tuberculosis control in man and animals. St. Louis, MO: Warren H. Green.
3. Sjöland, L. 1995. Regional and country status reports. Sweden, 1968-1992. *In* C. O. Thoen and J. H. Steele (ed.), *Mycobacterium bovis* Infection in Animals and Humans. Ames: Iowa State University Press, 248-49.

4. Bölske, G., L. Englund, H. Wahlström, G. W. de Lisle, D. M. Collins, and P. S. Croston. 1995. Bovine tuberculosis in deer farms: epidemiological investigations and tracing using restriction fragment analysis. *Vet Rec* 136:414-17.
5. Wahlström, H. 2004. Bovine tuberculosis in Swedish farmed deer. Ph.D. thesis, Department of Clinical Sciences, Swedish University of Agricultural Sciences, Uppsala.
6. Szewzyk, R., S. B. Svensson, S. E. Hoffner, G Bölske, H. Wahlström, L Englund, A. Engvall, and G. Källenius. 1995. Molecular epidemiological studies of *Mycobacterium bovis* infections in man and animals in Sweden. *J Clin Microbiol* 33:3183-85.
7. Wahlström, H., T. Carpenter, J. Giesecke, M. Andersson, L. Englund, and I. Vågsholm. 2000. Herd-based monitoring for tuberculosis in extensive Swedish deer herds by culling and meat inspection rather than by intradermal tuberculin testing. *Prev Vet Med* 43:103-16.

Chapter 11

Benefit and Cost Assessment of the U.S. Bovine Tuberculosis Eradication Program

M.J. Gilsdorf, DVM, MS, E.D. Ebel, DVM, MS, and T.W. Disney, PhD

Introduction

Historically, the National Tuberculosis (TB; *Mycobacterium bovis*) eradication campaign in the United States is an economic and animal health success. The success of the past is manifest in the low occurrence of TB in U.S. cattle, bison, captive cervids, and swine today. The reduction or elimination of TB's burden is a perpetual benefit that all subsequent generations realize.

The U.S. TB eradication program has improved the welfare of consumers and producers alike. When the program began in 1917, bovine TB occurred within a substantial proportion of cattle. There can be no doubt that the TB pathogen was withdrawing value from the U.S. cattle industry at that time. This agent was also inflicting terrible consequences on humans via unpasteurized milk.

To summarize the accomplishments of the U.S. TB eradication campaign, the annual benefits and costs of the program are evaluated from its inception to 2003.

Annual Benefits

The benefit of reducing the occurrence of TB among cattle is a reduction in losses caused by the TB bacterium. Most of these losses can be assessed at the individual animal level. The total cost (reduced benefit) of TB from these productivity losses is, therefore, proportional to the prevalence of infection among all U.S. cattle.

To estimate the annual benefits, the downward trend in animal prevalence is estimated first. Next, the productivity costs associated with TB infection are estimated. Finally, these productivity costs for each year are compared to a scenario in which TB is not controlled.

The existence of TB in the United States also influences the international trade of cattle and public health. These additional economic losses are not considered in the following analysis but would increase benefits beyond what we have shown.

The international trade costs caused by TB are complex and difficult to estimate. Although the productivity losses of TB represent a direct cost to U.S. producers, international trade losses for U.S. producers represent a transfer of benefits to other countries. If the U.S. experiences a loss in trade, then another country undoubtedly benefits. Nevertheless, the existence of TB in the United States also creates inefficiencies in the world market that are corrected by control or eradication.

For example, if country A prefers to purchase cattle from country B but does not because of the existence of TB in country B, then country A may not be as prosperous or successful if they must purchase from another country other than country B. Country A hypothetically prefers country B cattle because of price or quality factors. Nevertheless, the other country experiences a benefit from country B and country A's loss. The trade benefits from the U.S. eradication program represent improvements in market efficiency and losses to countries whose cattle are preferred less than those of the United States.

Although public and animal health were synergistic motivations for the U.S. TB program, the public health benefits that were subsequently realized, especially outside of the agricultural communities, were more the result of pasteurization than of reduction in the prevalence of TB in cattle (1). Between 1901 and 1933, *M. bovis* was responsible for 158 (13%) of 1200 human cases of tuberculosis in the United States (1). Nevertheless, the progressive implementation of milk pasteurization, beginning about 1908, nearly eliminated human illnesses caused by *M. bovis*. Between 1954 and 1968, *M. bovis* was responsible for 6 (0.2%) of 2086 human cases of tuberculosis in the Unites States (1). The direct transmission of TB from cattle to humans is an important public health hazard, and as long as TB occurs among U.S. livestock, it remains a public health risk.

Prevalence Trend

Since 1917, the estimated prevalence of infected U.S. cattle has declined from about 5% to about 0.001%. Estimates of TB prevalence during the intervening years have been previously reported (2–6). Early estimates of prevalence were primarily based on individual-animal testing results. The program was focused on individual-animal testing from 1917 through 1959, and prevalence was estimated as the number of reactors detected divided by the number of cattle tested in a given year. Since 1959, TB surveillance has shifted to a much greater reliance on slaughter inspection of carcasses. Estimates of cattle prevalence since that time are commonly calculated as the number of TB-positive cattle detected among all of the cattle slaughtered in the United States for a given year.

The trend in prevalence of TB-infected cattle is downward and log-linear (Fig. 11.1). Such a pattern is consistent with a program that experiences diminishing returns. Early success is dramatic as the program more easily identifies and eliminates infected cattle. As prevalence decreases, however, its rate of decline decreases because infected cattle are more difficult to detect and eliminate. Therefore, the exponential relationship between prevalence and time in the program is expected.

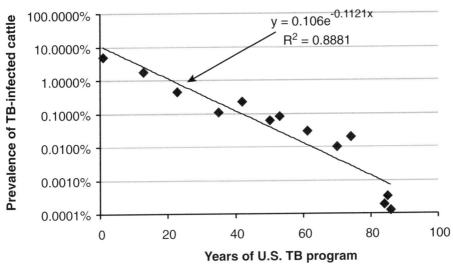

Figure 11.1.   Relationship between the prevalence of tuberculosis-infected cattle and the number of years the tuberculosis program has been operating in the United States. The data points shown are the available reported estimates of prevalence at different times in the program. The trend line was estimated using regression, and the best-fitting equation is shown (Microsoft Excel 2000 TM).

The log-linear trend illustrated in Figure 11.1 is a graphical representation of this relationship, where the *y*-axis is shown in $\log_{10}$ units.

The log-linear trend indicates that the prevalence of TB-infected cattle has decreased by 90% for each 20 years of the program. For example, between the 20th year of the program (1937) and the 40th year of the program (1957), the prevalence decreased 90%, from approximately 1% to 0.1%.

Although the trend line seems reasonably accurate through the first 40 years of the program, the estimated prevalence levels for more recent years are less consistent with this log-linear relationship. For example, the trend line consistently underestimates prevalence relative to reported prevalence during the period between the 40th (1957) and 80th (1997) years. However, recent estimates for the 84th–86th years of the program (2001–2003) suggest dramatically lower prevalence levels than the trend predicts. These recent reductions in prevalence may be directly attributable to increased vigilance in the national TB program.

Discrepancies between the data points and the trend line should not be overinterpreted, but it is interesting to note that reported prevalence exceeds the predicted prevalence for much of the time (after 1959) that slaughter surveillance has been emphasized. It is also important to note that most of the TB-infected cattle detected at slaughter for the last decade were ultimately determined to be steers that originated in Mexico. Therefore, the trend and data illustrated in Figure 11.1 are only a rough estimate of the true prevalence of infected cattle in the United States. Despite the potential inaccuracies, however, this trend in prevalence is useful for estimating the benefits that have accumulated through the efforts of the U.S. TB eradication program.

Benefits Are Foregone Costs

As the TB program progressed through the years, the benefits accruing to the Unites States were the costs not experienced because of TB prevalence, and more important, the number of infected animals was decreasing. These benefits are typically referred to as "foregone" costs.

The productivity losses from TB infection have been estimated in previous analyses (7,8). These direct losses are categorized into slaughter and on-farm losses. Slaughter losses apply to infected cattle that are condemned or retained at slaughter. On-farm losses include reduced milk production for infected dairy cattle, as well as decreased reproductive capacity and replacement costs for infected beef and dairy cattle.

To estimate slaughter losses, the methods of Kryder et al. (7) are used. Infected cattle that are slaughtered can be classified as condemned (12%), retained (45%), or neither retained or condemned (43%). The loss from a condemned carcass is essentially the purchased value of a slaughter animal. The loss from a retained carcass is some fraction of the value of a carcass. This retained carcass cost was assumed to be approximately $10 in 1970 dollars (7).

To estimate on-farm losses, a combination of previous methods is used (7,8). It is assumed that TB is responsible for a 10% decline in milk production among infected dairy cattle, a 20% reduction in calf weight, and a 5% opportunity cost from replacing infected cattle. Opportunity cost is calculated as 5% of the difference between the value of a purchased replacement animal and the value of a slaughtered animal. In other words, this estimate assumes one-quarter year of lost production in a typical 5-year productive life. These values have been calculated to be between 5% and 20% (7,8). The lower value is used in this assessment to generate conservative benefit estimates.

To measure the total annual cost of TB infection, the average cost per infected animal is calculated (Table 11.1). The average on-farm cost per infected animal per year comprises milk loss, calf loss, and replacement loss. For an average infected dairy cow, the milk cost ranges between $55.66 and $258.74 (10% × [4033–18749 pounds] × $0.14). For both dairy and beef cows, the cost of calf loss is $22.40 (20% × $112.00). The cost from early replacement is $39.86 and $24.66 (5% × [$1390–592.80] or [$1086–592.90]) for dairy and beef cows, respectively. The average on-farm cost per infected cow is further adjusted to account for culling (7). An infected cow that is culled would only accrue, on average, one-half the farm-level losses. Therefore, average on-farm cost for infected dairy cows is calculated as

$$70\% \times [\text{Total Average Cost}] + 30\% \times \left[\frac{\text{Total Average Cost}}{2} \right], \qquad (11.1)$$

where the culling fraction is 30%. This cost is similarly calculated for beef cows, except a 20% culling fraction is used.

Average slaughter cost per infected cow comprises losses from condemnation and carcass retention. The average cost from condemnation is $21.34 (30% × 12% × $592.90) per infected dairy cow and $14.23 (20% × 12% × $592.90) per infected beef cow. Retention costs are similarly calculated.

Table 11.1. Prices and production effects used to determine annual average cost of tuberculosis infection per infected cow. Prices are adapted from USDA-NASS,[1] assuming an average weight of 1200 pounds for cull cows and beef cow replacements, except that the cost of carcass retention is from Kryder et al. (7) and adjusted for inflation.

Prices (2003 dollars)	Dairy	Beef
Cull cow slaughter price	$592.80	$592.80
Replacement cow price	$1390.00	$1086.00
Milk price per lb.	$0.14	$0.00
Calf price	$112.00	$112.00
Retained carcass cost	$47.42	$47.42

[1]http://usda.mannlib.cornell.edu/reports/nassr/price/pap-bb/2004/agpr0104.txt

The total cost of TB per year is calculated as

$$P \times N_{dairy} \times [\text{Avg. cost } per \text{ infected cow}_{dairy}]$$
$$+P \times N_{beef} \times [\text{Avg. cost } per \text{ infected cow}_{beef}], \quad (11.2)$$

where P is the prevalence of TB infection and N is the number of cows. Prevalence decreases as a function of years in the program (Fig. 11.1). The number of dairy and beef cows also changes with time in the program, as does the average milk production per dairy cow (Fig. 11.2). Prevalence is held constant at about 5% between 1917 and 1921 to avoid the upward bias for these early years estimated by the equation in Figure 11.1.

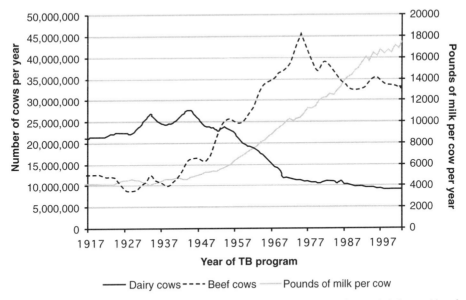

Figure 11.2. Time series information shows the pattern in numbers of dairy and beef cows, and milk production per cow, between 1917 and 2003. Beef cow data were only available back to 1920, so the 1920 inventory was assumed for 1917–1919. Similarly, milk production data were only available back to 1924, so the 1924 production level was assumed for 1917–1923. Source: USDA-NASS (http://www.nass.usda.gov:81/ipedb/).

To calculate the annual benefits of the TB eradication program, the foregone costs per year are estimated. The TB program results in a declining prevalence across time. The question that could be asked is, What would the U.S. cattle industry look like today if there had been no TB program? Experience, in the TB program in monitoring prevalence, within the United States and areas that were deficient in meeting the U.S. TB eradication program minimum standards, has shown that if the disease is left uncontrolled, it will increase to a level higher than 5%. Therefore, the number of infected animals in 1917 would remain constant, or increase, between 1917 and 2003 if there were no program. If the number of infected cattle is held constant, then the total cost estimated in 1917 (using 2003 dollars) is the point of reference for calculating the foregone costs for subsequent years of the program. In other words, the benefits experienced in year$_t$ are equal to the total cost of TB in 1917 minus the total cost of TB in year$_t$.

Stipulating that the total number of infected cows would remain constant at 1917 levels had there been no TB program, the annual benefits of the TB eradication program increase from zero in 1917 to more than $180 million by 1951 (Fig. 11.3). These benefits stabilize at nearly $190 million per year through 2003. Nevertheless, it seems more likely that the number of infected cows would increase between 1917 and 2003 if there had been no TB program. If TB occurrences increased across time, then the benefit stream shown in Figure 11.3 represents a lower-bound estimate of the actual annual benefits the United States experienced between 1917 and 2003. The benefits shown in Figure 11.3 are further reduced because the on-farm cost from replacement of infected cows is based on the 5% estimate of Bernues et al. (8) instead of the 20% estimate of Kryder et al. (7). If this 20% estimate is used, the total benefit per year stabilizes around $350 million.

The benefit from the TB eradication program might be almost $2 billion per year if the reference point for measuring foregone costs is an increasing prevalence between 1917 and 2003. To assess how TB infection might have increased from 1917, a simple Reed-Frost transmission model was constructed using the demographic data in Figure 11.2. This simple model indicates that if there is just one infective contact per year, then prevalence levels increase to, and stabilize around, 30% after 1960. One study has estimated an average of 2.2 infective contacts per year (9). At this contact rate, the prevalence stabilizes around 50%–60% by 1930 and remains at that level indefinitely. If these substantially higher prevalence levels were to apply to the benefit model we have constructed, the calculated benefits could be 5 to 10 times larger than shown in Figure 11.3.

Annual Costs

The costs of the TB eradication program comprise the cost of government personnel and equipment involved in the daily operations of the program, the costs of laboratory resources, and the cost of compensating owners for animals depopulated because of the eradication effort. On an annual basis, these costs are paid by federal and state governments. There are also producer's costs, such as labor costs in gathering and handling cattle, as well as loss in milk or meat production because of handling stress. Producer costs are difficult to estimate and are not included in this estimate. It is thought, however, that such costs represent a small fraction of the total annual cost of the eradication program.

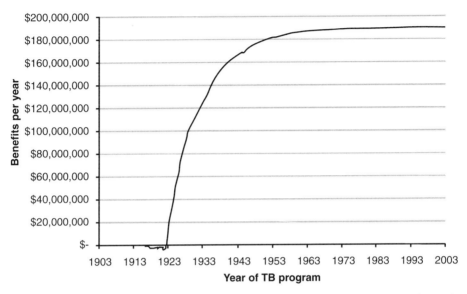

Figure 11.3. Lower-bound estimate of the benefits per year of the tuberculosis eradication program is shown.

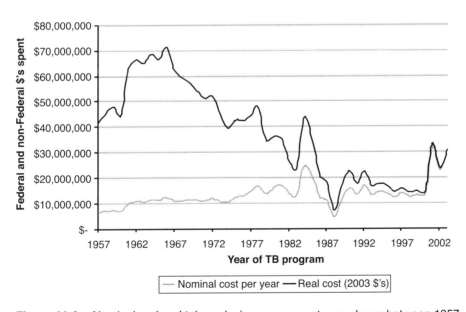

Figure 11.4. Nominal and real tuberculosis program costs are shown between 1957 and 2003. Real costs were estimated from nominal costs using the consumer price index (U.S. Department of Labor, Bureau of Labor Statistics).

Annual Government Costs

The annual TB expenditure by federal and nonfederal governments has been summarized in nominal values since 1957 (Fig. 11.4). The consumer price index is
used to estimate the annual expenditures in 2003 dollars. Although the nominal
costs per year appear to increase slightly between 1957 and 2003, the trend in real
costs appears to be generally downward. Nevertheless, these are substantial fluctu-
ations in annual costs. For example, real cost increases from just over $40 million
in 1957 to above $70 million in 1967. Although the reasons for this dramatic change
are uncertain, it is likely that there was a deemphasis in the TB program in the
mid-1950s that was corrected by the late 1960s. A reduction in TB program intensity around this time was noted by Frye (2).

Although empiric information is available between 1957 and 2003, no such evidence is available between 1917 and 1957. To estimate the early-year costs, an
exponential function was used in calculating the average cost-per-cow data (Fig.
11.5). The average cost per cow was estimated for 1957–2003 by dividing the real
program cost per year by the total inventory of cows per year. The trend in these data
is downward. Exponential predictions result in larger program costs than the linear
predictions. In keeping with the conservative approach of this analysis, the exponential relationship is used because smaller net benefits result using the exponential
prediction.

Since the TB program began, the total cost of the program has declined while
its total benefits have increased (Fig. 11.6). Total cost of the TB program is calculated for each year by multiplying the estimated average cost per cow by the total

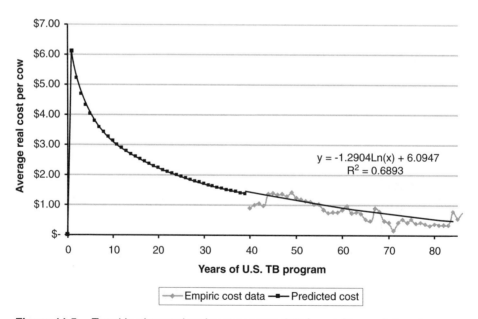

Figure 11.5. Trend in observed real cost per cow data is used to predict cost per
cow levels from 1917 to 1957 (the 40th year of the program). The trend line and its
equation are also shown.

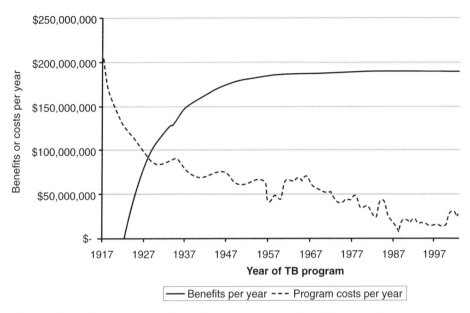

Figure 11.6. Estimated benefits and costs per year of the TB eradication program—from 1917 through 2003—are shown. Benefits and costs are conservatively estimated such that benefits represent lower-bound estimates, while costs represent upper-bound estimates.

inventory of cows in the United States. The estimated cost of the program equaled its benefit in about 1927, and after that time, benefits have steadily outpaced costs, such that in 2003 the net benefit of the TB program (i.e., Total Benefits per Year − Total Costs per Year) is about $159 million.

Present Value of Net Benefits

The net benefit for each year of the program is the difference between benefits and costs. For the first 10 years of the program, net benefits were negative. For example, in 1917 it is estimated that almost $206 million were spent without any appreciable reduction in TB. Following 1927, however, net benefits became positive as the benefits of the program began exceeding its cost (Fig. 11.6).

Net benefits experienced in the past are reinvested into other activities during subsequent years. These alternative activities reasonably gain in value with time. Therefore, the present value of the net benefits between 1917 and 2003 is calculated as

$$Total\ Net\ Benefits = \sum_{1917}^{2003} NB_t (1+i)^{2003-t}, \qquad (11.3)$$

where NB_t is the net benefit calculated for year t and is the social discount rate. This social discount rate is conservatively assumed to be 3% historically.

Despite the conservative assumptions made in the analysis, the total net benefits of the TB program are valued at $13.1 billion. In other words, the TB program has returned over $13 billion to the U.S. economy since it began. These monies were gained by controlling disease losses that otherwise would have been experienced within the cattle industry.

The true economic return of the TB program could be substantially greater than $13 billion. For example, if the Kryder et al. (7) assumption of a 20% replacement loss is used, and all other assumptions are held constant, the total net benefit of the TB program since 1917 is almost $55 billion. Modest reductions in the annual costs of the program during its early years could also substantially increase the total net benefits. Similarly, allowing for increasing numbers of infected cattle in lieu of a TB program would dramatically increase the benefits of control.

Net benefits can be reduced by decreasing TB's expected production effects on infected cattle. For example, if the percentage decline in calf value is decreased from 20% to 10%, then the present value of net benefits is reduced from $13 billion to $6.9 billion. Similarly, if the percentage decline in milk production is decreased from 10% to 5%, then the present value of net benefits is reduced to $6.2 billion.

The break-even values for the three production-effect inputs are the levels at which the present value of net benefits equals zero. These break-even values are about 0%, 1%, and 1% for the percentage decline in calf value, percent replacement loss, and percentage decline in milk production, respectively. These findings indicate that the economic valuation of the TB program is most sensitive to the assumed percentage replacement loss because this input can only be reduced from 5% to 1% before the present value of net benefits equals zero. The present value of net benefits is moderately sensitive to the percentage decline in milk production because this input must be reduced from 10% to 1% before a zero value is obtained. The percentage decline in calf value is the least sensitive input because it can be reduced from 20% to 0%, whereas the present value of net benefits remains greater than zero.

Summary

This historical analysis used available data to assess the economic benefits and costs of the U.S. TB program. More sophisticated methods, such as welfare economic methods that estimate consumer and producer surplus, might generate different estimates than derived here. Nevertheless, the essential nature of disease loss—and mitigation of disease loss—is captured in the analysis described in this report. For livestock diseases, the economic consequence of living with infection is reduced livestock performance caused by the pathogen. To combat the losses imposed by a pathogen such as TB requires a coordinated effort on the part of industry and government. This effort involves substantial investment of public funds. The true economic return of the TB program, as discussed above, is estimated to be between $13 and $55 billion.

As shown in this analysis, the U.S. TB program has been a highly beneficial campaign. Furthermore, there are additional trade benefits resulting from reduced TB occurrence that have not been included in this analysis. These trade benefits for the U.S. are potentially substantial and could be increased as the U.S. achieves eradication of bovine TB.

References

1. Banwart, G. J. 1979. Basic Food Microbiology. Westport, CT: AVI.
2. Frye, G. H. 1995. Bovine tuberculosis eradication: The Program in the United States. In *Mycobacterium bovis* Infection in Animals and Humans. Ames: Iowa State University Press, 119-130.
3. Martin, S. W., R. A. Dietrich, P. Genho, et al.. 1994. Evaluation of the cooperative state-federal bovine tuberculosis eradication program Livestock Disease Eradication, Committee on Bovine Tuberculosis, Board on Agriculture, National Research Council. Washington, DC: National Academy Press.
4. Meyer, R. and VanTiem, J. 2001. Status of surveillance for bovine TB in the United States. Proceedings of the One Hundred and Fifth Annual Meeting of the U.S. Animal Health Association, U.S. Animal Health Association, Richmond, VA, 490-500.
5. Meyer, R. 2002. Status of surveillance for bovine TB in the United States, Proceedings of the One Hundred and Sixth Annual Meeting of the U.S. Animal Health Association, U.S. Animal Health Association, Richmond, VA, 590-600.
6. Beals, T. and R. Meyer. 2003. Status of the State-Federal-Industry Cooperative Bovine Tuberculosis Program, fiscal year 2003, in Proceedings of the One Hundred and Seventh Annual Meeting of the U.S. Animal Health Association, U.S. Animal Health Association, Richmond, VA, 558-590.
7. Kryder, H. A., J. D. Roswurm, and V. C. Beal. 1970. Model—tuberculosis eradication. Hyattsville, MD: U.S. Department of Agriculture, Animal Health Division and Agricultural Research Service.
8. Bernues, A., E. Manrique, and M. T. Maza. 1997. Economic evaluation of bovine brucellosis and tuberculosis eradication programmes in a mountain area of Spain. *Prev Vet Med* 30:137-49.
9. Perez, A. M., M. P. Ward, and A. Charmandarian, and V. Ritacco. 2002, Simulation model of within-herd transmission of bovine tuberculosis in Argentine dairy herds. *Prev Vet Med* 54:361-72.

Chapter 12

The Fall and Rise of Bovine Tuberculosis in Great Britain

T. Goodchild, DVM, and R. Clifton-Hadley, DVM

Despite a steady decrease in the prevalence of bovine tuberculosis (BTB) between 1935 and 1980 (the number of cattle slaughtered annually decreased from 23,000 to less than 1000), since then there has been a many-fold increase, with 24,000 head being slaughtered annually between 2002 and 2004, of which 19,700 a year were reactors to the skin test. The role of the badger in the epidemiology of BTB was not acted on until 1975. Despite badger control program halving the incidence of BTB in cattle in 4 years, a further 18 years of control did not prevent a rise in incidence. Since 1990, the number of BTB-lesioned or BTB-infected animals has doubled every 4 years.

The cost of control has increased in parallel with the incidence of BTB because of an increasing number of routine tests and tests of restricted herds and an increase in the rates of compensation paid to farmers. The cost of research is also edging upward, with at least half being spent on work to understand the role of the badger. There is an ever-increasing urgency to develop precise methods for detecting infected animals, the ability to distinguish strains for epidemiological and pathogenesis studies, vaccines for cattle and wildlife, and cost-effective policies.

It is possible that husbandry trends have contributed to the rate of increase in BTB, including increasing herd sizes and changes in cattle genotypes. Whether these account for all of the increase in BTB incidence in the country is an unsettled question.

History of Bovine Tuberculosis in Great Britain

From the Beginning of the Eradication Program

The extent and zoonotic effect of BTB in cattle was recognized in the 1930s, when as many as 40% of cattle in Great Britain were infected (1). It led to a program of progressively skin-testing herds, slaughtering animals that reacted to the test, and accrediting herds in which the disease had been controlled. In 1960, after the slaughter of some 2.2 million cattle (Fig. 12.1), some 240,000 herds became accredited. In all years, animals other than test reactors have been slaughtered for the sake of BTB control, but these animals have been a minority. The number of cattle slaughtered annually continued to decrease until the late 1970s, stayed constant until the mid-1980s, and then commenced the present pattern of doubling every 4 years (Figs. 12.1 and 12.2).

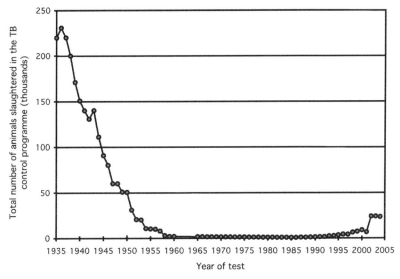

Figure 12.1. Number of animals slaughtered in the bovine tuberculosis control program, 1935–2004. Data for 1951–1964 (- - - -) were unreliable and have been interpolated; the small number removed in 2001 was a result of the Foot and Mouth Disease epidemic.

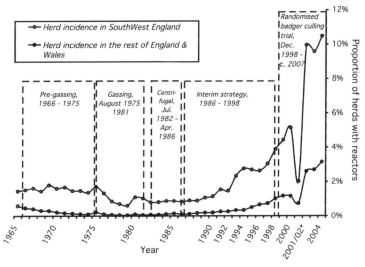

Figure 12.2. Herds with reactors as a proportion of all herds in Southwest England and the rest of England and Wales (extended from Krebs *et al.* 1997). The incidence for 2001 and 2002 has been averaged and shown as one point. Boxes surrounded by broken lines show various badger control strategies.

Pattern of Spread, 1986 to Date

The increase in number of animals slaughtered in the BTB control program in the last 20 years (Fig. 12.1) has largely resulted from the increased number of herds affected (Fig. 12.2), although an increase in the number of reactors in each incident has made a contribution (Table 12.1). The large numbers of animals slaughtered between 2001 and 2004 offer no clear evidence that the national rate of increase of new infections has been affected by the 8 months' suspension of testing in 2001. There was also no sign of a national effect of the change in compensation rate from 75% to 100% in 1997–1998.

Fronts of Prevalence that Move with Time

So-called hot spots are areas of long-established BTB prevalence in cattle in which there is a large risk of local transmission. They are sometimes referred to as endemic areas. If test-reactor cattle with typical slaughterhouse lesions or cattle from which *Mycobacterium bovis* has been isolated are assumed to have BTB, the most direct measurement is incidence (the rate that animals with BTB are detected), rather than prevalence (the proportion of live cattle infected with BTB). Starting in 1986, Fig. 12.3 maps the years in which the incidence of BTB reached 2.5 visibly lesioned (VL) bovines per 5 × 5 km square (i.e. 0.1 VL/km^2). Hot spots represent isolated clusters with expanding fronts of infection. In areas in which BTB is sporadic, isolated points tend to remain isolated, sometimes representing a potential hot spot that failed to develop (Fig. 12.3). Some patterns, such as those in Scotland and Northern England, are intermediate between the hot spot and sporadic type, indicating that longer-distance spread from the focal cluster may have occurred.

Each of the hot spots shown in Fig. 12.3 accounts for between 5% and 20% of the current incidence of BTB in Great Britain. Although each spot started as isolated clusters of incidents, there have been many more clusters than there now are hotspots. The benefit of preventing each new hot spot is potentially considerable, and there is a range of possible preventive methods from which to choose, such as preempting the initial cluster (through tracing and premovement testing) or assessing the risk that a cluster may expand and preventing this (through neighborhood testing and wildlife surveys).

Table 12.1. The total number confirmed bovine tuberculosis incidents and average numbers of reactors or slaughterhouse cases taken, in three representative years

Year	Number of Confirmed Incidents	Proportion of Confirmed Incidents with More Than One Skin-Test Reactor	Mean Number of Skin-Test Reactors or Slaughterhouse Cases per Confirmed Incident
1990	162	59.9%	4.1
2000	1128	67.5%	7.0
2003	1778	76.1%	8.0

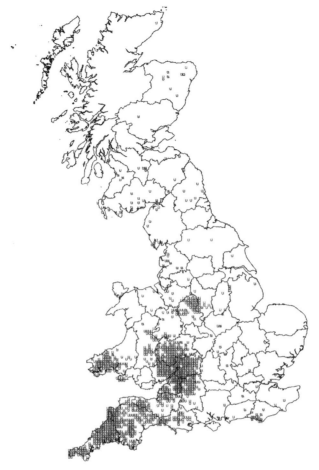

Figure 12.3. Year (during the period 1986–2004) in which the cumulative number of visibly lesioned animals first reached 0.1 per square kilometer.

Next Year's Prevalence as a Function of the Previous Year's Prevalence

The older established map squares (Fig. 12.3) are either surrounded by more recent squares (BTB hotspots) or not (sporadic BTB). The progress of BTB within a 5 × 5 km map square also depends on the history of BTB for that square. The number of VL animals in the next calendar year tends to increase with the number of VL animals already recorded in the same map square (Fig. 12.4). Where 2.0 or fewer VL animals have been recorded since 1986 in a square, it is rare for that square to have more than 1.0 VL in the following year. Where more than 4.0 VL animals have been recorded, it is 10%–50% probable that more than 1.0 VL will be found in the next year. The progress of BTB in each square may be described as autocatalytic, where a certain prevalence of BTB is necessary before epidemic local spread can be sustained.

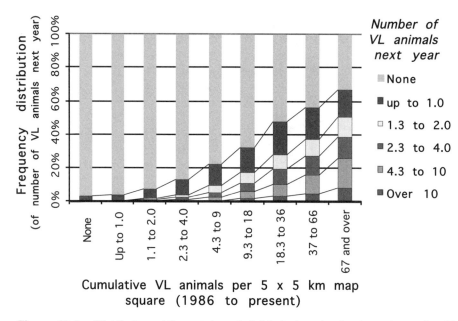

Figure 12.4. Distribution of the number of visibly lesioned animals next year for different cumulative numbers of visibly lesioned animals, for each 5 × 5 km map square. Non–visibly lesioned animals have been treated as the equivalent of 0.33 visibly lesioned animals.

The three processes—expansion of hotspots, increasing incidence in endemic areas, and appearance of potential new hotspots in sporadic areas—together describe the exponential increase in BTB in Great Britain since the mid-1980s.

The Role of Wildlife

Wildlife and the Transmission of BTB to Cattle

The role of the badger in the epidemiology of BTB in cattle was recognized by the U.K. government in the early 1970s (2). The presence of badger setts and finding badger carcasses are significant risk factors for BTB infection of cattle herds in Northern Ireland (3). Badger control program in Great Britain commenced in 1975 and were focussed on areas where a proportion of culled badgers had signs of BTB. The badger control program continued until 1998, but they were not associated with any decrease in the BTB incidence in cattle except in the first 4 years after 1975 (Fig. 12.2).

Widespread Culling of Badgers

The program of badger gassing from 1975 to 1981 coincided with a halving of the incidence of BTB in the first 4 years, followed by a small increasing trend (Fig. 12.2). Interpretation of the reduction has been contentious, as in 1975 the strain from which mammalian tuberculin was made changed from *M. tuberculosis* to *M.*

bovis AN5. This increased specificity and so reduced false-positive reactions. Nevertheless, confirmed incidence decreased substantially as well during the gassing program (4). Removal of badgers from wide areas in the Republic of Ireland with endemic badger BTB has reduced the incidence of disease in cattle, with most of the effect developing in the first 3 years (5). The Krebs Report (1) recommended a Randomized Badger Culling Trial (RBCT), 10 replicates of which commenced between 1999 and 2003. At the date of writing, however, a conclusive result for the effects of culling badgers in widespread areas (about 100 km^2) has not been published and may not be expected very much before 2007 (6).

Reactive Culling of Badgers

Following the program of gassing (1975–1981), and until 1998, badger control targeted farms on which infected cattle had been found. In centrifugal ("clean ring") culling (1982–1986), badgers were first removed from setts close to the infected herd, followed by their removal from successively distant setts until the prevalence of BTB in badgers was low. The average size of these areas was 7 km^2. The "interim strategy" (1986–1998) employed smaller culling areas, often less than 1 km^2, as only the land used by the reactor cattle was targeted. These culling strategies were associated—not necessarily causally—with the start of an exponential trend in the number of herds affected with BTB in the late 1980s (Fig. 12.2).

One of the now-suspended treatments in the RBCT, the reactive cull, had much in common with the culls of badgers around affected farms that commenced in 1982. In the autumn of 2003, the data indicated that the incidence of BTB in herds in treatment areas with reactive badger culling increased in comparison with areas without culling (7), but the statistical significance was marginal (6). It was hypothesized that this increase was attributed in part to a change in badger social behavior called perturbation. Perturbation can result in enlarged social group ranges that overlap considerably, are difficult to define (8), and could result in an increased risk of transmission of BTB between badgers that had formerly been living in separate territories.

The Role of Deer

Although an estimate of the prevalence of *M. bovis* in deer (Cervidae) is on the order of 1%, this figure derives from limited areas in the Southwest of England, where prevalence in cattle is high and prevalence in badgers can be even higher. There is variation between locations and species of deer (Central Science Laboratory, 2004, unpublished data). It is hypothesized that fallow deer are at increased risk from infection through their feeding preferences (grazing rather than browsing), and they do appear to have a prevalence that is about five times as high as that in red deer (Central Science Laboratory, 2004, unpublished data). Fallow deer also do not establish territories outside the rutting season (Deer-UK, unpublished data). As a result, fallow and other deer have larger feeding ranges than badgers. Deer may enhance the role of badgers in the geographical spread of BTB by acting as the longer-distance links in "small-world" networks (9).

Control Methods for Bovine TB

Regular Test and Cull

In Great Britain, veterinarians in the State Veterinary Service oversee the control of tuberculosis, and they normally take responsibility for disease control in herds in which BTB is suspected or demonstrated, including performing skin testing, organizing the removal of culls, and performing slaughterhouse inspection. The herds are initially detected by surveillance skin tests generally performed by a network of private veterinary surgeons or by routine veterinarian-supervised inspection of carcasses and offal from apparently healthy herds. The State Veterinary Service is organized into 24 divisional offices (Fig. 12.5), each of which is responsible for the control of notifiable diseases in around a third of a million cattle.

Interpretation of Test Results

The single intradermal comparative cervical tuberculin test measures 72-hour hypersensitivity reactions to two antigens injected into the dermis of the neck. The antigens used in the British Isles are proteins (tuberculins, also known a purified protein derivative) secreted by cultures of *M. bovis* (strain AN5, 100 μg) and of *Mycobacterium avium* (50 μg). The test compares the responses to the two tuberculins to increase discrimination between sensitization to BTB antigens and sensitization to other mycobacteria (specificity). It assumes that infection with *M. bovis* promotes a larger response to *M. bovis* tuberculin than to *M. avium* tuberculin, and that infections with other types of mycobacteria promote the reverse relationship (10). This assumption is a statistical one (Fig. 12.6) and is to some extent flawed, in that the hypersensitivity response to avian tuberculin in the field equalled or exceeded the response to bovine tuberculin in 5 of 58 animals infected with BTB (12). This fact was commented on by Morrison et al. (13) and has been observed

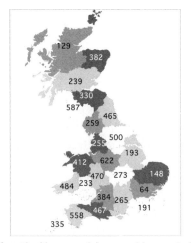

Figure 12.5. Number of cattle (thousands) served by each Animal Health Divisional Office. Divisions are contrasted by shading. Great Britain, mid-2004.

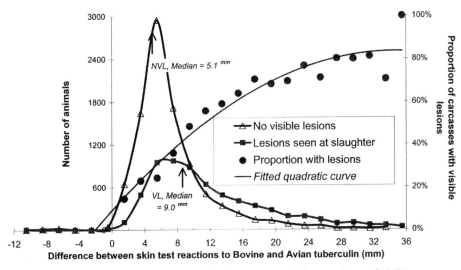

Figure 12.6. Frequency distribution of skin-test results for numbers of visibly lesioned and non–visibly lesioned carcasses, and the ratio between the two. Disclosing tests, 2002 and 2003; data are truncated where animals were not slaughtered.

on a wide scale in the national database. It is a main reason for the single intradermal comparative cervical tuberculin test being recommended as a herd screening test rather than a check test for individual animals.

Intervals between Routine Tests

Routine skin testing in Great Britain follows European Union guidelines (14), varying in frequency according to risk of infection. In the year ending 2004, about 26% of cattle were tested yearly, 13% in alternate years, and 61% at 3- or 4-year intervals. There has been a rapid annual increase in the number of herds tested annually, most of which were formerly tested in alternate years (Table 12.2). The distribution of testing intervals at the time of writing is shown in Figure 12.7.

The effectiveness of the testing intervals can be estimated indirectly. One of the most damaging aspects to farming of a BTB incident is its duration (15). The testing interval did not significantly affect the proportion of herds in which the duration of restriction was longer than 200 days (Table 12.3) or the duration of movement restrictions (except in 1990, when yearly testing was unable to keep duration in check). As the years progressed, the proportion of incidents that were long, their average duration, and the variability of the duration increased. One may conclude that the testing intervals, together with other measures, have distributed testing resources efficiently. As a result, farms are not disproportionately burdened by the duration of restrictions under any particular testing frequency.

The proportion of confirmed incidents with more than one reactor may be about 20 percentage units larger in yearly tested incidents than in 4-yearly tested incidents; differences were highly significant. The average number of reactors per confirmed incident has doubled over 13 years, but it has not steadily varied with testing

Table 12.2. Number of herds and cattle in parishes, with different testing intervals and changes with time

Parish Testing Interval	Herds (thousands)					Cattle (millions)			
	1990	2000	Annual Increase[a]	Autumn 2004		1990	2000	Annual increase[a]	Autumn 2004
1 year	7.5	11.3	+4.1%	22.8		0.48	0.98	+7.1%	2.16
2 years	29.2	9.0	$-411.7%	12.7		2.01	0.76	−9.7%	1.08
3 or 4 years	110.5	86.9	−2.4%	57.5		7.37	7.12	−0.4%	5.04
All GB	147.2	107.2	−3.2%	93.1		9.86	8.85	−1.1%	8.27

[a]Exponential rate of increase between 1990 and 2000.

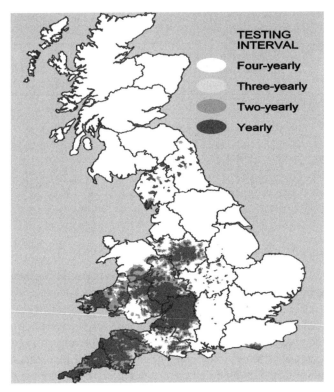

Figure 12.7. Testing intervals in force in Great Britain at the end of 2004.

interval in any of the years (Table 12.4). This, again, is evidence that the distribution of effort between testing intervals is broadly appropriate. Recently (16), there has been a change in the procedure for deciding testing intervals for each parish, but this must be seen as a precautionary response to the predicted spread of BTB (Table 12.3), rather than retrospectively reflecting the geographical pattern of BTB.

Table 12.3. Distribution of the lengths of time that confirmed incidents ending in one of 3 years remained under restriction, by testing interval in force at the end of the incident

Testing Interval	Percentage of Incidents Restricted for Longer than 200 Days			Length of Time under Restriction, Days (with standard deviation)		
	1990	2000	2003	1990	2000	2003
Yearly	14.3%	41.8%	63.8%	226 (108)	198 (92)	264 (172)
Two yearly	8.0%	34.2%	59.1%	115 (46)	158 (50)	230 (104)
Three yearly	0.0%	27.3%	66.7%	137 (49)	200 (100)	274 (177)
Four yearly	49.4%	37.5%	58.1%	149 (51)	213 (112)	289 (177)
All GB	28.2%	39.7%	62.1%	179 (95)	208 (107)	282 (176)

The herds have been classified by their testing intervals at the time of restriction.

Table 12.4. Total number of reactors taken in each confirmed incident: percentage distribution by testing interval

Testing Interval	Percentage of Incidents with More Than One Reactor[a]			Incidents with More (with standard deviation)		
	1990	2000	2003	1990	2000	2003
Yearly	40.7%	60.0%	65.5%	4.4 (10.6)	7.0 (12.3)	8.2 (12.1)
Two yearly	34.1%	47.7%	59.2%	3.8 (4.6)	7.7 (18.6)	7.3 (10.4)
Three yearly	34.0%	40.9%	56.5%	4.0 (5.3)	3.5 (6.4)	10.5 (12.7)
Four yearly	12.5%	36.2%	43.8%	1.0 (—)	6.8 (19.9)	7.9 (13.2)
All GB	35.8%	52.5%	60.1%	4.1 (8.0)	7.0 (14.5)	8.0 (12.0)

[a]As a percentage of all confirmed incidents.

Routine Slaughterhouse Inspection

Another monitor of the efficiency of testing intervals is the proportion of confirmed incidents that were not detected at routine herd testing but were disclosed when animals with lesions were slaughtered for reasons other than BTB control. Because cattle can be infected with BTB at any time during the intertest period, the longer this period, the greater proportion of cattle that could be missed in routine testing, even if the testing was highly efficient. The proportion of incidents first disclosed at slaughterhouse inspection would be expected to increase with the period of time between tests; it may not be a direct proportion, as it takes on average about 5 months for a reactor to progress to infectiousness (17). However, the testing interval for the parish does not apply to some herds, such as some beef fattening herds (not routinely tested) and herds that retail their own milk (tested every year). In actual fact, the proportion of confirmed incidents disclosed at slaughterhouse inspection rather than skin testing conforms closely to the parish testing interval (Fig. 12.8).

Herd Characteristics and TB

Several phenomena have occurred simultaneously with the rise in BTB. A causal relationship cannot be inferred, but in some cases the association is statistically significant and causality is theoretically possible.

Herd Size and Incident Duration

The incident duration almost doubles between a herd size of 1–20 cattle and a size of more than 350 animals (Table 12.5).

Herd Size and Herd Type

Although there are large differences between herd types in the average incidence of BTB, these can be explained by differences in herd size distributions (Table 12.6).

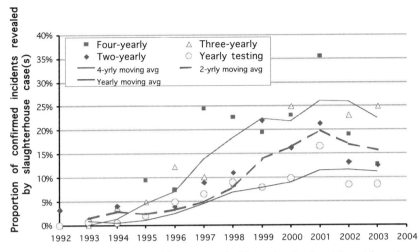

Figure 12.8. Confirmed incidents revealed by animals slaughtered from herds not suspected as being infected, as a proportion of the total number of incidents for each parish testing interval.

Table 12.5. Distribution of the lengths of time that confirmed incidents ending in 2003 have been under movement restriction, by herd size

Herd Size	Mean Duration, Days (with standard deviation)	Proportion Longer Than 200 Days
1–20	200 (95)	38%
21–50	228 (122)	48%
51–100	240 (139)	55%
101–350	294 (177)	65%
Over 350	360 (220)	78%
All herds	281.7 (176.0)	62.0%

Table 12.6. Number of confirmed incidents in three types of herd according to herd size categories in the year 2003

| Herd Size Category | Herd Type | | |
	Beef	Dairy	Other
1–20	0.3%	0.8%	0.3%
21–50	1.1%	0.9%	1.0%
51–100	2.2%	1.8%	1.8%
101–350	3.6%	4.0%	4.2%
Over 350	5.0%	7.0%	7.2%
Mean for herd type	1.43%	3.31%	1.09%
Mean for GB		1.78%	

Table 12.7. Number of confirmed bovine tuberculosis incidents per 100 herds in 2003, where herd size, testing interval, and herd type were adjusted for the other two factors by means of logistic regression

Herd Size[a] (adjusted for testing interval and herd type)	Confirmed Bovine Tuberculosis Incidents per 100 Herds (and standard error)	Testing Interval (adjusted for herd size and type)	Tuberculosis Incidents per 100 Herds (and standard error)	Confirmed Bovine Type of Herd (adjusted for herd size and testing interval)	Confirmed Bovine Tuberculosis Incidents per 100 herds (and standard error)
1–20	0.3% (0.04%)	Four yearly	0.3% (0.02%)	Beef	1.8% (0.06%)
21–50	1.1% (0.84%)	Three yearly	1.5% (0.34%)	Dairy	1.6% (0.06%)
51–100	2.0% (0.11%)	Two yearly	3.2% (0.17%)	Other	1.8% (0.15%)
101–350	3.8% (0.13%)	Yearly	8.3% (0.23%)		
Over 350	6.7% (0.41%)				

VetNet data (acknowledgments: Robin Sayers, VLA, 2004).
[a]The numbers of herds in each size group (thousands) were 23.0, 14.2, 14.9, 25.3, and 3.6.

Herd Size, Testing Interval, and Herd Type

Both herd size and testing interval affected the incidence of BTB (Table 12.7).

Association with Previous TB History

From 2000, some herds have shown recurrence of BTB as much as three times in 3 years (Table 12.8).

Number of Reactors and Testing Interval

The frequency distribution of the number of reactors is similar, whatever the parish testing interval. Large numbers of reactors are possible in any testing interval in all three time periods studied (Figure 12.9).

Table 12.8. History of confirmed bovine tuberculosis in the previous 3 years of herds having a confirmed incident in 1990, 2000, or 2003

Year	Number of Confirmed Incidents in the Year	Number of Confirmed Incidents in the Previous 36 Months, %			
		None	One	Two	Three
1990	162	94.4%	5.6%	0.0%	0.0%
2000	1128	75.5%	20.7%	3.3%	0.5%
2003	1777	76.8%	19.7%	3.3%	0.2%

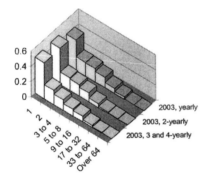

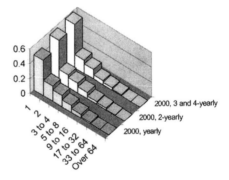

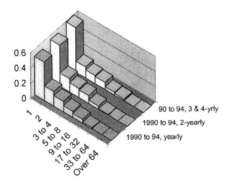

Figure 12.9. Frequency distribution of numbers of reactors and slaughterhouse cases in the disclosing tests of confirmed incidents in 2003 (top left), 2000 (top right), and 1990–1994 (bottom left).

Table 12.9. Average annual costs of the bovine tuberculosis control program in Great Britain, 1996–2003 (millions of pounds)

	Average Costs in 1996–2000	Costs in 2001	Average Costs in 2002 and 2003	Percentages of Total, 2002 and 2003
Tuberculin testing by PVS[a]	6.98	3.57	11.92	14.7%
Net compensation[b]	3.47	9.24	32.75	40.4%
Net compensation per animal culled (GBP)[c]	516	1,367	1,358	
SVS veterinary and administrative staff costs[d]	5.60	1.88	17.87	22.0%
Tuberculin production and laboratory diagnosis[e]	2.14	3.67	4.70	5.8%
Badger control and RBCT[f]	3.20	6.00	6.87	8.5%
Other research[g]	3.05	6.11	6.95	8.6%
Total	24.45	30.48	81.05	100.0%

Source: MAFF (1999) and J. Montague (personal communication).

[a]The cost of paying private veterinary surgeons (PVS) to carry out routine testing. As average intervals between tests decrease, the number of animals routinely tested tends to increase.

[b]After compulsory slaughter (including Reactor, slaughtered Inconclusive Reactor, and Contact animals), but not including the salvage obtained from sale of parts of the carcasses deemed to be fit for human consumption.

[c]The salvage value is passed on to the farmer, who will thereby receive an average of GBP 250 more than this figure.

[d]Staff costs are those for arranging, monitoring, recording, and assessing tests, as well as conducting investigations of incident herds, veterinary advice, and administration of BTB policy.

[e]Provided by the Veterinary Laboratories Agency.

[f]Badger removal was part of the bovine tuberculosis control policy before 1998. Thereafter, it was almost entirely confined to a research project, the Randomised Badger Culling Trial (RBCT).

[g]All MAFF-funded research on bovine tuberculosis in cattle and badgers other than the RBCT.

Cost of Control Methods

BTB control legislation in Great Britain intends for the state to bear the costs, through providing a testing and implementation service and through compensation payments to farmers for each animal removed. The actual costs of the control program are incurred for each herd, for each animal tested, and for each animal culled. The unit costs (per herd, animal, or cull) vary by production system, season of the year, and to some extent amount of pedigree breeding effort expended on herds (15,17). Because the costs not borne directly by the state are paid to farmers through a compensation system that depends solely on valuations of animals culled, it is almost impossible for each and every farmer to receive accurate compensation for all components of costs (18).

In the late 1990s, the government's net disbursement of compensation to farmers was about one-seventh of the total cost to government of BTB control; the absolute amount increased about tenfold after the foot-and-mouth disease epidemic of 2001 (Table 12.9). In the late 1990s, by far the largest cost was that of the State Veterinary Service and their veterinarian subcontractors—over 50% of the total—but since the epidemic of foot-and-mouth disease, this cost has been overtaken by the cost of compensation. Laboratory costs and badger control and research, being 10%–13% of the total cost in the late 1990s, have now doubled in absolute cost but are a smaller proportion of the total. Badger control (or the RBCT) has cost about the same as non-RBCT research in all years.

Conclusions

In response to the increasing incidence of TB, Defra developed a 5-point plan incorporating the recommendations of the Krebs Review (1). More recently, a consultation process has been undertaken by Defra as a preliminary step toward a new bovine TB control strategy for Great Britain (16). It is to be hoped that this process, combined with the results from the extensive research program now in place in Great Britain and other countries, will be able to reverse the TB trends of the last 20 years.

References

1. Krebs, J. R., R. Anderson, T. Clutton-Brock, I. Morrison, D. Young, and C. Donnelly. 1997. *Bovine Tuberculosis in Cattle and Badgers.* Report to the Rt. Hon. Dr. Jack Cunningham. MAFF publications PB 3423, London.
2. McInerney, J. P. 1986. Bovine tuberculosis and badgers—technical, economic and political aspects of a disease control programme. *J Agric Soc Univ College Wales* 67:136-67.
3. Denny, G. O. and J. W. Wilesmith. 1999. Bovine tuberculosis in Northern Ireland: a case-control study of herd risk factors. *Vet Rec* 144:305-10.
4. Clifton-Hadley, R. S., J. W. Wilesmith, M. S. Richards, P. Upton, and S. Johnston. 1995. The occurrence of *Mycobacterium bovis* infection in and around an area subject to extensive badger (*Meles meles*) control. *Epidemiol Infect* 114:179-93.

5. Griffin, J. M. 2000. A field trial to assess the impact of badger removal on tuberculosis levels in cattle in four geographical areas in Ireland. Paper presented at the International Conference on *Mycobacterium bovis*, Cambridge, August 2000.

6. Godfrey, H. C. J., R. N. Curnow, C. Dye, D. Pfeiffer, W. J. Sutherland, and M. E. J. Woolhouse. 2004. Independent scientific review of the Randomised Badger Culling Trial and associated epidemiological research. Report to Mr. Ben Bradshaw, MP, March 4, 2004. Available at: http://defraweb/science/publications/2004/GodfreyReport_Bovine TBEpidemiology.pdf.

7. Donnelly, C. A., R. Woodroffe, D. R. Cox, J. Bourne, G. Gettinby, A. M. Le Fevre, J. P. McInerney, and W. I. Morrison. 2003. Impact of localized badger culling on tuberculosis incidence in British cattle. *Nature* 426:834-37.

8. Tuyttens, F. A. M., R. J. Delahay, D. W. MacDonald, C. L. Cheeseman, B. Long, and C. A. Donnelly. 2000. Spatial perturbation caused by a badger (*Meles meles*) culling operation: implications for the function of territoriality and the control of bovine tuberculosis (*Mycobacterium bovis*). *J Anim Ecol* 69:815-28.

10. Watts, D. J. and S. H. Strogatz. 1998. Collective dynamics of "small-world" networks. *Nature* 393:440-42.

11. Lesslie, I. W. and C. N. Hebert. 1975. Comparison of the specificity of human and bovine tuberculin PPD for testing cattle. 3. National trial in Great Britain. *Vet Rec* 96:338-341.

12. Morrison, W. I., F. J. Bourne, D. R. Cox, C. A. Donnelly, G., J. P. McInerney, and R. Woodroffe. 2000. Pathogenesis and diagnosis of infections with *Mycobacterium bovis* in cattle. *Vet Rec* 146:236-42.

13. European Economic Community. 1964. Council Directive of 26 June 1964 on animal health problems affecting intra-community trade in bovine animals and swine (64/432/ EEC, as amended). Available at:
http://europa.eu.int/eur-lex/en/consleg/main/1964/en_1964L0432_index.html.

14. Temple, M. and S. M. Tuer. 2000. The cost at farm level of consequential losses from tuberculosis control measures. TB Forum Paper 34. Bovine TB and Zoonoses Division, MAFF, London. Available at:
http://www.defra.gov.uk/animalh/tb/forum/papers/tbf34.pdf.

15. Department for Environment, Food and Rural Affairs. 2004. *Preparing for a new GB strategy on bovine tuberculosis*. PB9066. London: Nobel House, Department for Environment, Food and Rural Affairs.

16. Barlow, N. D., J. M. Kean, G. Hickling, P. G. Livingstone and A. B. Robson. 1997. A simulation model for the spread of bovine tuberculosis within New Zealand cattle herds. *Prev Vet Med* 32:57-75.

17. Bennett, R. M. and R. Cooke. 2004. Assessment of the economic impacts of TB and alternative control policies (SE3112) final report. Defra Science Directorate, London. Available at:
http://defraweb/science/project_data/DocumentLibrary/SE3112/SE3112_1428_FRP.doc.

Chapter 13

Economic Significance of Bovine Tuberculosis in Italy and Effect of *M. bovis* Infection in Wild Swine

A. Dondo, DVM, E. Ferroglio, DVM, PhD, M. Goria, Dr of Sci, G. Moda, DVM, L. Ruocco, DVM, and P. Vignetta, DVM

Bovine Tuberculosis Eradication Plans in Italy

In Italy, measures against bovine tuberculosis (TB) were enforced for the first time in 1954, with compulsory slaughtering of bovines showing clinical evidence of TB. Eradication plans on a voluntary basis took place in 1964. Since 1977, the eradication scheme has been made compulsory in every breeding herd with the exception of specialized and separated fattening units. Compared with other European countries, this program indicates a medium delay of 12 years, which was one of the reasons for the higher TB prevalence in the years following 1977 (Tables 13.1 and 13.2) (1).

Nevertheless, during the years of the required compulsory control, and particularly after the reform law that enhanced the veterinary public health services was passed in 1978, some improvements were obtained. Since 1995, a more severe regulation, in accordance with the European Community requirements, has made the

Table 13.1. Tuberculosis eradication plans in different European countries

Country	U.K.	France	Italy
Compulsory slaughtering of bovines with clinical tuberculosis	1925	1933	1954
Voluntary slaughtering of tuberculosis reactors	1950	1954	1964
Compulsory slaughtering of tuberculosis reactors all over the country	Before 1960	1965	1977

Table 13.2 Tuberculosis annual herd prevalence in different European countries (1961–1978)

Country	1961	1970	1978
U.K.	0.16	0.045	0.019
France	2.5	0.25	0.26
Italy	13.7	3.87	1.01

eradication scheme more effective. The main measures adopted to strengthen the organization of the plan were the following:

- Programs on a 3-year basis
- Better identification of premises and bovines
- Requirements for introducing animals in fattening herds and specific surveillance programs
- Summer grazing limited to officially free herds
- Tracing back of TB visible lesions at slaughter
- Epidemiological investigation in outbreaks
- TB test in newly introduced cattle
- Periodical controls on dealers
- Stamping out in highly infected premises
- No compensation or public contribution to breeders that do not cooperate in controls
- Controls against illegal antitubercular drugs and frauds.

From 1995 to 2001, the annual herd prevalence dropped from 1.31% to 0.63%. In the same time, the percentage of TB reactors decreased from 0.31% to 0.16% (Fig. 13.1).

The Italian eradication scheme includes an annual single intradermal test with bovine PPD injection in the medial third region of the neck of every bovine aged more than 6 weeks, lower frequencies in free areas, a higher frequency of tests in infected premises (6–8 weeks interval), and slaughtering of TB reactors within 30 days with partial governmental compensation of the value of the animal.

Diagnosis is performed by official veterinarians of the Local Veterinary Units belonging to the National Health System, and the prescriptive measures are adopted forcibly by the municipality.

Since 1996, in some still seriously infected herds and areas of northern Italy (Piemonte), the gamma interferon assay, properly adapted and validated, was successfully used as a complementary test, receiving the final approval of the Commission of the European Community in 2002 (EU Reg. 8/7/2002 N.1226/2002) (2).

In 2003, the herd national prevalence of the disease was 0.98%, but it has to be pointed out that the value is mainly a result of the exceptionally widespread presence of the disease in Sicilia (5.94%). On a total number of 4,775,000 cattle submitted to periodical controls, 6573 were found to be positive, half of them in Sicilia.

Apart from bovines, TB is diagnosed rarely in goats, which are raised in strict contact with infected bovines.

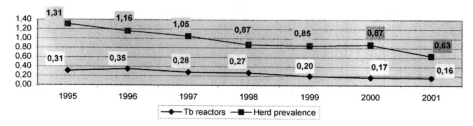

Figure 13.1   Annual tuberculosis prevalence in Italy (years 1995–2001).

TB seems to have a low impact also in Italian buffalos, which are mainly bred in Lazio and Campania: In the last year, out of 319,000 buffalo, only 109 were positive to tuberculinization.

Thanks to the progresses made, seven provinces in northern and central Italy have had official recognition of their free status from the European community. This requires an uninterrupted period of 6 years with a prevalence of 0.1% infected herds and with 99.9% officially free herds. The qualification is not granted if the rate of herds controlled by tuberculinization is less than 100%.

Mycobacterium bovis Infection in Wild Boar

Mycobacteriosis in wild boar is caused both by *Mycobacterium tuberculosis* and by *Mycobacterium avium* complex.

Mycobacterium bovis was reported in wild boar (*Sus scrofa*) for the first time in Germany in the 1930s, and it has been lately found in many European countries, in North America, and in Oceania. The vast majority of cases refer to sporadic cases or situations with low prevalence in wild boar or feral pig populations. Reports rarely refer to a high prevalence of infection in free-ranging wild boar or feral pig populations. In northwest Australia, prevalence dropped from 31% in the 1960s to 4.9% in the 1980s and to a mere 0.25% in the 1990s (3,4). This decrease was a result of the reduction of infection in buffaloes, which are considered the source of infection in the feral pig populations (4). The same reduction occurred in California in the 1960s, when after the restocking of cattle herds with TB-free animals, TB disappeared from feral pigs. In New Zealand, the infection is reported from free-ranging feral pigs, but these animals are considered as dead-end hosts that contract the infection scavenging infected carcasses of possums (6).

In Italy, a focus of TB was determined in the late 1990s to be wild boars from the Liguria region. Prevalence was high: Up to 12% of wild boars presented lesions in mandibular lymph nodes, but only 4.5% of animals tested positive at the *Mycobacterium tuberculosis* complex probe.

Lesions are localized in the head lymph nodes, and TB nodules in lymph nodes seem to evolve from the necrotic to the fibronecrotic-calcified form with the "sterilization" of nodules (7).

Nodules are never open, so that wild boars do not eliminate *M. bovis* in the environment, as happens with other wild reservoirs of infection such as possums or badgers. Another confirmation of the self-limiting process of TB infection in wild boar lymph nodes arises from the fact that although the prevalence of lesions increases significantly with the wild boar's age, positive results upon DNA probing actually decrease with the animal's age. In the area under consideration, TB in domestic cattle was still high, and it is possible that wild boars of the area became infected by scavenging infected cattle carcasses or during rooting by ingestion of *M. bovis* present in the soil (8).

Wild boars that are reported to be infected by *M. bovis* show lesions at necroscopy. Very rarely, *M. bovis* isolation occurs from wild boar carcasses with no lesion at necroscopy, as happens in other animal species (i.e. in cattle). On contrast, the presence of lesions is not sufficient to diagnose the infection correctly: diagnosis must be confirmed by a panel of laboratory tests, including bacteriological and histopathological techniques and, nowadays, with the aid of biomolecular methods. The implementation of molecular assays in addition to the traditional microbiological techniques has permitted the realization of diagnostic protocols to accelerate the demonstration of the agent, the typing of isolated strains, and the characterization of their genome. As well as in TB control strategies for domestic animals, the implementation of diagnostic tests has improved the knowledge about the role of wild boar in the epidemiology of TB infections, allowing the enhancement of the regional surveillance scheme on wildlife diseases as realized in Piemonte, in areas close to the outbreak in the Liguria Region (7).

Diagnosis of Mycobacteriosis in Wild Boar

A diagnostic protocol was formulated by the aid of research projects aimed to evaluate its efficacy by the comparison and the exchange of experience among several centers involved in mycobacterial disease diagnosis in both the human and animal fields. To apply the diagnostic protocol correctly, lymph nodes or organs with suspected lesions are cleaned from connective and adipose tissue, and the specimens are homogenized and then submitted to decontamination procedures, mainly based on alkali (2%–4% NaOH) and hexadecylpyridinium chloride (1.5% HPC). Subsequently, each aliquot is seeded in selective culture media according to the OIE Manual of Diagnostic Test and Vaccines for Terrestrial Animals, 5th edition (2004). Slopes are examined weekly for either occurring gross contamination or Ziehl-Neelsen staining of suspected grown colonies.

Usually, mycobacteria culture from wild boar samples require a longer incubation time (at least 90–120 days), as often the growth is very slow.

Every isolated strain must be submitted to identification procedures to determine its cultural and biochemical properties, together with molecular characterization.

Molecular methods can also be applied to recognize the presence of mycobacteria DNA directly in tissue specimens from domestic and wild animals as well as to identify and characterize, by the genomic way, mycobacteria previously isolated by selective culture media.

Mycobacteria identification is thus obtained by the traditional microbiological assays (biochemical profile) and by genomic analysis of specific gene targets (mostly IS*6110* genes for *M. tuberculosis* complex, Oxy-R analysis, spoligotyping for DR locus polymorphism analysis, Variable Number of Tandem Repeats/VNTR polymorphism analysis, etc.). Moreover, molecular DNA analysis could also provide intraspecific characterization of strains, which represents a very helpful tool to enrich epidemiological investigations with objective and proofing information.

Concerning mycobacteriosis etiology, it is important to report that many studies are still ongoing in wild boar to detect mycobacteria that could infect or lodge in. Data collected during the last 5 years (2000/04) reported that mycobacteria other than *M. bovis* are often isolated from wild boar, and sometimes they show unusual biochemical and molecular profiles (Table 13.3).

Table 13.3 Mycobacteria detection in wild boar specimens during the period 2000–2004 in Northwestern Italy

Mycobacteria bovis	Mycobacteria tuberculosis Complex Strains of Uncertain Classification	M. avium	Mycobacterium spp	Negative Samples	Total Tested Samples
10	37	8	74	532	661

By means of molecular techniques, DNA from TB complex mycobacteria could be detected, particularly from tissue samples (lymph nodes, organs) of hunted wild boars in particular restricted geographic areas in northwestern Italy. The direct detection by heminested polymerase chain reaction technique recognizes the presence of the IS*6110* gene, which represents a specific target gene of the TB complex mycobacteria genome. This target gene, widely investigated by restriction fragment length polymorphism analysis, was usually found in a high number of copies (10–12) in *M. tuberculosis* strains and in a very low number of copies (one to two) in *M. bovis* strains.

In domestic animal species, the detection of IS*6110* by polymerase chain reaction analysis is very often confirmed by the isolation of *M. bovis* strains on selective culture media. On the contrary, in wild boars, a very high frequency is registered in IS*6110* polymerase chain reaction detection, followed only in a few cases with isolation of TB complex mycobacteria strains. These strains are commonly very slow growers, and they show a biochemical profile not sufficiently defined to allow the proper attribution to specific species identification for *M. tuberculosis* or *M. bovis*. In the light of most well-established tests applied for the characterization of TB complex, the resulting genomic profile does not allow a definite identification of a species: it still remains an open, rising question.

The analysis of published reports and the results of experiences in Italy seem to indicate that wild boars, or the feral pig population, are not an effective reservoir of *M. bovis*. The role of wild boars appears, rather, to be that of a sentry species that, because of its omnivorous feeding habit, can contract *M. bovis* from infected soil during rooting or, in particular circumstances unusual in our country, by scavenging infected carcasses.

Evidence of *M. bovis* Cattle-to-Human Transmission

One of the main concerns about the presence of *M. bovis* in domestic animals and wildlife is its capability to be transmitted to man.

Despite the well-known idea that *M. bovis* is able to induce a disease in humans that is indistinguishable with regard to clinical findings, lesions, and evolution to that caused by *M. tuberculosis*, human infections caused by *M. bovis* are rarely reported (9). Specimens from TB patients are not submitted to identification of the causal agent, and as a consequence, TB caused by *M. bovis* is detected in humans only by specifically dedicated surveillance systems (10).

Therefore, estimation of the losses caused by animal-to-man transmission is always difficult. However, in areas with a high prevalence of the disease, TB has been repeatedly diagnosed in owners of herds with a history of bovine TB. The application of molecular techniques of strain typing has recently confirmed three cases in Piemonte, bringing to evidence the suspicion that bovine TB is an occupational disease that is not rare, and that is already demonstrated in veterinarians working in the same area (11).

Other Losses Resulting from Bovine TB

Apart from the serious consequences of the disease in humans, of great relevance with regard to food safety and public health, bovine TB is responsible for a series of damages and losses resulting from both the direct effects of the disease (morbidity and diminution of the productivity of infected animals, mortality, and reduction of the productive life span) and the regulatory restrictions on infected herds.

With the actual prevalence rates, most of the extra expenses resulting from the presence of TB in domestic animals falls more on the breeding system than on the food industry. According to the current national and European Union law, cattle positive to the tuberculin test are slaughtered separately and submitted to post-mortem examination. Carcasses are not ordinarily destroyed and are declared fit for consumption with the same rules as other slaughtered animals. The entire carcass is considered unfit for human consumption only in the case of generalized or disseminated TB: localized lesions only require the discharge of the lesioned offal. The major losses in meat production are caused by the anticipated elimination of infected cattle suffered by the breeder. However, the reduced income for the meat industry is usually less important.

Second, the milk of infected animals has to be destroyed. However, milk coming from negative heads of an infected herd cannot be destined directly to consumers (it requires preliminary pasteurization), nor is it allowed in raw-milk productions and high-quality products.

The residue rates of tubercular infection are still a major concern for the breeding system. The risk of reinfections in officially free herds is, in theory, a result of infected bovine herds and wildlife reservoirs. The main source of risk is actually represented by the vicious circle set up in case of persistence of the disease even in a small percentage of bovine herds. A few infected herds that are undetected because of fraud or that are lacking or have low-frequency controls can cause more damage than a higher number of promptly detected infected herds (1).

Infected herds are severely restricted, and selling bovines from these herds is not allowed, except for slaughter. This restriction impedes or hampers the full development of the breeding industry in still-infected areas, reducing the potentiality in national and international trade of local breeds and of Italian cattle.

The evidence indicating the minor importance of the wild boar as reservoir, the gradual elimination of TB from bovines, and cobred goats suggests that, at least for some years after eradication in domestic species, active surveillance plans on wildlife should be maintained (11).

References

1. Piedmont Regional Working Group on Bovine Tuberculosis. 1991. Eradicazione della tubercolosi bovina: aspetti attuali di una battaglia non ancora conclusa. *Ed. Regione Piemonte. Torino. 15-16.*

2. Dondo, A., M. Goria, G. Moda, L. Cesano, A. Garanzini, M. Giammarino, G. Minola, E. Morioni, G. Porta, P. Banchio, and G. Marmo. 1996. La prova del gamma interferone per la diagnosi della tubercolosi bovina: determinazione della sensibilità e della specificità in prove di campo. *Med Vet Prev* 13:14-18.

3. Corner, L. A., R. H. Barrett, A. W. D. Lepper, V. Lewis, and C. W. Pearson. 1981. A survey of mycobacteriosis of feral pigs in the Northern Territory. *Aust Vet J* 57:537-42.

4. McInerney, J., K. J. Small, and P. Caley. 1995. Prevalence of Mycobacterium bovis infection in feral pigs in the Northern Territory. *Aust Vet J* 72:448-51.

5. Paterson, B. M. and R. S. Morris. 1995. Interactions between beef and simulated tuberculous possums on pasture. *N Z Vet J* 43:289-93.

6. Bollo, E., E. Ferroglio, V. Dini, W. Mignone, B. Biolatti, and L. Rossi. 2000. Detection of *Mycobacterium tuberculosis* complex in lymph nodes of wild boar (*Sus scrofa*) by a target-amplified test system. *J Vet Med B* 47:337-42.

7. Ferroglio, E. 1998. Epidemiologia della tubercolosi e della brucellosi in ambiente silvestre. PhD Thesis, University of Bologna.

8. Moda, G. and M. Valpreda. 1994. Bovine tuberculosis eradication: need of collaboration between physicians and veterinarians. *Alpe Adria Microbiol J* 3:296-97.

9. Moda, G., C. J. Daborn, J. M. Grange, and O. Cosivi. 1996. The zoonotic importance of *M. bovis. Tubercle Lung Dis* 77:103-108.

10. Ara, G., P. Brunoventre, S. Bonora, A. Dondo, M. Goria, A. Malabaila, and L. Sala. 2003. Tubercolosi come zoonosi. *Med Vet Prev* 25:12-14.

11. Dondo, A., S. Squadrone, C. Grattarola, and M. Goria. 2000. Wild boar and TB in North-Western Italy. *Proceedings of the Third International Conference on* Mycobacterium bovis. Cambridge, 56.

Chapter 14

The Effect of Wildlife Reservoirs of *Mycobacterium bovis* on Programs for the Eradication of Tuberculosis in Cattle in Ireland

P.J. Quinn, MVB, PhD, MRCVS, and J.D. Collins, MVB, MVM, MS, Dipl. ECVPH, PhD, MRCVS

Diseases in domestic animals caused by mycobacteria include tuberculosis in avian and mammalian species, paratuberculosis in ruminants, and feline leprosy. Bovine tuberculosis, caused by *Mycobacterium bovis*, occurs worldwide. Despite the fact that cattle are considered to be the natural hosts of *M. bovis*, this pathogen has an exceptionally wide host range, with most warm-blooded animals and humans susceptible to infection.

Although there are a number of ways whereby *M. bovis* can spread in cattle populations (Fig. 14.1), there is general acceptance that airborne transmission is the most common method of pathogen transfer. In tuberculous cattle, lesions in the respiratory tract occur much more frequently than in the alimentary tract (1). Because of the low occurrence of generalized tuberculosis in cattle in developed countries, shedding of *M. bovis* in milk, urine, feces, and exudates is considered to be a relatively infrequent mode of transmission of these pathogenic mycobacteria.

Because of the zoonotic implications of the disease and the production losses caused by its chronic progressive nature, tuberculosis eradication programs have been implemented in many countries. The incidence of human infection with *M. bovis* has been reduced to low levels in countries in which tuberculosis eradication programs for cattle have been implemented. In addition, pasteurization of milk has eliminated the exposure of humans to infection from dairy products. Bovine tuberculosis eradication programs, however, have had limited success in countries in which transmission of *M. bovis* from domestic to wild animals has led to the emergence of wildlife reservoirs of this disease. As a consequence, in many countries, persistence of tuberculosis in cattle populations has been attributed to reservoirs of *M. bovis* in wildlife or feral animals. Only a small proportion of wildlife species that become infected with *M. bovis*, however, can act as maintenance hosts for this pathogen. Examples include brushtail possums, badgers, bison, deer, and African buffalos. Once infection spills over into animal species that can become maintenance hosts, conventional control and eradication measures for bovine tuberculosis are no longer effective.

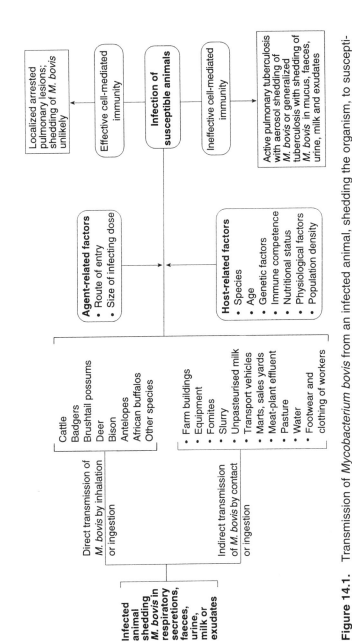

Figure 14.1. Transmission of *Mycobacterium bovis* from an infected animal, shedding the organism, to susceptible animals. Factors that can influence the outcome of exposure of susceptible animals may be agent or host related. Human exposure to *M. bovis* can occur under similar circumstances.

Among wildlife species, brushtail possums, badgers, deer, and African buffalos constitute important reservoirs of *M. bovis* in defined geographical regions throughout the world. In Ireland and the United Kingdom, the European badger *(Meles meles)* is a species of particular importance, and in New Zealand, brushtail possums *(Trichosurus vulpecula)* and feral deer are important reservoirs of *M. bovis*. African buffalos *(Syncerus caffer)* act as maintenance hosts for *M. bovis* in South Africa and transmit infection not only to predators and scavengers but also to other wildlife species and livestock in the same environment (2). Wildlife reservoirs of *M. bovis* in North America include deer and bison.

The socioeconomic importance of *M. bovis* infection in wild animals relates to their ability to act as maintenance hosts and to transmit infection to cattle and other wildlife species. Reinfection of herds in Ireland can be linked to the presence of infected badger colonies in close proximity to grazing cattle, with evidence of transfer from badgers to cattle. Restriction fragment length polymorphism analysis and spoligotyping of 452 isolates of *M. bovis* in Ireland, most of which were obtained from cattle, badgers, and deer, demonstrated the same range and geographical distribution of strains in all three species (3). These findings indicate that transmission of infection occurred between these three species. Brushtail possums are recognized as the most important wildlife reservoirs of *M. bovis* in New Zealand (4). In defined geographical regions of North America, tuberculosis is reported to be endemic in wood bison *(Bison bison athabascae)* herds (5), and the disease is recognized as an increasing problem in white-tailed deer *(Odocoileus virginianus)* (6).

Herd Breakdowns with Tuberculosis

Factors that contribute to herd breakdowns with tuberculosis include lateral spread from contiguous herds with established *M. bovis* infection and purchase of replacement animals with undetected infection. It is recognized that recently infected cattle fail to react to tuberculin, as reactivity is not usually apparent until at least 30 days following infection. False-negative reactions to the tuberculin test may relate to reduced potency of tuberculin, injection of an insufficient quantity of tuberculin, desensitization following recent intradermal testing, immunosuppression relating to the physiological state of the animals under test, and errors in reading and recording test results (7).

The intradermal test may fail to detect infection in old anergic cattle, and such animals may shed *M. bovis* in their secretions or excretions for long periods of time. In areas of Ireland in which tuberculosis affects multiple or contiguous herds, involvement of *M. bovis*–infected badgers is often suspected as the source of infection. Contamination of farm buildings, pasture, and feed by badger excretions or secretions containing large numbers of *M. bovis* is a possible source of infection for cattle. The fact that *M. bovis* can survive for long intervals in cattle slurry suggests the possibility of prolonged environmental contamination as a consequence of shedding of *M. bovis* by wildlife reservoir hosts (8).

Transmission of *M. bovis*

M. bovis shed in respiratory secretions, feces, urine, milk, or exudates by infected domestic or wild animals may be transmitted directly to susceptible animals. Typically, infection is acquired by inhalation or ingestion (Fig. 14.1). Alternatively, infection may be acquired indirectly from a contaminated environment. Because of the modes of transmission of *M. bovis* and the ability of this pathogen to infect a wide range of domestic animals including cattle, sheep, pigs, horses, dogs, and cats, there are many opportunities for wild animals to become infected through contact with domestic animals shedding *M. bovis*. Likewise, the opportunity for domestic animals to acquire infection from wildlife species is enhanced through the wildlife–livestock interface.

Farms bordering game reserves, national parks, or other lands designated for the preservation of wildlife species provide an opportunity for common grazing by domestic and wild ruminants. Badgers and possums, which live either on farms or in close proximity to grazing land, may share the same general environment as grazing cattle. Transfer of infection from terminally ill badgers or possums to cattle may occur through licking, sniffing, or biting moribund animals on pasture. Cattle shedding *M. bovis* into the environment can indirectly infect badgers and possums with agent-related and dose-related factors that determine the severity of infection (Fig. 14.1). In possums, tuberculosis is usually progressive and fatal (9). More than 80% of tuberculous possums have lung lesions, indicating that infection was acquired by the respiratory route. The lungs and kidneys are two common sites of lesions in tuberculous badgers, with high concentrations of *M. bovis* recorded in the urine and sputum of infected animals (10). The interactive behavior of cattle and infected badgers at pasture indicates that direct transmission of *M. bovis* through inhalation by cattle of expired aerosols from infected badgers is unlikely (11). Most cattle avoided grass contaminated with badger feces and urine, but when grass was scarce, individual cattle inhaled and grazed close to badger excretions on pasture. In this study, it was noted that badgers were attracted to and ate cattle food throughout the year.

Nocturnal observations, radio telemetry, and time-lapse camera surveillance of an estimated 26 identifiable badgers from two social groups were used to investigate visits by these nocturnal animals to two cattle farms (12). The badgers, which included three individuals infected with *M. bovis*, frequented cowsheds, feed sheds, barns, haystacks, slurry pits, and cattle troughs in their search for food. Among the observations, it was noted that contamination of cattle feed with badger feces occurred and that badgers also came into close contact with cattle. During the course of the study, outbreaks of tuberculosis occurred on both farms on which the badger surveillance took place.

In some animal species, a change in behavior may occur in the advanced stages of tuberculosis. It has been noted that brushtail possums, which are normally nocturnal, may become active during daylight. Such behavioral changes may be important in the transmission of infection to other animals. It has been reported also that cattle and farmed deer at pasture may become infected as a result of direct or close contact with brushtail possums that are terminally ill with tuberculosis.

Detection of Tuberculosis in Wildlife

Tuberculosis caused by *M. bovis* is a chronic, progressive disease, and the majority of infected animals show few characteristic clinical signs. The most common clinical sign of tuberculosis in most wildlife species is weight loss, but this change becomes evident only in the advanced stage of the disease. In common with many other microbial infections, the specificity of immune-based tests for the diagnosis of *M. bovis* infection depends on the antigens employed in such tests. Formerly, only complex mixtures of antigens such as purified protein derivative were available for diagnostic procedures—usually the tuberculin skin test. The availability of purified mycobacterial antigens has improved the number and specificity of tests for the diagnosis of tuberculosis not only in cattle but also in wildlife species.

Diagnostic Tests Based on Cell-Mediated Responses

The intradermal tuberculin test, which has been a standard test for identifying tuberculous cattle in many countries for decades, has serious limitations when applied to wild animals. Practical difficulties include reexamination of sites injected with tuberculin between 48 and 96 hours and the necessity for standardization of the tuberculin dose for each species. The potential immunosuppressive effect of the stress arising from capture may adversely affect delayed-type hypersensitivity responses in some wildlife species. Diagnostic tests yielding results in less than 24 hours would allow retention of animals until test results were known. Some *in vitro* cell-mediated tests require restraint on only one occasion. Lymphocyte proliferation assays, which offer this advantage, have been employed in a number of wildlife species including brushtail possums and badgers. The requirement for viable white blood cells, collected within 24 hours, and technical difficulties relating to standardization have restricted the application of this method to research trials. An assay based on the detection of interferon γ (IFN-γ) in purified protein derivative-stimulated white blood cells has been used for some time in cattle, with considerable success. Levels of IFN-γ are measured using an ELISA capture assay employing monoclonal antibody. The success of this assay system has stimulated interest in developing similar reagents for badgers, deer, and other wildlife species. The requirement for species-specific monoclonal antibodies adds to the cost of such test systems. A further refinement of the IFN-γ test for cattle, which involves the use of the purified antigens ESAT-6 and CFP10 derived from *M. tuberculosis*, is reported to enhance the specificity of this convenient *in vitro* test. It is likely that additional purified antigens derived from *M. bovis* and *M. tuberculosis* will improve the specificity of cell-mediated tests for use in wildlife, a group of animals in which nonspecific infections sometimes limit the reliability of test procedures.

Serological Tests

Many serological tests have been employed for the detection of tuberculosis in different host species, with limited success. As high levels of antibody to mycobacterial antigens are usually present in the advanced stages of tuberculosis when acid-fast bacteria are numerous, many of the serological tests developed for use in wildlife species have a low level of sensitivity. Serological tests for identifying tuberculosis in badgers have been refined in recent years. A blocking ELISA test using monoclonal antibody to an antigenic determinant on *M. bovis* that is immunodominant in badgers had high specificity but low sensitivity (13). Similar low levels of sensitivity have been obtained in brushtail possums. It is reported that few possums with subclinical tuberculosis produce detectable antibodies, but animals with advanced disease can be detected using serological tests.

Both domestic and wild ruminants with advanced tuberculosis sometimes exhibit anergy, a state in which they are unresponsive to the intradermal tuberculin test because of suppressed or weak cellular immune responses. Such animals, however, may have moderate or high levels of circulating antibody. A combination of lymphocyte proliferation assay and ELISA has been used to detect tuberculosis in deer (13). Prior intradermal skin testing of deer boosted the levels of specific antibody detected by ELISA in this species.

Postmortem Diagnosis

The distribution of lesions in an animal with tuberculosis depends on the route by which infection was acquired and whether or not dissemination of *M. bovis* has occurred. Animals with lesions in the thoracic cavity are presumed to have acquired infection by inhalation of aerosols containing *M. bovis*. Lesions in the mesenteric lymph nodes are consistent with infection acquired by the oral route. The sites in which lesions occur may point to the likely route of transmission of infection to in-contact animals. Kidney lesions occur in approximately 25% of tuberculous badgers with tuberculosis (10), and accordingly, contaminated urine has been identified as a further means of spreading *M. bovis* in the environment.

A presumptive diagnosis of tuberculosis in cattle is often made on the basis of characteristic macroscopic lesions, followed by histopathology. The appearance, nature, and distribution of tuberculous lesions in wildlife species are sometimes different from those observed in cattle. In brushtail possums and badgers, fibrosis is not a feature of tuberculous lesions, and mineralization is uncommon. High numbers of acid-fast bacilli are usually observed in tuberculous lesions in brushtail possums and badgers. In contrast, the number of acid-fast bacteria in bovine lesions is usually low, and Ziehl-Neelsen-stained smears require careful examination to confirm the presence of these bacteria in smears from lesions.

Microbiology

Although a presumptive diagnosis of tuberculosis can be arrived at by the detection of acid-fast bacilli in a smear from a suspect lesion, culture of *M. bovis* is required for confirmation. Bacterial isolation, although a sensitive and specific method, requires weeks to months for final identification of pathogenic mycobacteria. A number of DNA amplification methods for the detection of *M. bovis*, including the polymerase chain reaction, have been developed in recent years. These methods, which are potentially specific, sensitive, and rapid, require rigorous procedures to minimize sample contamination. Typing systems, employing DNA fingerprinting, are widely used for studying the epidemiology of tuberculosis in domestic animals and wildlife species. Restriction endonuclease analysis has been used extensively as part of such epidemiological investigations of tuberculosis in cattle. Other DNA typing methods that have been used for comparing isolates of *M. bovis* from cattle and wildlife include restriction fragment length polymorphism and spoligotyping (3).

Immunity to *M. bovis*

Much of our current understanding of immunity to *M. bovis* derives from studies in experimental animals, and mostly laboratory animals. Although the information derived from such studies may not be directly applicable to tuberculous cattle or infected wildlife species, it is probable that many common mechanisms of immunity to *M. bovis* apply in most mammalian species.

In common with many other intracellular pathogens, immunity to *M. bovis* involves immune responses at two levels; namely, innate or nonspecific immune mechanisms—the first line of defense—and specific cell-mediated responses that require the active participation of T lymphocytes and macrophages. Components of the functional elements of the immune system that operate in a nonspecific manner include anatomical structures such as skin and mucous membranes that hinder the entry of microbial pathogens, inhibitory secretions such as gastric hydrochloric acid and bile, and antimicrobial factors present in blood and secretions, including lysozyme, complement, and interferons. Phagocytic cells, particularly neutrophils and macrophages, contribute to the removal of microbial pathogens from the tissues and their destruction within the phagolysosomes. A notable virulence factor of *M. bovis* is its ability to survive within phagocytic cells and to later replicate in these cells before specific immune responses develop. Before specific immunity develops, natural killer cells contribute to body defenses by killing bacilli-laden macrophages and producing IFN-γ, which activates macrophages and stimulates a T_H1 cytokine immune response in preference to a T_H2 response. Macrophages and dendritic cells, stimulated by microbial products, produce interleukin (IL) 12. Both natural killer cells and T_H1 lymphocytes are activated by IL-12 (14). Subsequently, IL-12 induces IL-10 production in lymphocytes and macrophages. Lymphocytes provide the immunological specificity for the host's cell-mediated response to tubercle bacilli. When exposed to specific antigens, T and B lymphocytes undergo clonal proliferation, with T cells responsible for cell-mediated responses and B cells for humoral immune responses.

In the early stages of tuberculosis, cell-mediated responses predominate, with macrophage participation limiting the intracellular multiplication of these pathogenic mycobacteria. In contrast, humoral immunity does not affect the survival of these intracellular bacteria in infected animals, and high antibody levels occur only in advanced stages of tuberculosis when large numbers of acid-fast bacteria are present. T cells have two important functions in animals infected with *M. bovis*; namely, producing cytokines that activate macrophages so that those phagocytic cells can kill or inhibit the growth of tubercle bacilli, and killing weakly activated macrophages in which pathogenic mycobacteria are multiplying. On the basis of the cytokines that they produce, CD4+ T cells can be divided into two subsets, T_H1 and T_H2. The T_H1 subset produces IL-2, which promotes T-cell proliferation, and also IFN-γ and tumor necrosis factor β, both of which activate macrophages. The T_H2 subset produces IL-4, IL-5, IL-6, IL-9, IL-10, and IL-13, which promote antibody production. The cytokines IL-4, IL-10, and IL-13 down-regulate T_H1 responses. Cytokines provide two-way communication between macrophages and T cells. Macrophages and dendritic cells are the principal producers of IL-12, especially when macrophages have engulfed tubercle bacilli. IL-12 is one of the major cytokines involved in the specific expansion of the T_H1 population and in up-regulating its diverse functions. Accordingly, IL-12 plays a central role in promoting cell-mediated immune responses to *M. bovis* and in regulating delayed-type hypersensitivity responses that ultimately determine the pathogenesis of tuberculosis.

In tuberculous cattle, antigen-responsive T-cell clones of CD4+, CD8+, and WC1+ phenotypes have been isolated (15). *In vitro* studies of antigen-stimulated bovine lymphocytes have shown that CD8+ T cells are capable of releasing metabolically active *M. bovis* from infected macrophages, indicating that cytolytic activity is a feature of cell-mediated immunity in bovine tuberculosis.

The number of pathogenic mycobacteria in the infecting dose, the route of entry into the host, and the ability of the infected animal to deal with the organisms at the site of entry often determine the outcome of infection, and ultimately whether or not shedding of *M. bovis* occurs (Fig. 14.1).

Vaccination against *M. bovis*

Protection of cattle against infection with *M. bovis* through vaccination is likely to be considered an important control strategy in some countries in which persistence of mycobacteria in wildlife results in reinfection of cattle. Vaccination of wildlife reservoirs of *M. bovis* is ecologically and politically a more attractive option than depopulation of such maintenance hosts in countries in which eradication of tuberculosis in cattle, using test and slaughter programs, has not succeeded.

Induction of protective immunity to pathogenic mycobacteria presents many challenges. In the human population, the use of live attenuated *M. bovis* Bacille Calmette-Güerin (BCG) for the prevention of infection with *M. tuberculosis* has yielded inconsistent results. Vaccination studies in brushtail possums and badgers using BCG vaccine have shown promising results when vaccinated animals were challenged with virulent *M. bovis*. In possums, BCG delivered as an intranasal aerosol induced a protective immune response that persisted for 12 months after vaccination (9). Revaccination of opossums enhanced protection, and conjunctival vaccination proved as effective as an intranasal aerosol. Oral baits are readily accepted by brushtail possums and badgers, but delivery of live vaccines by the oral route has serious limitations because of the adverse effects of gastric acidity on live bacteria. Microencapsulation of the BCG vaccine may overcome this difficulty. Despite the potential usefulness of the BCG vaccine for inducing immunity to *M. bovis*, studies in mice have shown that animals exposed to certain environmental bacteria produce an immune response that controlled the replication of BCG, thereby curtailing the vaccine-induced immune response before it developed. In mice sensitized to live environmental mycobacteria before exposure to BCG, the vaccine elicited only a transient immune response with a low frequency of myco-bacterium-specific cells and no protective immunity against challenge with *M. tuberculosis* (16).

Apart from the BCG vaccine, attempts are being made to develop new vaccines through the deletion of virulence genes in *M. bovis*. The efficacy of a range of non-living vaccines including inactivated mycobacteria, subunits of mycobacterial proteins, and DNA vaccines for use in domestic and wild animals are being evaluated at present. Live attenuated vaccines, however, offer several potential advantages over inactivated or subunit vaccines for the induction of immunity to pathogenic mycobacteria. Because these pathogens can replicate intracellularly, live vaccines, which promote strong cell-mediated immune responses, are often preferred over inactivated vaccines. Furthermore, in comparison with inactivated or subunit my-cobacterial vaccines, live attenuated vaccines usually require only a single admin-istration for the induction of long-lasting protective immunity, a point of particular importance when dealing with wildlife species.

In small animal models, mycobacterial DNA vaccines have yielded encourag-ing results (17). Studies in mice have shown that DNA vaccines encoding a single protein or epitope can stimulate IFN-γ and cytotoxic T-cell responses. Improved protection was achieved with mycobacterial vaccines encoding several proteins or epitopes and incorporating adjuvant. Using murine models, it has been demon-strated that mycobacterial DNA vaccines can also contribute to the elimination of existing infections. Diagnostic reagents capable of differentiating infected from vac-cinated animals are necessary for the practical development and utilization of a vaccine against tuberculosis in cattle and also in wildlife. Recent studies have de-monstrated that diagnostic peptide cocktails, based either on recombinant proteins or on peptides derived from antigens expressed in *M. bovis* but not in BCG, can distinguish between vaccinated and infected cattle, using lymphocyte transforma-tion and IFN-γ assays (18).

Concluding Comments

Until more reliable methods for the diagnosis of *M. bovis* infection in wildlife species are available, control of tuberculosis in free-ranging wildlife in a manner similar to the test-and-slaughter policies used for eradication of tuberculosis in cat-tle are unlikely to be successful. Even if reliable antemortem tests for wildlife species were available, sampling sufficient numbers of animals to determine their health status presents many logistical challenges. An additional complication is the legal status of some wildlife species within a country. The control of badgers by depopulation has resulted in much public debate, as this species is statutorily pro-tected in a number of countries, including Ireland.

Control measures for tuberculosis in domestic animals must include considera-tion of all sources of infection, including wildlife reservoirs (Fig. 14.2). Culling of

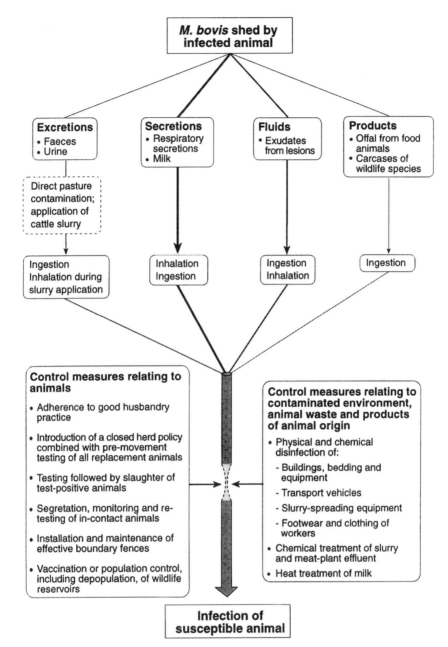

Figure 14.2.   Modes of transmission of *Mycobacterium bovis* from infected to susceptible animals and relevant control measures relating to animals and the environment.

selected wildlife species, principally brushtail possums in defined areas of New Zealand, resulted in the eradication of *M. bovis* from both domestic animals and wildlife. Depopulation studies of badgers in areas of the United Kingdom and Ireland where the incidence of tuberculosis in cattle herds was high demonstrated a substantial decline in the occurrence of confirmed cases of tuberculosis in such herds. Despite the data obtained from these studies, it is uncertain whether public opinion would support large-scale culling of badgers for the control and eradication of tuberculosis in cattle. However, different wildlife reservoirs of *M. bovis* are present in many countries and, accordingly, the species of animals implicated often require different control strategies.

Awareness of the importance of tuberculosis in wildlife, not only as a potential reservoir of infection for domestic animals but also as a threat to the endangered wildlife species involved, has increased in recent years. Surveillance of the health status of wildlife species should form a central part of national programs for the eradication of tuberculosis from the cattle population. Control programs should be carefully balanced to reflect the ecological importance of many wildlife species. Substantial research investment may be required to devise effective control measures such as vaccination, which can be applied to wildlife reservoirs of *M. bovis*, but ultimately the benefits derived from such investment may assist in the elimination of tuberculosis from national herds in many countries.

References

1   Neill, S. D., D. G. Bryson, and J. M. Pollock. 2001. Pathogenesis of tuberculosis in cattle. *Tuberculosis* 81:79-86.
2. Michel, A. L. 2002. Implications of tuberculosis in African wildlife and livestock. *Ann N Y Acad Sci* 969:251-55.
3. Costello, E., D. O'Grady, O. Flynn, R. O'Brien, M. Rogers, F. Quigley, J. Egan, and J. Griffin. 1999. Study of restriction fragment length polymorphism analysis and spoligotyping for epidemiological investigation of *Mycobacterium bovis* infection. *J Clin Microbiol* 37:3217-22.
4. Morris, R. S. and D. U. Pfeiffer. 1995. Directions and issues in bovine tuberculosis epidemiology and control in New Zealand. *N Z Vet J* 43:256-65.
5. Nishi, J. S., C. Stephen, and B. T. Elkin. 2002. Implications of agricultural and wildlife policy on management and eradication of bovine tuberculosis and brucellosis in free-ranging wood bison of northern Canada. *Ann N Y Acad Sci* 969:236-44.
6. Schmitt, S. M., D. J. O'Brien, C. S. Bruning-Fann, and S. D. Fitzgerald. 2002. Bovine tuberculosis in Michigan wildlife and livestock. *Ann N Y Acad Sci* 969:262-68.
7. Monaghan, M. L., M. L. Doherty, J. D. Collins, J. F. Kazda, and P. J. Quinn. 1994. The tuberculin test. *Vet Microbiol* 40:111-24.
8. Scanlon, M. P. and P. J. Quinn. 2000. The survival of *Mycobacterium bovis* in sterilized cattle slurry and its relevance to the persistence of this pathogen in the environment. *Irish Vet J* 53:412-15.
9. Corner, L. A. L. 2001. Bovine tuberculosis in brushtail possums *(Trichosurus vulpecula)*: Studies on vaccination, experimental infection, and disease transmission. Ph.D thesis, Massey University, New Zealand.
10. Gallagher, J. and R. S. Clifton-Hadley. 2000. Tuberculosis in badgers; a review of the disease and its significance for other animals. *Res Vet Sci* 69:203-17.
11. Benham, P. F. J. 1993. The interactive behaviour of cattle and badgers with reference to transmission of bovine tuberculosis. *In* T. J. Hayden (ed.), The Badger. Dublin: Royal Irish Academy, 189-95.

12. Garnett, B. T., R. J. Delahay, and T. J. Roper. 2002. Use of cattle farm resources by badgers *(Meles meles)* and risk of bovine tuberculosis *(Mycobacterium bovis)* transmission to cattle. *Proc R Soc Lond B* 269:1487-91.

13. de Lisle, G. W., R. G. Bengis, S. M. Schmitt, and D. J. O'Brien. 2002. Tuberculosis in free-ranging wildlife: detection, diagnosis and management. *Rev Sci Tech Off Int Epiz* 21:317-34.

14. Dannenberg, A. M. 1999. Immunology of tuberculosis. *In* D. Schlossberg (ed.), Tuberculosis and Nontuberculous Mycobacterial Infection. Philadelphia: W.B. Saunders, 29-41.

15. Pollock, J. M., J. McNair, M. D. Welsh, R. M. Girvin, H. E. Kennedy, D. P. Mackie, and S. D. Neill. 2001. Immune responses in bovine tuberculosis. *Tuberculosis* 81:103-107.

16. Brandt, L., J. F., A. W. Olsen, B. Chilima, P. Hirsch, R. Appelberg, and P. Andersen. 2002. Failure of the *Mycobacterium bovis* BCG vaccine: some species of environmental mycobacteria block multiplication of BCG and induction of protective immunity to tuberculosis. *Infect Immun* 70:672-78.

17. Buddle, B. M. 2001. Vaccination of cattle against *Mycobacterium bovis*. *Tuberculosis* 81:125-32.

18. Vordermeier, H. M., P. J. Cockle, A. O. Whelan, S. Rhodes, and R. G. Hewinson. 2000. Towards the development of diagnostic assays to discriminate between *Mycobacterium bovis* infection and Bacille Calmette-Guérin vaccination in cattle. *Clin Infect Dis* 30:S291-298.

Chapter 15
Control and Eradication of Bovine Tuberculosis in Central Europe

I. Pavlik, DVM, MVDr, CSc

Introduction

This chapter is devoted especially to bovine tuberculosis in animals and human beings in seven Central European countries (Bosnia and Herzegovina, Croatia, the Czech Republic, Hungary, Poland, Slovakia, and Slovenia). These countries, lying between the Baltic and the Adriatic seas, cover an area of 661,635 km^2, with 72.030 million inhabitants. Until 1995, a total of 13.040 million head of cattle were kept in this area, of which 6.001 million were cows (Table 15.1).

Bovine Tuberculosis in Cattle

With the framework of the national bovine tuberculosis control programs of the seven above-mentioned Central European countries, bovine tuberculosis was successfully eliminated between the years 1953 and 1980 (Table 15.1). During the postelimination period, the incidence of bovine tuberculosis decreased.

Bovine Tuberculosis in Cattle in the Czech Republic

In the Czech Republic (1), the incidence of bovine tuberculosis in cattle was recorded following the postelimination period (1969–1996), when incidence reached 12–16 outbreaks per year during the years 1969–1978. During the next decade (1979–1988), however, this incidence decreased to from one to nine outbreaks per year, with a consequent decline to zero outbreaks in the years 1981, 1987, and 1988. Nevertheless, bovine tuberculosis of cattle was observed sporadically (from one to two infected herds per year), and the last outbreak was reported in 1995 (2). In the years 1989, 1990, 1993, and 1996–2003, however, no bovine tuberculosis was reported in cattle at all (3,4; unpublished statistical data, State Veterinary Administration, Prague, the Czech Republic). Subsequently, on 31 March 2004, the Czech Republic was declared a bovine tuberculosis–free country by the European Union (Commission Decision 2004/320/EC, OJ NO. L102, 07.04.2004, p. 75).

Table 15.1. Bovine tuberculosis in cattle herds in seven Central European countries (3)

Country	Data about the country[a]	No. of	herds	1990	1991	1992	1993	1994	1995	1996	1997	1998	1999	Total
Bosnia and Herzegovina	1962–1973[b]	Small[1]	n[4]	N[4]	n[4]	n[4]	n[4]	n[4]	n[4]	1	0	1	0	2
	51,233 km²	Large[2]	n[4]	N[4]	n[4]	n[4]	n[4]	n[4]	n[4]	0	0	0	0	0
	250,000[5] cows	Total	n[4]	N[4]	n[4]	n[4]	n[4]	n[4]	n[4]	1	0	1	0	2
	4.0[5] mil. inhab.	%	n[4]	N[4]	n[4]	n[4]	n[4]	n[4]	n[4]	n[4]	n[4]	n[4]	n[4]	
Croatia	1953–1966[b]	Small[1]	n[4]	3	1	7	3	4	6	3	1	3	0	31
	56,538 km²	Large[2]	n[4]	0	0	0	0	0	0	1	0	0	0	1
	330,000 cows	Total	n[4]	3	1	7	3	4	6	4	1	3	0	32
	4.5 mil. inhab.	%	n[4]	n[4]	n[4]	n[4]	n[4]	n[4]	n[4]	n[4]	n[4]	n[4]	n[4]	
Czech Republic	1959–1968[b]	Small[1]	n[4]	0	0	1	0	0	1	0	0	0	0	2
	78,864 km²	Large[2]	n[4]	0	2	1	0	2	0	0	0	0	0	5
	830,000 cows	Total	5 410[3]	0	2	2	0	2	1	0	0	0	0	7
	10.3 mil. inhab.	%	100	0	0.036	0.036	0	0.036	0.018	0	0	0	0	
Hungary	1962–1980[b]	Small[1]	n[4]	0	3	3	2	5	0	2	5	3	5	28
	93,031 km²	Large[2]	n[4]	2	3	3	2	3	0	4	3	3	0	23
	420,000 cows	Total	50 936[3]	2	6	6	4	8	0	6	8	6	5	51
	10.2 mil. inhab.	%	100	0.004	0.012	0.012	0.008	0.016	0	0.012	0.016	0.012	0.010	
Poland	1959–1965[b]	Small[1]	n[4]	134	101	142	126	134	70	61	54	51	32	905
	312,683 km²	Large[2]	n[4]	21	14	17	11	7	3	2	0	0	0	75
	3,763,000 cows	Total	1 373 500[3]	155	115	159	137	141	73	63	54	51	32	980
	35.7 mil. inhab.	%	100	0.011	0.008	0.012	0.010	0.010	0.005	0.005	0.004	0.004	0.002	
Slovakia	1959–1968[b]	Small[1]	n[4]	0	0	1	2	0	0	0	0	0	0	3
	49,035 km²	Large[2]	n[4]	2	1	1	1	0	0	0	0	0	0	5
	348,000 cows	Total	1 369[3]	2	1	2	3	0	0	0	0	0	0	8
	5.4 mil. Inhab.	%	100	0.146	0.073	0.146	0.219	0	0	0	0	0	0	

Continues

Table 15.1. (Continued)

Country	Data about the country[a]	No. of	herds	1990	1991	1992	1993	1994	1995	1996	1997	1998	1999	Total
Slovenia	1962–1973[b]	Small[1]	n[4]	1	0	1	2	0	0	0	0	0	0	4
	20,251 km²	Large[2]	n[4]	0	0	0	0	0	0	0	0	0	0	0
	210,000 cows	Total	n[4]	1	0	1	2	0	0	0	0	0	0	4
	1.9 mil. Inhab.	%	n[4]	n[4]	N[4]	n[4]	n[4]	n[4]	n[4]	n[4]	n[4]	n[4]	n[4]	
Total	1953–1980[b]	Small[1]	n[4]	138	105	155	135	143	77	67	60	58	37	975
	661,635 km²	Large[2]	n[4]	25	20	22	14	12	3	7	3	3	0	109
	6 051 000 cows	Herds	n[4]	163	125	177	149	155	80	74	63	61	37	1 084
	72.0 mil. inhab.	%		15.0	11.5	16.3	13.8	14.3	7.4	6.9	5.8	5.6	3.4	

[1]Small cattle herd (≤10 cows).

[2]Large cattle herd (>10 cows).

[3]No. of establishmentts in 1997: OIE, 1998, World animal health in 1997. Parts 1 and 2, OIE, Paris - France, ISBN 92-9044-454-1, 754 pp.

[4]Official data not available.

[a]Official data from 1995: WHO (http://who.int), Surveillance of Tuberculosis in Europe (http://www.ceses.org/eurotb/eurotb.htm) and *FAO-OIE-WHO, 1997, Animal Health Yearbook*, Rome, Italy, 280 pp.

[b]National control programs against bovine tuberculosis.

Bovine Tuberculosis in Other Central European Countries

In the other Central European countries, the postelimination epizootiological situation of the disease in cattle was analogous to that in the Czech Republic (Table 15.1; 3). During the study period (1990–1999), bovine tuberculosis was diagnosed in 1084 herds of cattle. In 975 (89.9%) small herds (≤10 cows) outbreaks of infection were found, whereas in large herds (≥10 cows), this number reached only 109 (10.1%). The incidence of bovine tuberculosis reached its maximum peak (16.3%) in 1992; nevertheless, the incidence of infection decreased in the following years, with the 1999 incidence rate (3.4%) attaining the minimum (Table 15.1).

During the last decade of the last century (1990–1999), the last outbreak of bovine tuberculosis in cattle was diagnosed in Slovakia, Slovenia, the Czech Republic, Croatia, and Bosnia and Herzegovina in the years 1993, 1994, 1995, 1998, and 1999, respectively (Table 15.2). Bovine tuberculosis was diagnosed as a result of the proper quarantine in Slovenia of 37 fattening bulls imported from two foreign European countries before the animals were introduced to the targeting farms (3).

As preventive measures, all animals up to the age of 2 years are subject to an intravital skin test for bovine tuberculin at least once every 2 years in all study countries except Bosnia and Herzegovina, where this test was performed, because of the war, after 1996. Six to 8 weeks later, all reactor animals to the first single intradermal skin test are further tested by a simultaneous intradermal inoculation of bovine and avian tuberculin. As a consequence, animals with repeated positive skin test results to bovine tuberculin are slaughtered, and direct microscopy, histological, and culture examinations are performed. The same diagnostic procedure is applied to examine tuberculous lesions found during routine abattoir meat inspection (3,4).

Tuberculous Lesions in Cattle Caused By Other Causal Agents than *Mycobacterium bovis* or *Mycobacterium caprae*

Although in the Czech Republic bovine tuberculosis was controlled in domestic animals including cattle and pigs in 1995 (2), tuberculous lesions were still being found, above all, in the intestinal and lung lymph nodes of cattle. During the years 1990–1999, mycobacteria were isolated from the organs of cattle only in 561 (17.5%) of 3202 culturally examined animals. *M. bovis* only was isolated from 48 (8.6%) animals, originating from seven herds (two infected herds in each year in 1991, 1992, and 1994, and one infected herd in the year 1995): Four outbreaks were detected by annual skin testing, one outbreak by movement tuberculin skin testing, and two outbreaks by the detection of tuberculous lesions at slaughter (4).

During the years 1990–1999, in the Czech Republic *M. avium* complex isolates of serotypes 1, 2, and 3 and of genotype IS*901*+ and IS*1245*+ (*M. avium* subsp. *avium* according to the current taxonomy) were detected in 331 (59.0%) slaughter cattle, and isolates of serotypes 4–6, 8–11, and 21, and of genotype IS*901*− and

Table 15.2. Incidence of bovine tuberculosis in other animals than cattle in six Central European countries (9)

Country	Animals from	1990	1991	1992	1993	1994	1995	1996	1997	1998	1999	Total	%
Croatia	Free nature	0	0	1[a]	0	0	0	0	0	0	0	1[a]	100
	Subtotal	0	0	1[a]	0	0	0	0	0	0	0	1[a]	100
Czech Republic	Free nature	0	1[b]	0	0	0	0	0	0	0	0	1[b]	7.1
	Game park	0	1[c]	0	0	0	0	0	0	0	0	1[c]	7.1
	Zoological garden	0	0	0	1[d]	2[e,f]	2[e]	0	0	0	0	5[d,e,f]	35.8
	Cattle farm	0	0	0	0	0	5[g]	0	0	0	0	5[g]	35.8
	Cervid farm	0	0	0	0	0	0	0	0	0	1[h]	1[h]	7.1
	Circus	0	0	1[i]	0	0	0	0	0	0	0[i]	1	7.1
	Subtotal	0	2	1	1	2	7	0	0	0	1	14	100
Hungary	Free nature	0	0	0	0	0	0	1[a]	0	0	0	1[a]	33.3
	Zoological garden	0	0	0	0	0	0	0	0	0	1[j]	1[j]	33.3
	Cervid farm	0	0	0	0	0	0	0	0	0	1[h]	1[h]	33.4
	Subtotal	0	0	0	0	0	0	1	0	0	2	3	100
Poland	Free nature	0	8[l,m]	1[l]	0	0	0	0	2[j]	0	1[j]	12[j]	24.5
	Zoological garden	0	0	0	4[n]	4[m,o]	4[m,o,p]	2[d]	2[e]	7[j]	1	24[d,e,k,l,m,n,o]	49.0
	Cattle farm	3[h,r]	0	0	0	0	0	1[h]	9[h,r,s]	0	0	13[g,p,r]	26.5
	Subtotal	3	8	1	4	4	4	3	13	7	2	49	100
Slovakia	Free nature	0	0	3[a]	0	0	0	0	0	0	0	3[a]	100
	Subtotal	0	0	3	0	0	0	0	0	0	0	3	100
Slovenia	Free nature	0	0	0	0	0	0	0	0	0	0	0	0
	Subtotal	0	0	0	0	0	0	0	0	0	0	0	0
Subtotal	Free nature	0	9	5	0	0	0	1	2	0	1	18	25.7
	Zoological garden	0	0	0	5	6	6	2	2	7	2	30	42.9
	Cattle farm	3	0	0	0	0	5	1	9	0	0	18	25.7
	Cervid farm	0	0	0	0	0	0	0	0	0	2	2	2.9
	Game park	0	1	0	0	0	0	0	0	0	0	1	1.4
	Circus	0	0	1	0	0	0	0	0	0	0	1	1.4
Total No. of animals		3	10	6	5	6	11	4	13	7	5	70	100
%		4.3	14.3	8.6	7.1	8.6	15.7	5.7	18.6	10.0	7.1		

140

[a]Wild boar (*Sus scrofa scrofa*).
[b]Red deer (*Cervus elaphus*).
[c]European wild goat (*Capra aegagrus*).
[d]Bison (*Bison bison*).
[e]Tapir (*Tapirus terrestris*).
[f]Cassowary (*Casuarius casuarius*).
[g]Domestic pig (*Sus scrofa f. domestica*).
[h]Red deer (*Cervus elaphus*).
[i]Bactrian camel(*Camelus ferus*).
[j]Puma (*Puma concolor*).
[k]European bison (*Bison bonasus*).
[l]Sitatunga (*Tragelaphus spekei*).
[m]Reticulated giraffe (*Giraffa camelopardalis reticulata*).
[n]Elands (*Taurotragus oryx*).
[o]Gnu (*Connochaetes taurinus*).
[p]Vietnamese pot-bellied pig (*Sus bucculentus*).
[r]Domestic sheep (*Ovis ammon f. aries*).
[s]Dog (*Canis lupus f. familiaris*).

141

IS*1245*+ (*M. avium* subsp. *hominissuis* according to the current taxonomy) were detected in 132 (23.5%) slaughter cattle. Potentially pathogenic mycobacteria like *Mycobacterium terrae, Mycobacterium chelonae, Mycobacterium phlei,* and *Mycobacterium triviale* were isolated from 50 (8.9%) heads of cattle (4).

From the tuberculous lesions of cattle, except those of mycobacteria, *Rhodococcus equi* and other species of bacteria were commonly isolated (4,5). IS*901* restriction fragment length polymorphism analysis of *Ma avium* isolates in the Czech Republic showed high heterogeneity of sources of infection for cattle, which develop tuberculous lesions in lymph nodes, leading to economic losses (6). Because of the risk of transmission of *M. avium* complex infections to the human population, in which avian mycobacterioses are considered as serious and difficult-to-treat infections (7,8), attention should be paid to these infections.

Current Risk Factors for the Spread of Bovine Tuberculosis

The possible risk factors for new infection of cattle in the Central European countries with causal agents of bovine tuberculosis can be as follows (1,3): cattle kept on pasture in an extensive farming condition may acquire infection from natural reservoirs by direct or indirect contact with infected wild animals; import of animals from countries with prevalence of bovine tuberculosis and uncontrollable shift of infected animals from farm to farm without the knowledge of veterinary services personnel and failure to perform required bovine tuberculin tests may account for the hazardous source of new infections—animal auction centers and artificial insemination sites, where animals from different herds interact, are places where animals may contract infection; attendants who are involved in the management practice of caring for animals should be tuberculin test negative; and the impairment of the immune system of animal caretakers, at advanced age, with chronic lesions of bovine tuberculosis may lead to overt tuberculosis. These individuals are the potential source of infection for food-producing animals via sputum, urine, and direct exhalation.

Bovine Tuberculosis and Tuberculous Lesions Caused By Other Causal Agents in Domestic Pigs

The elimination of the major source of causal agents of bovine tuberculosis represented by infected cattle was accompanied by decreasing incidence of this infection in other domestic animal species in all Central European countries (Table 15.1; 1,9,10).

During the veterinary meat-inspection of pigs slaughtered, however, tuberculous lesions were still being found in the head and intestinal lymph nodes. Parts of the adjacent organs (or on occasion the whole body of the pig) were then assessed according to valid veterinary regulations to ensure that the consumer was protected against mycobacterial infection. For this reason, some organs were condemned, and the whole bodies of animals were adjudged to be conditionally edible after processing (i.e., only for heat-treated products). Pig breeders of animals affected in this way suffered major economic losses. In the Czech Republic, the resulting financial losses were 6% from confiscating the head, intestines, and stomach, and 22%–24% for assessing meat as conditionally edible after processing (i.e., intended only for heat-processed products, 11).

The most common isolates obtained from pig lymph nodes with tuberculous lesions were of the *M. avium* complex and, less commonly, atypical mycobacteria—and also *Rhodococcus equi* (5,11). In the monitored period (1990–1999) in the Czech Republic, higher incidence of tuberculous lesions in pigs was recorded in two peaks: the first increase occurred in the mid-1990s, when enzymatically (e.g., using Envistim) split sawdust began to be more commonly used in pig rearing as deep bedding; this sawdust was often contaminated with *Ma hominissuis* (12). The second peak occurred at the end of the 1990s, when peat and kaolin often contaminated with *Ma hominissuis* began to be used as an addition to feed for piglets for 2 and up to 4 weeks after birth (12,13).

The infection of pig herds by *M. avium* complex members is represented by the transmission of *Ma avium*, the causal agent of avian tuberculosis, by free-living wild birds, especially in smaller herds, using traditional feed technology (13). In the autumn, at the time when these small terrestrial mammals migrate into the barns of pigs, they evidently may become vectors for the transmission of pathogenic mycobacterial species for pigs (14). In large herds of pigs, contact between pigs and wild or domestic birds is made impossible. However, contact between pigs and nonvertebrates, which may also be infected with *M. avium* complex members or atypical mycobacteria cannot always be ruled out (13,15).

Bovine Tuberculosis in Animal Species Other than Cattle and Domestic Pig

With regard to the distribution of the disease in other species of animals than cattle, higher incidence was observed especially in zoological gardens (Table 15.2; 1,9). Diagnosed bovine tuberculosis in free-living European bison, red deer, and wild boar (1,9,10) can represent risk factors that can dramatically change the current extremely low incidence of bovine tuberculosis in domestic ruminants in the above mentioned Central European countries.

Molecular Epidemiology of Bovine Tuberculosis

Spoligotyping and/or IS*6110* RFLP analysis were used to examine randomly selected *M. bovis* and *M. caprae* isolates from Croatia, the Czech Republic, Hungary, Poland, Slovakia, and Slovenia (2,16,17). The results confirm an effective control of bovine tuberculosis in cattle in this area, because previously circulating spoligotypes were successfully eradicated. The data also indicated that *M. caprae* belongs to an often-isolated causal agent of bovine tuberculosis in Central European countries in animal and human populations and that other reservoirs of bovine tuberculosis may exist among free-living wild animals.

Bovine Tuberculosis in the Human Population

A reduction in the incidence of bovine tuberculosis in the human population was enhanced by an improved understanding of the pathogenesis of the disease, introduction of milk pasteurization, and meat inspection at abattoirs. Other preventive veterinary hygiene measures in agriculture were also introduced to reduce the risk of infection to humans working with infected animals. As a result, tuberculosis in human population caused by the causal agent of bovine tuberculosis gradually decreased in Central Europe to the current low level, compared to the relatively high occurrence of *M. tuberculosis* cases (18).

A survey on bovine and human tuberculosis in human populations has been performed in four Central European countries (Croatia, the Czech Republic, Slovakia, and Slovenia), with 22.135 million inhabitants during the years 1990–1999 (18). During the studied period, new cases of tuberculosis were bacteriologically diagnosed in 47,516 patients. *M. tuberculosis* infection was detected in 47,461 (99.88%) cases, and bovine tuberculosis was found only in 55 (0.12%) patients. The rate of infection with bovine tuberculosis in humans did not exceed 0.29% in the study countries. The annual incidence of bacteriologically confirmed bovine tuberculosis did not exceed 0.1 per 100,000 inhabitants (Table 15.3).

The data obtained for 44 patients infected with *M. bovis* in the Czech Republic, Slovakia, and Slovenia indicate that the ratio of infection in men and women was 1:4. The number of infected individuals varied among age categories, with none of the patients being under 30 years of age. Twelve (27%) patients were in the age group of 31–60 years, and the remaining 32 (73%) were between the ages of 61 and 90 years. Thirty (83%) of the 36 patients in the Czech Republic were either inhabitants of the rural area or had at least lived in the countryside and worked in farms in their youth (18).

Although bovine tuberculosis is eradicated from the cattle population of the Central European countries, considerable attention should also be given to the following risk factors: infected wild animals manifesting clinical signs of weakness and a loss of timidity may become a source of causal agent of bovine tuberculosis for their self-sacrificing rescuers; wild animals kept in captivity at zoological gardens, and domestic animals like cats, horses, dogs, and others, may pose the risk of infection for humans; refugees from Third World countries infected with a causal agent of bovine tuberculosis and working on farms may also represent a risk in spreading the infection; and products from infected animals, such as milk and milk products processed from unpasteurized milk, and the total absence of or inconsistent meat inspections in slaughterhouses, as well as inadequate laboratory examination of organs with tuberculous alterations, may leave a dangerous window of infection for humans.

Infection Caused By *M. tuberculosis* in Domestic and Wild Animals

Another risk could be presented by the animals that have tuberculous lesions—found at the veterinary meat inspections—that are caused by *M. tuberculosis*. The

Table 15.3. Incidence of bacteriological confirmed *Mycobacterium tuberculosis* and *Mycobacterium bovis* infections in human populations in four Central European countries (18)

	Croatia				Czech Republic				Slovakia			
	M. tuberculosis		*M. bovis*		*M. tuberculosis*		*M. bovis*		*M. tuberculosis*		*M. bovis*	
Year	Abs.[1]	Rel.[2]	Abs.[1]	Rel.[2]	Abs.[1]	Rel.[2]	Abs.[1]	Rel.[2]	Abs.[1]	Rel.[2]	Abs.[1]	Rel.[2]/
1990	2576	55.0	0	0	1 505	14.5	7	0.07	1 191	22.7	2	0.04
1991	2158	45.0	0	0	1 549	14.9	6	0.06	1 197	22.7	1	0.02
1992	2185	46.0	2	0.04	1 420	13.8	8	0.08	1 180	22.6	0	0
1993	2279	48.0	5	0.10	1 222	11.8	4	0.04	1 139	22.4	1	0.02
1994	2217	46.0	2	0.04	1 161	11.2	3	0.03	1 165	22.5	0	0
1995	2114	44.0	0	0	1 188	11.5	1	0.01	961	17.9	2	0.04
1996	2174	45.0	1	0.02	1 095	10.6	2	0.02	849	15.8	1	0.02
1997	2054	43.0	1	0.02	1 047	10.2	1	0.01	783	14.5	0	0
1998	2118	44.0	0	0	1 065	10.3	1	0.01	744	13.8	0	0
1999	1770	37.0	0	0	0 999	9.6	3	0.03	651	12.9	0	0
Total	21,649		11		12,242		36		9860		7	

	Slovenia				Total No. of patients with tuberculosis caused by		
	M. tuberculosis		*M. bovis*				
Year	Abs.[1]	Rel.[2]	Abs.[1]	Rel.[2]	*M. tuberculosis*	*M. bovis*	%[3]
1990	419	22.1	0	0	5 691	9	0.16
1991	363	19.1	0	0	5 267	7	0.13
1992	388	20.4	1	0.05	5 173	11	0.21
1993	420	22.1	0	0	5 060	10	0.20
1994	334	17.6	0	0	4 877	5	0.10
1995	345	18.2	0	0	4 608	3	0.07
1996	423	22.3	0	0	4 541	4	0.09
1997	356	18.7	0	0	4 240	2	0.05
1998	346	18.2	0	0	4 273	1	0.02
1999	316	16.6	0	0	3 727	3	0.08
Total	3710		1		47 461	55	0.12

[1] Absolute number of bacteriological confirmed case.
[2] Relative number of bacteriological confirmed cases per 100,000 inhabitants.
[3] Percentage of patients infected with *M. bovis*.

detection of causal agent of human tuberculosis in animals was analyzed in six Central European countries (Croatia, the Czech Republic, Hungary, Poland, Slovakia, and Slovenia). In the monitoring period, 1990–1999, *M. tuberculosis* from animals was isolated only in two countries (Poland and Slovakia), from 16 animals with tuberculous lesions (11). These 16 animals comprise nine head of cattle (*Bos taurus*), four domestic pigs (*Sus scrofa* f. *domestica*), and three wild animals: an African elephant (*Loxodonta africana*), an agouti (*Dasyprocta aguti*), and a terrestrial tapir (*Tapirus terrestris*), originating from a zoological garden in Gdansk in Poland. In January 2004, one 5.5-year-old dog, after 4 months of contact with its owner, who was suffering open tuberculosis, was found to be infected with *M. tuberculosis* in the lung and mesenteric lymph nodes in the Czech Republic (unpublished data).

The steady decrease in the incidence of tuberculosis in humans was recorded during the monitoring period in all countries. The human population of the study countries was 68.03 million. In the period monitored, infection caused by *M. tuberculosis* was identified in a total of 241,079 patients, with a decreasing incidence of tuberculosis found in all countries. The lowest relative bacteriologically confirmed disease was found in the Czech Republic, Slovakia, and Slovenia. Given the low number of infected domestic and wild animals, the epidemiological and epizootiological situation may be considered auspicious (19).

However, domestic and wild animals kept in captivity are most frequently put at risk of infection from infected attendants or from visitors who feed animals with food often contaminated with their secretions, saliva, and nasal discharges. As people are most frequently infected with *M. tuberculosis,* they may act as the primary source of infection for animals in zoological gardens. In this way, animals kept, for example, in zoological gardens, national parks, and other establishments are put at risk of *M. tuberculosis* infection not only from attendants but also from visitors (18).

Conclusions

The epidemiological situation of bovine tuberculosis in animal and human populations could be considered as stable and promising. From tuberculous lesions from cattle, pigs, and other domestic and wild animals, other mycobacterial isolates (esp. *M. avium* species) than members of *M. tuberculosis* complex were received. Rarely, *Ma paratuberculosis* (a causal agent from paratuberculosis or Johne's disease) was isolated from tuberculoid lesions in mesenteric lymph nodes in the Czech Republic (6).

Paratuberculosis has become the most serious chronically bacterial infection for which prevalence is increasing following the socioeconomic and agricultural reforms that took place in the end of the 1980s in all Central European countries. Agricultural transformation brought about the disintegration of large-scale state and collectively owned farms into small holdings as a result of restitution of state-seized properties, especially in the Czech Republic, Hungary, Slovakia, and Slovenia. Previously, the countries restricted animal importation, but in the 1980s, the low paratuberculosis prevalence restrictions were lifted, giving way to the introduction of various purebred dairy and beef cattle from Western European countries with a relatively high prevalence of paratuberculosis (20).

References

1. Pavlik, I., J. Bartl, I. Parmova, M. Havelkova, M. Kubin, and J. Bazant. 1998. Occurrence of bovine tuberculosis in animals and humans in the Czech Republic in the years 1969 to 1996. *Vet Med* 43:221-31.
2. Pavlik, I., F. Bures, P. Janovsky, P. Pecinka, M. Bartos, L. Dvorska, L. Matlova, K. Kremer, and D. Van Soolingen. 2002. The last outbreak of bovine tuberculosis in cattle in the Czech Republic in 1995 was caused by *Mycobacterium bovis* subspecies *caprae*. *Vet Med* 47:251-63. Available at: http://www.vri.cz/docs/vetmed/47-9-251.pdf.
3. Pavlik, I., W. Y. Ayele, I. Parmova, I. Melicharek, M. Hanzlikova, B. Körmendy, G. Nagy, Z. Cvetnic, M. Ocepek, N. Fejzic, and M. Lipiec. 2002. Incidence of bovine tuberculosis in cattle in seven Central European countries during the years 1990-1999. *Vet Med* 47:45-51. Available at: http://www.vri.cz/docs/vetmed/47-3-45.pdf.
4. Pavlik, I., L. Dvorska, L. Matlova, P. Svastova, I. Parmova, J. Bazant, and J. Veleba. 2002. Mycobacterial infections in cattle in the Czech Republic during 1990-1999. *Vet Med* 47:241-50. Available at: http://www.vri.cz/docs/vetmed/47-9-241.pdf.
5. Dvorska, L., I. Parmova, M. Lavickova, J. Bartl, V. Vrbas, and I. Pavlik. 1999. Isolation of *Rhodococcus equi* and atypical mycobacteria from lymph nodes of pigs and cattle in herds with the occurrence of tuberculoid gross changes in the Czech Republic over the period 1996, 1998. *Vet Med* 44:321-30.
6. Dvorska, L., L. Matlova, M. Bartos, I. Parmova, J. Bartl, P. Svastova, T. J. Bull, and I. Pavlik. 2004. Study of *Mycobacterium avium* complex strains isolated from cattle in the Czech Republic between 1996 and 2000. *Vet Microbiol* 99:239-50.
7. Dvorska, L., M. Bartos, O. Ostadal, J. Kaustova, L. Matlova, and I. Pavlik. 2002. IS*1311* and IS*1245* restriction fragment length polymorphism analyses, serotypes, and drug susceptibilities of *Mycobacterium avium* complex isolates obtained from a human immunodeficiency virus-negative patient. *J Clin Microbiol* 40:3712-19.
8. Bartos, M., J. O. Falkinham III, and I. Pavlik. 2004. Mycobacterial catalases, peroxidases, and superoxide dismutase and their effects on virulence and isoniazid-susceptibility in mycobacteria. *Vet Med* 49:161-70. Available at: http://www.vri.cz/docs/vetmed/49-5-161.pdf.
9. Pavlik, I., M. Machackova, W. Y. Ayele, J. Lamka, I. Parmova, I. Melicharek, M. Hanzlikova, B. Körmendy, G. Nagy, Z. Cvetnic, M. Ocepek, and M. Lipiec. 2002. Incidence of bovine tuberculosis in domestic animals other than cattle and in wild animals in six Central European countries during 1990-1999. *Vet Med* 47:122-31. Available at: http://www.vri.cz/docs/vetmed/47-5-122.pdf.
10. Machackova, M., L. Matlova, J. Lamka, J. Smolik, I. Melicharek, M. Hanzlikova, J. Docekal, Z. Cvetnic, G. Nagy, M. Lipiec, M. Ocepek, and I. Pavlik. 2003. Wild boar (*Sus scrofa*) as a possible vector of mycobacterial infections: review of literature and critical analysis of data from Central Europe between 1983 to 2001. *Vet Med* 48:51-65. Available at: http://www.vri.cz/docs/vetmed/48-3-51.pdf.
11. Pavlik, I., L. Matlova, L. Dvorska, J. Bartl, L. Oktabcova, J. Docekal, and I. Parmova. 2003. Tuberculous lesions in pigs in the Czech Republic during 1990-1999: occurrence, causal factors and economic loses. *Vet Med* 48:113-25. Available at: http://www.vri.cz/docs/vetmed/48-5-113.pdf.

12. Matlova, L., L. Dvorska, M. Bartos, J. Docekal, M. Trckova, and I. Pavlik. 2004. Tuberculous lesions in pig lymph nodes caused by kaolin fed as supplement. *Vet Med* 49:379-88. Available at: http://www.vri.cz/docs/vetmed/49-10-379.pdf.

13. Matlova, L., L. Dvorska, J. Bartl, M. Bartos, W. Y. Ayele, M. Alexa, and I. Pavlik. 2003. Mycobacteria isolated from the environment of pig farms in the Czech Republic during the years 1996 to 2002. *Vet Med* 48:343-57. Available at: http://www.vri.cz/docs/vetmed/48-12-343.pdf.

14. Fischer, O., L. Matlova, J. Bartl, L. Dvorska, I. Melicharek, and I. Pavlik. 2000. Findings of Mycobacteria in insectivores and small rodents. *Folia Microbiol.* 45:147-52.

15. Fischer, O., L. Matlova, L. Dvorska, P. Svastova, J. Bartl, I. Melicharek, R. T. Weston, and I. Pavlik. 2001. Diptera as vectors of mycobacterial infections in cattle and pigs. *Med Vet Entomol* 15:208-11.

16. Pavlik, I., L. Dvorska, M. Bartos, I. Parmova, I. Melicharek, A. Jesenska, M. Havelkova, M. Slosarek, I. Putova, G. Martin, W. Erler, K. Kremer, and D. Van Soolingen. 2002. Molecular epidemiology of bovine tuberculosis in the Czech Republic and Slovakia in the period 1965-2001 studied by spoligotyping. *Vet Med* 47:181-94. Available at: http://www.vri.cz/docs/vetmed/47-7-181.pdf.

17. Erler, W., G. Martin, K. Sachse, L. Naumann, D. Kahlau, J. Beer, M. Bartos, G. Nagy, Z. Cvetnic, M. Zolnir-Dovc, and I. Pavlik. 2004. Molecular fingerprinting of *Mycobacterium bovis* subsp. *caprae* isolates from Central Europe. *J Clin Microbiol* 42: 2234-38.

18. Pavlik, I., W. Y. Ayele, M. Havelkova, M. Svejnochova, V. Katalinic-Jankovic, and M. Zolnir-Dovc. 2003. *Mycobacterium bovis* infection in human population in four Central European countries during 1990-1999. *Vet Med* 48:90-98. Available at: http://www.vri.cz/docs/vetmed/48-4-90.pdf.

19. Pavlik, I., W. Y. Ayele, I. Parmova, I. Melicharek, M. Hanzlikova, B. Körmendy, G. Nagy, Z. Cvetnic, V. Katalinic-Jankovic, M. Ocepek, M. Zolnir-Dovc, and M. Lipiec. 2003b. *Mycobacterium tuberculosis* in animal and human populations in six Central European countries during 1990-1999. *Vet Med* 48:83-89. Available at: http://www.vri.cz/docs/vetmed/48-4-83.pdf.

20. Kennedy, D. J. and G. Benedictus. 2001. Control of *Mycobacterium avium* subsp. *paratuberculosis* infection in agricultural species. *Rev Sci Tech Off Int Epiz* 20:151-79.

Chapter 16
Bovine Tuberculosis in Latin America and the Caribbean

V. Ritacco, MD, PhD, P. Torres, DVM, M.D. Sequeira, MSc, A. Reniero, PhD, and I.N. de Kantor, PhD

By 1992–1994, control measures for bovine tuberculosis (TB) based on a test-and-slaughter policy and disease notification were applied in 11 countries: Argentina, Uruguay, Paraguay, Peru, Venezuela, Cuba, Guatemala, El Salvador, Dominican Republic, and two Caribbean isles. The regional prevalence of bovine TB was at that time estimated to be 1% and higher in 67% of the total cattle population, and 0.1%–0.9% in a further 7% of the population; the remaining 26% were free of the disease or approaching the point of elimination.(1)

In 1998, of 34 Latin American and Caribbean countries, 12 had reported bovine TB as having sporadic/low occurrence (Brazil, Ecuador, Paraguay, Uruguay, Cuba, Mexico, Belize, Honduras, Nicaragua, Costa Rica, Montserrat, and Trinidad-Tobago), eight reported it as enzootic (Argentina, Chile, Bolivia, Peru, Venezuela, Guatemala, El Salvador, and Dominican Republic), and another 12 countries had not reported any bovine TB, among them Colombia, Panama, and several Caribbean isles. No data were available from Guyana and Surinam. Almost 76% of the cattle population was at that time—and continues to be—in countries where bovine TB is notifiable and a test-and-slaughter policy is used. Thus, approximately 24% of the cattle population in this region is either only partly controlled for bovine TB or not controlled at all (2). Cosivi et al. estimated that 60% of the human population lives in countries where cattle undergo no control or only limited control for bovine TB (2).

In 1999–2000, the Pan American Health Organization/World Health Organization (PAHO/WHO) conducted a survey on brucellosis and TB in domestic mammalian species including bovines, swine, and goats, recording information from 23 Latin American and Caribbean countries (3,4).

Table 16.1 presents information concerning the compulsory notification of TB in these species; this requirement has been established in most of these countries.

Control activities are based on tuberculin testing and veterinary inspection in official abattoirs, followed in certain cases by microbiological and histopathological confirmation of macroscopic lesions of suspected TB (5–9).

In 21 of the 23 countries included in the PAHO/WHO survey, tuberculin testing must be performed on cattle from herds either suspected or confirmed to be TB

Table 16.1. Compulsory notification of TB in bovines, swine, and goats (Source: PAHO/WHO survey, 2000) (3,4)

Subregion	Countries (No.)	Bovines	Swine	Goats
North America	1 (Mexico)	1	1	1
Central America	5	5	4	4
South America	12	10	6	3
The Caribbean	5	5	3	3
Total	23	21	14	11

infected, and 16 of these countries reportedly follow a test-and-slaughter policy on bovine positive reactors to the tuberculin test. Nevertheless, this policy may not be applied in all cases. At present, there are constrictions in the availability of purified protein derivatives (PPD). Several countries import the product from Europe (Netherlands). Other countries (Dominican Republic, Honduras, Mexico, Brazil, Uruguay, Paraguay, Colombia, Cuba, Argentina, and Venezuela) are producing this biological in official or private laboratories, in different amounts (7,8).

A national quality-control system is available at least in Brazil, Mexico, and Argentina. The Regional Reference Laboratory Control Service (Instituto Panamericano de Protección de Alimentos y Zoonosis, PAHO/WHO), as well as the production of reference bovine and avian PPD for the region, were discontinued in 1999. The Brazilian Reference Laboratory (Laboratorio Regional de Apoio Animal, Minas Gerais), produces the PPD batch used as the PAHO/WHO reference. The lab also performs external quality control of PPD batches produced by national laboratories in other countries of the region.

Significant differences in the units per dose, as required by the countries' national standards for the caudal bovine PPD test in cattle, were observed (Table 16.2), as well as diversity in the positivity criteria: in some countries, any reaction to the intradermal PPD is considered positive, whereas in others, a diameter of 2 mm or more—3, 4, or even 5 mm—are required for defining a positive reactor. Regional standardization is still lacking, and so is the comparability of results for different countries in the region (3,4).

Surveillance in Abattoirs

An adequate system of epidemiological surveillance and control starts with surveillance in abattoirs, with an infrastructure of services and sufficient personnel trained for detecting macroscopic lesions compatible with TB in the sacrificed livestock, and with a mechanism to correlate each lesion with the animal and herd of origin (6).

Official inspection exists and is currently working in at least 22 countries. In 16 countries, the process depends on the Ministry of Agriculture, and in the rest it depends on the Ministry of Health or on the provincial or other local authority. In most of the countries, there is only one veterinary inspector per establishment, except in abattoirs and meat processing plants for export, where the conditions are better. This situation limits the sensitivity of postmortem examination. Taking this into account, the estimated rates of TB lesions per 10,000 bovines killed could be higher than those presented in Table 16.3.

Table 16.2. International Units in 0.1 mL of bovine PPD, as required in 23 different Latin American and Caribbean Countries (PAHO/WHO survey, 2000)(3,4)

Countries (No.)	I.U. per Doses, in 0.1 mL
1	500
2	2500
7	3250
3	5000
1	10000
9	Not reported

Table 16.3. TB lesions in bovines sacrificed under official inspection: annual rates/10,000 animals, 1994–1998 (PAHO/WHO survey, 2000)(3,4)

Country	Rate/10,000
Argentina	220
Paraguay	32
Chile	31
Mexico	10
Nicaragua	0.4
Jamaica	0.3
Panama	0.25
Cuba	0.04

In Guyana, El Salvador, Brazil and Dominican Republic, lesions apparently caused by TB were only sporadically observed. Rates there reported were, respectively, 99, 57, 9, and 3 per 10,000.

Laboratory Confirmation of Macroscopic Diagnosis

The laboratory confirmation by culture, followed by the identification of *Mycobacterium bovis,* is a basic component in the surveillance of TB infection in bovines.

Samples of tissues collected from animals inspected or submitted to necropsy are sent to the laboratory for histopathological and bacteriological examination. In areas free of bovine TB, a number of samples suspicious for TB or selected at random are sent to the laboratory. When *M. bovis* is detected in a sample, a trace-back to the origin should be made, followed by tuberculin testing of all the animals and herds considered to be contacts. In Table 16.4, the number and results obtained in samples submitted from the slaughterhouse are presented. Differences in positivity rates can be appreciated. For Cuba, a country that is nearing the eradication of TB, the rate of *M. bovis* isolations from samples submitted was approximately 1.5/100,000, whereas in other countries, like Paraguay, the only sample examined in the laboratory resulted positive for *M. bovis.*

Table 16.4. Bacteriological confirmation of *Mycobacterium bovis* in samples collected at the veterinary inspection in abattoirs, 1994-98. (PAHO/WHO survey, 2000)(3,4)

Country	Samples (No.)	Cases of Samples with *M. bovis* Isolated by Culture
Chile	579	161
Mexico	—	174
Uruguay	8	3
Cuba	196 943	3
Colombia	—	338
Paraguay	1	1
Panama	94	7
Nicaragua	18	2
Dominican R.	—	33
Bolivia	16	—
Jamaica	3	0
Trinidad-Tobago	6	0

Coverage of Surveillance

In eight of 23 countries (3,4), surveillance for bovine TB has a national coverage, and in another six countries it is limited to regions administered by official services. Finally, another eight countries were not reported to have any surveillance system implemented.

Projects for Certified Free Herds

In Table 16.5 information is presented on the projects for herds certified to be free from bovine TB in the region.

TB-Free Herds, Regions and Countries

Cuba (nearly 4 million head of cattle) and Jamaica (nearly 300,000 head) are considered to be free of bovine TB. Panama (1.5 million head), which had achieved this category in 1994, suffered a reinfection (Province Boca del Toro, 1997), and new cases were still being detected in 2001. In South America, even though there

Table 16.5. Bovine tuberculosis in cattle. Projects for certification of free herds: Latin American and Caribbean Region (PAHO/WHO Survey, 2000) (3,4)

Subregion	No. of Countries Included in the Survey	No. of Countries with Projects
North America	1*	1
Central America	5	5
South America	12	8
The Caribbean	5	2
Total	23	16

* Mexico.

Table 16.6. Bovine tuberculosis—free populations by regions or countries: Latin America and The Caribbean, 2000 (PAHO/WHO,3,4)

Subregion	Country/Zone	Free Population (Cattle)
The Caribbean	Jamaica	370,000
	Cuba	4,643,656
South America	Paraguay (J. E. Estigarribia)	49,295
	Venezuela (Cañada de Urdaneta, Zulia)	127,272

are not TB-free countries registered, there are TB-free zones: J.E. Estigarribia, in Paraguay, and Cañada de Urdaneta, Zulia State, in Venezuela (Table 16.6). Uruguay (11 million head), where control activities in dairy herds started at the beginning of the 1960s and a national campaign was launched in July 1996, is near achieving eradication.

Three groups of countries can be considered according to the information currently available (10): first, countries with prevalence less than 0.1% or null (Caribbean: Anguilla, Antigua, Bahamas, Barbados, Bermuda, Virgin Islands, Dominican Republic, Grenada, Guadeloupe, St. Kitts-Nevis, St. Lucia, St. Vincent-Grenadines, Trinidad-Tobago, Jamaica, and Cuba; Central America: Panama, Costa Rica, Honduras, and Belize; South America: Colombia, Surinam, Paraguay, Uruguay, and Venezuela); second, countries with a prevalence between 0.1 and 1.0% (only Dominican Republic in the Caribbean); and third, countries with prevalence greater than 1%, or with no information available (North America: Mexico; Caribbean: Haiti; Central America: El Salvador, Guatemala, and Nicaragua; South America: Argentina, Bolivia, Brazil, Chile, Ecuador, Peru, and Guyana).

Current Status of Infection and Programs

Central America

In the Central American countries (8), there is an increasing cooperation between PAHO/WHO, OIRSA (Regional Cooperation Agency), Universities and Ministries of Agriculture, specially in training activities, addressed to veterinary and laboratory professionals to improve diagnosis of animal brucellosis and TB.(10)

Dominican Republic (2.4 million cattle) started a national program for brucellosis and TB eradication in 1973. By 2001 the prevalence of tuberculin reactors was 0.36%, scattered around the country, which makes eradication quite difficult.

Costa Rica (1.4 million cattle) restarted the national program for brucellosis and TB eradication in 1999, in coordination with official authorities and cattle breeders associations, with the aim of achieving a brucellosis- and TB-free status. In 2001, 1.5% of 6969 animals that were tuberculin tested resulted in positive reactors.

Guatemala (2.1 million cattle) has suffered a weakening in the official veterinary services structure in the last decade. No recent information on TB infection status is available, mainly because of a shortfall in PPD supplied for tuberculin testing. PPD was previously imported from the United Kingdom, but this importation was discontinued for sanitary reasons.

Nicaragua (1.8 million cattle) also suffered a weakening in the official veterinary services similar to that of Guatemala. The Brucellosis and TB National Program started in 1998. In the first tuberculin survey, 0.45% of cattle tested resulted positive. It is now projected that Ometepe Island, in the Nicaragua Lake, with some 3000 cattle, will be declared free of brucellosis and TB.

Panama (1.5 million cattle) is the first country in Central America close to attaining a TB- and brucellosis-free status. Active epidemiological surveillance is based mainly on the control of cattle movement and disinfections. The polymerase chain reaction technique is being evaluated alongside conventional diagnostic methods for its potential use in the last stages of eradication. The National Direction of Animal Health, created in 1997, is in charge of sanitary campaigns for brucellosis, TB, and rabies eradication. TB infection was detected in 19.3% of cattle herds and in 0.61% of individual animals tested in 2001, restricted to Boca del Toro province on the Costa Rican border.

El Salvador (1.2 million cattle) started a national program for brucellosis and TB control in 1994, in coordination with cattle producers' associations. Even though 19% of herds were reported as being TB infected in the last decade, the rate of infected animals was low (0.7%). This situation of dispersion of the infection without achieving high rates of incidence has also been observed in Guatemala and Nicaragua (6).

North America

Mexico

In Mexico, with a cattle population composed of 29.5 million beef cattle and 1.2 million dairy cattle, eight states are in phase II (eradication)—North Baja California, Chihuahua, Coahuila, Durango, Nuevo Leon, Sonora, Tamaulipas, and Yucatan—and another nine states are in phase I—South Baja California, Colima, Jalisco, Nayarit, Quinatana Roo, San Luis de Potosí, Sinaloa, Tabasco, and Zacatecas (8,11).

TB infection seems to be confined to certain areas of the country, and particularly to dairy cattle. Several recent publications confirmed *M. bovis* in dairy cattle and also showed a very low prevalence in beef cattle from the northern states.

In Queretaro, from 1201 carcasses reviewed at slaughter, 17% presented gross TB lesions, of which 79% were positive for isolation of *M. bovis*. Most affected animals were females more than 2 years old. (12)

In samples received from Mexico and processed in the United States, *M. bovis* was identified by polymerase chain reaction in 32.6% of the samples of milk from 460 animals and in 56.2% of the nasal swabs ($n = 121$) from tuberculin-positive cattle (13).

In other investigations, tissue specimens with apparent TB lesions were collected during routine inspection at slaughterhouses. *M. bovis* was confirmed in 16% of 2500 cattle carcasses. Most cattle were adult females from large dairy herds and were not included in the Mexican TB control program (14).

In the situation in beef cattle, the TB control program has obtained important achievements in the northern states of Mexico. In an evaluation of TB prevalence, performed in Texas, on a sample of 65,000 adult beef cattle originating from different states in Mexico, it was concluded that overall prevalence of TB in adult beef cattle was approximately 0.5/1000, ranging from 0.07/1000 in cattle from Chihuahua to 1.81/1000 in cattle from Tamaulipas (15).

In a previous study conducted in Baja California to estimate the annual prevalence of TB in beef and dairy cattle, about 200,000 (95% beef, 5% dairy) cattle were examined postmortem, and apparent TB lesions were submitted to laboratory confirmation. Prevalence of TB in all slaughtered cattle was 0.12% and 0.46% in 1995 and 1996, respectively (beef cattle, 0.02% and 0.05%, respectively; dairy cattle, 2.0% and 8.3%, respectively) (16).

South America

In South America, Argentina, after some achievements in the control of Foot and Mouth Disease (1999–2000) has reformulated official rules and requirements to strengthen the campaign to control bovine TB (17,18). In Brazil, a second *Regulations Manual for the National Program, Control, and Eradication of Animal Brucellosis and Tuberculosis* was published in January 2001 (19).

Argentina

Out of the 53.5 million head of cattle that constitute the bovine population in Argentina, approximately 3 million are dairy cattle (20,21). The major milk-production areas of the country are located in the so-called "wet pampas," which include the Santa Fe and Buenos Aires provinces, where spatial clusters of bovine TB are found.(22)

Even before the launching of specific control policies, a decline was observed in the prevalence of bovine TB, probably resulting from modernization in farming management. In the period from 1969 to 2002, for an average of 10 million bovines annually killed in slaughterhouses and submitted to veterinary inspection, the percentage of animals suffering condemnation because of apparent TB lesions decreased from 6.7% to 1.3% (Fig. 16.1). Between March 1995 and February 1997, a survey was conducted among the 160 slaughterhouses with Federal Inspection, all over the country. Data collected from the 126 establishments that answered the questionnaire showed that 1.35% of 9.5 million cattle suffered condemnation caused by apparent TB lesions. TB condemnations were found in all regions, confirming that TB is widely distributed.

Only since 1999 has a compulsory program been implemented aimed to eliminate TB, based on test-and-cull strategies with no official compensation for culled animals. Since then, 3455 farms holding 1.2 million head have been officially declared free of the disease. Ninety percent of these TB-free animals belong to dairy herds (18), and the number of TB-free herds increased from 44 in 1995 to 3455 in 2003 (Fig. 16.2).

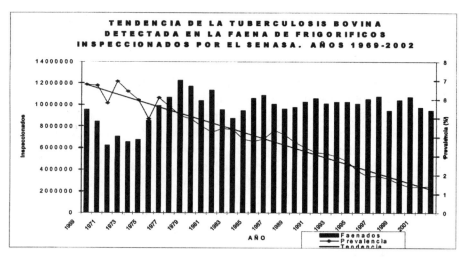

Figure 16.1. Argentina: trends of slaughterhouse condemnations, in percentage of cattle seizures for tuberculosis. Official veterinary inspection in abattoirs, SENASA, 1969–2002. Bars: cattle carcasses, submitted to official inspection, in millions. Values ranged between 6 and 12 million animals, indicated in the right scale. Points and black line indicate prevalence of animals with condemnations because of tuberculosis, in percentages of the total number submitted to the inspection, and its trend. Percentages decreased from near 7% in 1969 to 1.4% in 2002.

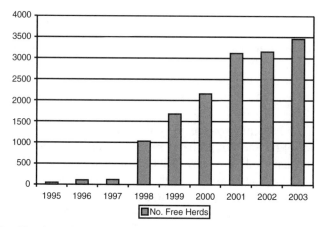

Figure 16.2. Number of herds free from bovine tuberculosis, Argentina, 1995–2003. (Source: SENASA, January 2004).

According to slaughterhouse condemnation, a parallel decline was observed in the prevalence of swine TB (Table 16.7). For an annual number ranging between 1.5 and 1.7 million carcasses inspected at slaughterhouses, the percentage of animals with condemnations varied between 8.4% in 1969 and 0.7% in 2002. The bovine bacilli are the mycobacteria most frequently isolated, and swine lesions are mainly found in the lymph nodes of the digestive tract, indicating that infection is acquired by the oral route (23). Hence, it can be inferred that in Argentina—in contrast

Table 16.7. Condemnations resulting from tuberculosis at slaughterhouses with federal inspection: Argentina 1990–1995–2000 (18)

Year	Cattle		Swine	
	Carcasses Examined (n)	With Tuberculous Lesions (%)	Carcasses examined (n)	With Tuberculous Lesions (%)
1990	10,280,981	3.44	1,327,274	4.40
1995	10,100,398	2.22	1,916,247	2.93
2000	9,480,492	1.79	1,783,349	0.78

with what is observed in many developed countries—bovine cattle are still the most probable source of mycobacterial infection for swine as a result of the practice of feeding hogs nonpasteurized dairy products (1).

Brazil

Harboring 182 million head of cattle, Brazil launched a nationwide program of control of TB in 2001 (Tables 16.8 and 16.9; 19,24). Compensation for culled cattle has been officially granted, and training courses for accredited veterinary doctors are being organized. Remarkably heterogeneous farming conditions challenge the endeavor throughout the country. In addition, the epidemiological situation regarding TB is uncertain in a vast part of the territory. The program proposes a stratification of areas and the design of different strategies according to the level of TB infection.

Table 16.8. Tuberculin skin testing of cattle: Brazil 1994–1998

Year	Herds		Animals	
	n	% positive	n	% positive
1994	16,974	4.0	411,904	0.9
1995	15,242	3.3	372,600	0.7
1996	19,061	4.3	454,108	0.8
1997	14,162	5.7	356,698	1.0
1998	14,464	7.1	343,441	1.3

Table 16.9. Tuberculin skin testing of cattle by region: Brazil 1998

Region	Herds		Animals	
	n	% Positive	n	% Positive
Northern	24	58.3	8,531	2.3
Northeastern	395	17.0	13,288	3.6
Southeastern	4,496	6.8	193,931	0.8
South	9,195	6.8	119,004	1.9
Central-Western	354	2.8	8,687	0.5
TOTAL	14,464	7.1	343,441	1.3

In 1999, in Minas Gerais state, 63,000 bovines from 1600 herds were tuberculin tested, recording an apparent prevalence of 0.8% (4). To assess the situation in this state, a statistically significant sample was designed in 2000 involving 1586 herds and 22,990 animals throughout the state. In such a study, 5% of the herds and 0.8% of the animals were infected according to tuberculin skin testing results (25). In another study, a total of 1632 animals from 13 dairy farms were tested, using the single cervical tuberculin test. Among those animals, about 15% of each herd, or 220 cattle in total, were positive. (26)

Chile

The total cattle population in Chile is 4.1 million head. During the 1990s, the Agricultural and Livestock Service developed a program of "certified free herds," particularly focused on dairy cattle, in the south. In 2000, with a new approach to the problem, a panel on which both the official and the private sectors were represented decided to implement a national program for bovine brucellosis and TB control on the basis of a feasibility analysis prepared by the Agricultural and Livestock Service. In 2001, out of 133 slaughterhouses existent in the country with official veterinary inspection, only 78 have a full-time inspection service. Mainly, efforts are being addressed to guarantee food hygiene in meatpacking plants (7,8).

Paraguay

Paraguay holds around 10 million head of cattle, 9% of which are dairy cattle. In 2000, 70,000 tuberculin tests were performed in cattle, detecting 650 positive animals (0.9%). In 2001 and 2002, the results of tuberculin skin testing were officially recorded in 16 out of the 18 districts of the country. Of nearly 11,000 animals investigated, positive tuberculin tests were detected in only 76 animals from 10 districts. In both consecutive years, the mean infection rate was 0.7%, ranging from 0% to 2.8%. No recent information is available on condemnation at slaughter (7,8).

Venezuela

Harboring nearly 4 million head of cattle, Venezuela is one of the South American countries with very low prevalence of TB infection in cattle (<0.1%). There is good continuity in the surveillance activities, based on meat inspection and tuberculin surveys performed by the caudal fold test. These surveys covered nearly 1,000,000 cattle annually, from 1989 to 1999 (7,8).

References

1. Kantor I.N. and V. Ritacco. 1994. Bovine tuberculosis in Latin America and the Caribbean: current status, control and eradication programs. *Vet Microbiol* 40:5-14.
2. Cosivi, O., J. M. Grange, C. J. Daborn, M. C. Raviglione, T. Fujikura, D. Cousins, R. A. Robinson, H. F. Huchzermeyer, I. de Kantor, and F. X. Meslin. 1998. Zoonotic

tuberculosis due to *Mycobacterium bovis* in developing countries. *Emer Inf Dis* 4: 59-70.

3. OPS/OMS. Brucelosis y tuberculosis (*Mycobacterium bovis*). Situación de los Programas en las Américas. Centro Panamericano de Fiebre Aftosa. Enero 2000.

4. OPS/OMS. Sistema Continental Integrado de Infecciones de Brucelosis y Tuberculosis en Zoonosis. Informe Semestral. Centro Panamericano de Fiebre Aftosa, 2000.

5. PAHO/WHO. Current status of bovine tuberculosis in Latin America and the Caribbean. Pan American Zoonoses Center, Buenos Aires, 1991.

6. PAHO/WHO. Plan of Action for the Eradication of Bovine Tuberculosis in the Americas. Phase I. HPV/TUB/113/92, Washington DC, 1992.

7. OPS/OMS. Reunión de Directores de Servicios de Sanidad Animal. Informe Final, San Salvador, 10-11 Julio 2001.

8. OPS/OMS. Seminario Taller de Vigilancia en Tuberculosis Bovina, Informe Final. Santa Cruz de la Sierra, Bolivia, Julio 2001.

9. PAHO/WHO. II Reunião Paises do Cone Sul, Tuberculose e Brucelose. Belo Horizonte. Gonçalves VS, Garin A, Cubillos V, Gutierrez-Pabello JA, Torres P. Situaçao dos Programas de Controle e Erradicaçao da Tuberculose Animal do Brasil, Uruguay, Chile, México e Argentina Mina Gerais, Brasil, 2002.

10. Cotrina, N. 2001. Meeting of Animal Health Directors, San Salvador, July 10-11, 2001; PAHO/WHO.

11. Secretaría de Agricultura, Ganadería y Desarrollo Rural. Proyecto de Norma Oficial Mexicana NOM-031-ZOO-1995, Campaña nacional contra la tuberculosis bovina (*Mycobacterium bovis*). Diario Oficial, 28 abril 1995, 12-32, primera sección. Diario Oficial 8 de enero 1996, 25-50.

12. Milian, F., L. M. Sanchez, P. Toledo, C. Ramirez, M. A. Santillan. 2000. Descriptive study of human and bovine tuberculosis in Queretaro, Mexico. *Rev Latinoam Microbiol* 42:13-9.

13. Sreevatsan, S., J. B. Bookout, F. Ringpis, V. S. Poumaalla, T. A. Ficht, L. Garry Adams, et al. 2000. A multiplex approach to molecular detection of *Brucella abortus* and/or *Mycobacterium bovis* infection in cattle. *J Clin Microbiol* 38:2602-10.

14. Milian-Suazo, F., M. D. Salman, C. Ramirez, J. B. Payeur, J. C. Rhyan, and M. Santillan. 2000. Identification of tuberculosis in cattle slaughtered in Mexico. *Am J Vet Res* 61:86-9.

15. Brown, W. H. and J. Hernandez de Anda. 1998. Tuberculosis in adult beef cattle of Mexican origin shipped direct-to-slaughter into Texas. *J Am Vet Med Assoc* 212:557-9.

16. Hernandez de Anda, J., T. Renteria Evangelista, G. Lopez Valencia, and M. Montano Hodgers. 1997. An abattoir monitoring system for diagnosis of tuberculosis in cattle in Baja California, Mexico. *J Am Vet Med Assoc* 211:709-11.

17. Secretaría de Agricultura. SENASA. Sub Comisión Nacional de Tuberculosis Bovina. Manual de Normas y Procedimientos. Anexo I (Resol. 1287/93), Buenos Aires, 1993.

18. Torres, P. Situación de la tuberculosis bovina en la República Argentina. SENASA, Buenos Aires, 2002.

19. Departamento de Defesa Animal. 2001. Programa Nacional de Controle e Erradicaçao da Brucelose e da Tuberculose (PNCEBT). Available at: http://www.agricultura.gov.br.

20. FAO-OIE-WHO. 2003. Information on cattle population for different countries.

21. Secretary Agriculture, Direction of Animal Health. 2003. Information on cattle population. Buenos Aires, Argentina.

22. Perez, A., M. Ward, P. Torres, and V. Ritacco. 2002. Use of spatial statistics and monitoring data to identify clustering of bovine tuberculosis in Argentina. *Prev Vet Med* 56:63-74.

23. Perez, A., R. Debenedetti, M. Martínez Vivot, A. Bernardelli, P. Torres, and V. Ritacco. 2002. Tendencia de la tuberculosis porcina y validez de la inspección bromatológica para su detección en áreas de producción intensiva de Argentina. *Rev Med Vet* 83: 14-18.
24. Ministerio da Agricultura e do Abastecimiento. Boletím de Defesa Sanitária Animal Edicǎo 2001 Vol 30 Dez 1998. Brasilia DF, Brasil.
25. Cunha Belchior, A. P. 2001. Prevalencia, distribuçao regional e fatores de risco de tuberculose bovine en Minas Gerais. Universidade Federal de Minas Gerais. Escola de Veterinaria. Programa de Pos-Graduaçao.
26. Lilenbaum, W., J. C. Schettini, G. N. Souza, E. R. Ribeiro, E. C. Moreira, and L. S. Fonseca. 1999. Comparison between a gamma-IFN assay and intradermal tuberculin test for the diagnosis of bovine tuberculosis in field trials in Brazil. *Zentralbl Veterinarmed B* 46:353-58

Chapter 17

The Status of *Mycobacterium bovis* in India

R. Verma, MSc, MVSc, PhD

The Indian Veterinary Research Institute (IVRI) has played a major role in bovine tuberculosis research. Bovine tuberculosis (TB) in cattle was considered a rare disease in India until 1916. The increase in the incidence of bovine TB in India since that time raises some important questions as to whether this low incidence of tuberculosis was the result of the relatively high resistance of the indigenous breed of cattle, a low virulence of infective organisms, or merely the natural limitations on the spread of the disease resulting from the husbandry practices of cattle in India.

Dr. M. B. Soparkar arrived at IVRI in 1923, and facilities were placed at his disposal to work on TB. In 1925, the Board of Agriculture in Pusa, India, passed a resolution providing authority to conduct research on bovine TB. The Indian Research Fund Association provided funds to institute a Bovine Tuberculosis Enquiry to be undertaken by Dr. Soparkar. The enquiry identified the following objectives to determine the susceptibility of bovines to TB in India: the virulence of strains of tubercle bacilli isolated from natural bovine lesions in India, the diagnostic reliability of TB by tuberculin testing, and the types of tubercle bacilli responsible for the disease in man and in animals in India.

A preliminary experiment was conducted between 1923 and 1924 on the relative susceptibilities of bovine bacillus on the indigenous breeds in comparison with a known European breed. Twelve calves, consisting of hill cattle, Plains cattle of the desi breed (mixed Hariana and Gangaparu breeds), and buffalo calves, were artificially infected. The results of this experiment showed that buffaloes were more resistant than the bovine/ox calves. However some of the ox calves of both breeds were found to exhibit nearly as high a degree of susceptibility as that possessed by the average British calf. The information about animal TB in India has been reviewed in greater detail by Verma and Gupta (1).

Additional TB information has been generated on the basis of postmortem examination and tuberculin testing of herds in various farms in different parts of India. The data generated by these two surveillance methods over a period of years confirmed that TB infection existed not only in cattle but also in different animal species. India is endowed with great genetic diversity in animals, and as such there is a wide range of animals infected with tubercle bacilli in both domesticated and wild

161

animal populations. Interest also remains in determining the type of tubercle bacilli found in humans and animals in view of zoonotic concerns. With the limited availability of media and conventional methods, mycobacteria were typed traditionally. The diagnostic procedures of *Mycobacterium bovis* in veterinary medicine have now been largely improved in the IVRI laboratory with the use of molecular techniques including polymerase chain reaction (PCR) assays, restriction fragment length polymorphism, random amplified polymorphic DNA, species-specific allele PCR assays, and PCR amplification of IS*6110* in paraffin-embedded tissue.

Incidence

Cattle and Buffaloes

Information at a glance on the occurrence of TB in animals, gathered from the published reports of slaughterhouse animal examinations, is provided in Table 17.1.

Tuberculin was standardized for subcutaneous use in cattle by the single intradermal test (SID) (2). This test was replaced by the double intradermal test (DID),

Table 17.1 Occurrence of TB in animals in India

Sl. No.	Species of Animal Examined	No. of Animals Examined	Percentage Positive for TB	State or Province of India	Year of Reports
1.	Cattle	416	17.54%	Punjab	1917
2.	Animals	1586	4.8%	Bombay	1927
3.	Cattle	614	16%	Punjab and Uttar Pradesh	1927
4.	Animals	1116	22.85%	Lahore (undivided India)	1931
5.	Bullock	1	1%	—	1932
6.	Buffaloes	250	2.4%	Uttar Pradesh	1932
		120	13.3%	Bombay	1944
		130	2.3%	Calcutta	1944
7.	Buffaloes	754	1.45%	Uttar Pradesh	1966
8.	Swine	100	37%	West Bengal	1097
9.	Swine	143	13%	Tamil Nadu	1975
10.	Cattle	1268 (from 1974 to 1984)	13.25%	Uttar Pradesh	1985
11.	Buffaloes	4010	0.24%	Punjab	1957
12.	Buffalo calves	603	1%	Haryana	1987
13.	Buffalo	2028	17 (0.84%)		1998
14.	Buffaloes	2028	0.84%	Assam	1998
15.	Cattle	141	59.57%	Uttar Pradesh	1998
16.	Cattle	1050	7.14%	Kolkatta	2001
16.	Cattle	3600 samples of lungs	0.97%	Kolkatta	2002

or Comparative Cervical Test, on the recommendation of the British Tuberculin Committee of the Medical Research Council (1925). Under field conditions in India, it was difficult to follow up on the animals for a second injection and for the final reading, and therefore tuberculin testing with SID was standardized, and a final reading was taken at 72 hours postinjection. A total of 20,197 cattle were tested both by DID and SID tests, using synthetic heat concentrated tuberculin prepared from synthetic media from three human strains of *Mycobacterium tuberculosis* (P_w, D_t, and C). Analysis of the data showed that SID was equally good but that the doubtful cases should be tested by the DID test. These tests on both cattle and buffalo farms showed that the percentage of reactors varied from herd to herd depending on the spread of the infection. There were a number of herds that were free of infection, whereas other herds had up to 30%–55% tuberculin reactors. The number of tuberculin tests conducted at different period of times is summarized in Table 17.2.

Sheep

Until 1932, not a single case of caprine or ovine TB was reported. However, the Royal Commission on Human and Animal Tuberculosis (1907) (2) reported that goats were susceptible to bovine bacilli. Iyer (8) reported six (0.64%) cases out of 943 goats examined postmortem (9). Eleven female and three male goats (0.87%) of 602 carcasses examined had TB lesions (10). Seven (3.7%) of 180 sheep at Breeding Farm in Guttal, Bombay, and 12 (6.3%) of 191 sheep at the Sheep Breeding Farm in Poona, India, showed doubtful or positive reaction to the tuberculin test (11). One sheep out of 222 belonging to Uttar Pradesh and Himachal Pradesh tested with the DID tuberculin test showed one reactor (12). Histopathological lesions of TB were also reported in sheep by Manisha et al.(13).

Goat

In India, there was a common view that goats were either immune to TB or free of TB, which prompted Unani and Ayurvedic physicians to prescribe goat's milk as a remedy for TB in the human subject, causing this view to gain public acceptance. The Royal Commission on Human and Animal Tuberculosis (1907), however, indicated that goats are also susceptible to even small doses of tubercle bacilli of bovine types. In 1932, Iyer (8), for the first time, detected the presence of TB in six (0.64%) of 943 goats examined, followed by a report of TB in goats in 1943 by Nanda and Gopal (14), as well as many others.

Horse

Four specimens from horses were diagnosed for TB by histopathological examination at IVRI between 1924 and 1954. It was observed that TB was not common among horses in India. However, the findings of TB lesions in the larynx and epiglottis of horses showing symptoms of roaring were especially noteworthy (1936–1937). A survey was conducted to find out the incidence of TB in 166 horses

Table 17.2. Results of tuberculin testing in animals in India[a]

Name of State and Place of Testing	Year	Species	Number Tested	Positive Reactors	Percentage (Reactors)
Andhra Pradesh					
Hyderabad					
Himalayatsagar	1953–1954	Cattle	—	—	4.14
Aurangabad		–do–	—	—	2.9
Bihar					
Patna	1952–1953	Cattle	14,705	232	1.6
Patna	1957–1958	Bovines	466	41	8.8
Gujarat					
Ahmedabad	1946–1947	Cattle	6521	1061	16.3
Saurashtra and Kutch	1956–1957	Buffalo	5558	1404	25.3
		Bovines	400	4	1.0
India					
All over the country (Organized Farms)	1967	Cattle, young adult	999	4	0.4
		buffaloes	3295	79	2.39
			87	0	0.0
			1211	83	6.85
Jammu and Kashmir					
All over the state	1956–1957	Bovines	1470	77	5.27
Kerala					
Kerala	1956–1957	–do–	61	1	1.64
Madhya Pradesh					
Jabalpur	1950–1951	Bovines	399	1	0.25
Jabalpur	1965–1971	Cattle	—	—	3.2
		Young adult buffalo	—	—	3.9
All over the state		Young adult bovines	—	—	0.99
		Cattle	—	—	15.5
		Buffaloes	1471	30	1.35
			359	23	6.40
Maharashtra					
Poona	1941–1943	Cattle buffaloes	200	0	0.0
Bombay	1944	Cattle and buffaloes	120	16	13.3
Bombay	1953–1957	Bovines	3000	180	6.0
Bombay	1956–1957	Cattle	38	0	0.0
Government Farms	1985		1820	24	1.6
Mysore					
Mysore	1957–1958	–do–	60	0	0.0
Pondicherry[5]					
—	2001	Cattle	41	21	51.2
Punjab					
Lahore	1946–1947	Cattle	3550	431	12.1
PEPSU	1956–1957	Bovines	1052	72	6.8

(Continued)

164

Table 17.2. *continued*

Name of State and Place of Testing	Year	Species	Number Tested	Positive Reactors	Percentage (Reactors)
Organized Farm	1976	Buffaloes	328	15	4.37
Rajasthan					
Goshala and Pinjrapole	1953–1954	Cattle	—	—	3.09
Organized farms	–do–	–do–	—	—	0.82
All over the state	1954–1955	–do–	—	—	2.16
All over the state	1969	Cattle and	1010	14	1.36 (20% in buffaloes)
Tamilnadu					
Madras	1941	Bovines and cattle	203	0	0.0
Madras	1957	Young adult buffalo	5817 / 11146	92 / 158	1.582 / 1.12
Madras	1957–1958	Young adult bovines	2141 / 4479	32 / 150	1.49 / 3.35
Organized dairy farm	1983	Cattle	142 / 2600	0 / 60	0.0
Uttar Pradesh					
Izatnagar	1944	Buffaloes	250	6	2.4
Allahabad	1953–1954	Cows	—	—	1.98
Mukteshwar	1957–1958	Buffaloes	—	—	0.0
Izatnagar	–do–	Bovines	175	0	0.0
Bareilly and Rampur[6]	1968	–do–	615	81	0.19
		Buffaloes	—	—	0.19
West Bengal					
Calcutta	1944	Buffaloes	130	3	2.3
Calcutta	1958	Bovines	1072	182	17

*Source: Chauhan et al. (3), with added recent references Iyer (4), Mukhopadhaya (5), Rathore and Singh (6), Tomar and Tripathi (7)

of the Mounted Military Police, Bihar, using a DID tuberculin test; of these animals, the scientists found nine to have quite distinct reactions. A further study on the incidence of tuberculin reactors in horses using mammalian and avian tuberculin obtained by the IVRI in Izatnagar was made by Singh and Kuppuswamy (15), in which 38 reactors were found, of 87 horses tested (34 reacted to mammalian and four to both avian and mammalian tuberculin), and seven of these animals were positive to the intradermal tuberculin test.

Dog

Ajwani and Venkataraman (16) described the first case of TB in dogs in a six-year-old female. The smears and histopathological sections made from the liver, hepatic lymphatic glands, kidneys, and lungs showed acid-fast bacilli. No attempt to isolate the organisms could be made as a result of the fixation of the material in formalin. Eight of 35 dogs tested were positive on the tuberculin test, and one was a doubtful reactor. Postmortem examinations of four positive dogs revealed lesions in kidneys and liver, except in one dog, which did not show any lesions. An Alsatian dog with an apparent acute respiratory condition was diagnosed radiographically to have a case of pericarditis with massive effusion. Necropsy later confirmed the case as tuberculous pericarditis (17).

Camel

Of 802 camels, seven had a positive reaction and four had a suspicious reaction with tuberculin; two had a positive reaction and one a suspicious reaction with avian tuberculin. Two reactor camels were destroyed, and lesion material from one of them showed the presence of tubercle bacilli (IVRI). Tuberculous lesions taken from bullocks showed bovine-type tubercle bacilli. The report of the Disease Investigation Office in Punjab, India, reported eight animals (4.5%) as positive reactors among 178 camels tested during 1966–1967. The incidence of TB in camels in Bikaner was reported as 2.6% (18).

Pig

Examination of 245 pigs at a slaughterhouse in Bombay showed suspicious lesions of TB in 98 pigs. Samples from 25 of 98 pigs subjected to a biological test (guinea pigs, rabbits, and poultry; IVRI) were positive. Datta (19) found that 4% of slaughtered pigs had TB (20). Bombay, Jullunder, and Rawalpindi reported 17.7%, 5.3%, and 7.4% TB infection in slaughtered pigs. Tuberculous bronchopneumonia in 6-month-old piglets was reported by Rao and Venkatanaryanan (21). One hundred pigs were examined at Tangra Pig Slaughter House in Calcutta to detect the incidence of TB in pigs. Of 11 pigs found to be positive to the tuberculin test, eight reacted to mammalian tuberculin and three to avian tuberculin. Thirty-seven pigs of the total 100 examined after slaughter had gross lesions in different lymph nodes, including one that had foci in the lungs and spleen that were indicative of TB. Mycobacteria were isolated from both tuberculin-positive and tuberculin-negative pigs. Sadana (22) detected TB in 11 of 2187 pig carcasses in Delhi, Haryana, and Punjab. Three of these animals showed lesions in the lungs and lymph nodes, and in the remaining pigs, only bronchial and mediastinal lymph nodes were involved.

Genital TB

The involvement of uterus, horns, salpinx, endometrium, or other cases of generalized TB involving genital organs has been reported in India. A case of metritis and genital TB in buffalo (23) have been reported. Two of 230 uteri from slaughtered bovines showed TB infection. Acid-fast bacilli were demonstrated in lentil sizes, glistening nodules containing yellowish mucoid exudates present on uteri and uterine horns. One and a half percent of the uteri from 64 cattle examined during postmortem showed TB. Rajkhowa (24) reported uterine TB in crossbred

Jersey cows. Whether the cow was infected from an infected bull or during contaminated artificial insemination has not been determined. Tuberculous endometri-
tis with involvement of the salpinx was reported. Genital TB was reported in both
a pregnant and a nonpregnant cow. Congenital transmission of TB in calves also
has been reported. There appears to be one report of urogenital TB in a 6-year-old
breeding Tharparkar bull, in which lesions of TB were present in prostrate gland
and testicles (25). *M. bovis* has been reported in bovine semen (26), but there probably is no report on the tuberculous infection of the ovaries in India. Cases of generalized TB in cows and congenital transmission to their calves were reported. A
study comprising 13 reactor cows and their calves, which died of TB, indicated that
TB of the udder and uterus is more prevalent and that prenatal infection from cattle infected with generalized TB may be a strong possibility (27).

Semen

One of 20 semen samples of one of three breeding bulls tested was shown by PCR
amplification to be positive, followed by Southern hybridization of the target sequence from the IS*1081* element of *M. tuberculosis* complex (26). This implies that
semen can be a potential source of TB.

Tuberculous Mastitis

Mills (28) reported the first case of tuberculous mastitis in a tuberculin-positive
cow, which later revealed typical tuberculous lesions in the lungs and udder. Six
hundred seventy-four milk samples were tested for the presence of TB. Forty-seven
(7.6%) showed the presence of acid-fast bacilli, but tubercle bacilli could not be
demonstrated by animal inoculation. Similar negative findings by animal inoculation were reported in 100 cow milk samples and milk samples from reactor cows
of all ages. A number of laboratories failed to demonstrate the presence of acid-fast
bacilli by guinea pig inoculation in milk samples obtained from the tuberculin-
positive reactors at Amritsar. However, lesions were reported in a buffalo calf with
generalized TB. Cases of TB lesions in the udder were further reported in other
articles (29); described a case of tuberculous mastitis in a Sahaiwal cow caused by
bovine-type organisms affecting one-quarter of the udder, leaving a caseous type
of mastitis. Singh and SenGupta (30) stated an overall 0.5% incidence of tuberculous mastitis in their review. Impression smears prepared from affected mammary
glands and inguinal and supramammary lymph nodes were positive for acid-fast
bacilli. Incidence of tuberculous mastitis in buffalo has also been reported (31).

No Visible Lesions

Virulent tubercle bacilli were isolated from the material of a reactor to subcutaneous tuberculin, but no naked-eye lesions were detected on slaughter (Datta[19]).
Twenty-one (16 cows, 2 buffaloes, 2 sheep, and 1 goat) of 3000 animals positive
to the tuberculin test were slaughtered. Only one cow had detectable lesions of TB

(32). Of 136 cattle positive for tuberculin, 65 (47.79%) cases revealed gross lesions of TB. Seventy-five of 77 cattle negative for tuberculin had lesions of TB (33).

First Level Infection Due to Bovine Bacilli in Humans

The experimental investigation showed that most of the cases of glandular and surgical TB of man in India were caused by infection with the human type of bacilli. The researchers involved failed to demonstrate the bovine type of bacilli in 100 cases of surgical TB. Soparkar (34) investigated 65 patients, 40 of which had cervical adenitis, 8 axillary gland TB, and 17 pulmonary disease, as well as 20 cases of glandular TB in children under 16 years of age. In no case was a bovine bacillus detected, and it was believed to play no important role in the causation of human TB in India. Tables 17.3 and 17.4 provide a summary of the investigation of *M. bovis* in humans and *M. tuberculosis* in animals.

Human Infection Caused By *M. tuberculosis* Complex

A 25-year-old woman developed a cervical lesion after the consumption of unpasteurized raw milk. A biopsy from a potato-sized cervical nodule and a milk sample of the cow both yielded *M. bovis* on culture. PCR on biopsy material using

Table 17.3 *M. bovis* in humans

SI. No.	Year	No. of Cultures Investigated	Finding(s)
		Human Infection Due to *M. bovis*	
1.	1927	90	*2 M. bovis*
2.	1932	60	None
3.	1936	26	None
4.	1942	62	None
5.	1946	21	None
6.	1942–1967	71	None
7.	1987	1	*M. bovis*
8.	2001	25	None

Table 17.4 *M. tuberculosis* in animals

SI. No.	Year	Source	Finding(s)	Reference
1.	1969	Cattle	*M.tuberculosis*	Chandrasekaranand Ramakrishnan[36]
2.	1987	Cattle	*M.tuberculosis* (niacin variant)	Verma et al.[37]
3.	1993	Captive wild herbivores	*M.tuberculosis*	Chakraborty et al.[38]
3.	2001	Cattle	*M. tuberculosis*	Verma and Srivastava[39]

IS*1081* for *M. bovis* showed a positive result on Southern hybridization. Both *M. bovis* isolates were found to be identical on genetic fingerprinting with a conserved insertion sequence, thus supporting a possible milk-borne infection (35); Table 17.3. This is probably an authentic report of the zoonotic spread of bovine TB.

Animal Infection Caused By *M. tuberculosis*

Distribution of *M. bovis* and *M. tuberculosis*

The information in Tables 17.5 and 17.6 shows the type of tubercle bacilli isolated and identified from different animals and humans.

The above reports indicate that the incidence of TB in humans in India resulting from the bovine tubercle bacilli is probably low but needs to be more thoroughly investigated by both medical and veterinary laboratories. This may be a result of the generally nonprogressive form of the disease in indigenous cattle and

Table 17.5   From 1942 to 1967 (Lall[12])

	Number of Cultures	Type of Tubercle Bacilli	
Source		Bovine	Human
Human beings	71+1*	1*	71
Pigs	22+4*	4+3*	16+1*
Cattle and buffaloes (mostly buffaloes)	40+1*	40	1*
Camel	1+1*	1+1*	—
Giraffe	1	—	—
Sheep and goats	5	5	—
Dogs	6	—	6
Monkey	2	—	2
Chimpanzee	1	—	1
Deer	1*	1*	—

* Indicates culture identification other than IVRI

Table 17.6   From 1987 to 1999 (Verma and Srivastava[39])

Animal Species	Sample	No	Positive	Percentage Positive	Mycobacteria Isolated
Bovine	Lung	24	11	45.8	*M. bovis* (7), *M. tuberculosis* (4)
Bovine	Lymph nodes	17	10	58.8	*M. bovis* (8), *M. tuberculosis* (2)
Bovine	Lung and lymph node	03	03	100	*M. bovis* (2), *M. tuberculosis* (1)
Swine	Lung	02	01	50	*M. tuberculosis* (1)
Black buck	Lymph node	02	01	50	*M. bovis* (1)
Total		48	26	54.16	

the universal practice of boiling milk before consumption by humans. There are also reports that indirectly report the possibility of zoonosis of *M. bovis*. A small survey simultaneously carried out in both men and animals in Hoogly District of Calcutta, India, showed a large number of human TB cases where tuberculin reactor animals were housed. Throat swabs from 60 reactors of 2600 cattle were subjected to the tuberculin testing, and 16 cultures were isolated. Two of the 16 cultures were identified as *M. tuberculosis*. Chest radiography of 35 animal attendants at the farm showed lung lesions in eight attendants (40). However, the fact that cattle and buffaloes may act as maintenance hosts for *M. bovis* should not be ignored. Hence, TB in cattle, if not eradicated, will continue to be a risk for human health in India.

Control

In India, the eradication plan proposed aimed at building up a clean herd and later clean areas by following a test-and-segregation policy, with slaughter in clinical cases (20). Krishnaswamy (40), using a tuberculin test and segregation of reactors, could reduce the prevalence of TB in a dairy herd of 150 cows from 20% to nil in a period of 2.5 years. The reasons for choosing a test-and-segregation policy in India may be that a high percentage of tuberculin-positive animals exist in several areas, that their wholesale destruction may reduce both working bullocks used as power for agricultural operations and milk animals, and that this may adversely affect the economy of Indian agriculture. Sahai conducted a postmortem examination of 324 tuberculin reactor indigenous breed cattle at the government cattle farm, Hisar, where the infection rate was very high (20.22%), and he found that the lesions of indigenous cattle were not severe—the lesions in the majority of these cases were confined to the mediastinal and bronchial lymph nodes.

Polding compared the course of the disease in European calves with that in Hariana calves. He found that a dose of *M. bovis*, which generally produced the progressive form of the disease in calves of European breeds, was insufficient to set up a similar type of the disease in Hariana calves. Lall autopsied 12 tuberculin-positive indigenous cattle and found that 11 of those animals had only localized lesions in the bronchial or mediastinal or suprapharyngeal lymph nodes. Cultures of tubercle bacilli isolated from these animals were found to conform to the characters of *M. bovis*. These reports indicate that a large percentage of tuberculin-positive animals of indigenous breeds do not develop a rapidly progressive form of the disease. The lesions found in Indian cattle were generally localized and restricted to a few lymph nodes, although cases showing generalized lesions have been reported occasionally.

According to the report of the National Commission on Agriculture (1976), an all-India project for the control of TB was prepared in 1962 by the Indian Council of Agriculture Research (ICAR) and was approved by the planning commission, who recommended a phased program for the control of TB among animals that would not interfere with the agricultural economy and normal progress of the animal industry.

Phase I—Systematic control of TB on organized farms. The test-and-slaughter policy would be most suitable for making farms free from TB. However, for economic and technical reasons and in consideration of the public against destruction of tuberculin-reactor cattle and buffalo that may otherwise look healthy, a test-and-segregation policy may be followed. In other species of animals (e.g., pigs, goats, and poultry) in which the extent of infection is low, only the test-and-slaughter policy is advocated.

Phase II—Extension of the control program to cover animals in the entire country. Phase III—Final eradication program. At this stage the test-and-slaughter policy should be followed, with payment of compensation for the animals destroyed.

To date, there has been no change in the above policy.

References

1. Verma, R., and B. R. Gupta. 1990. *Animal Tuberculosis*. Izatnagar: Indian Veterinary Research Institute, 34-37.
2. Royal Commission on Human and Animal Tuberculosis. 1907.
3. Chauhan, H. V. S., P. Dwivedi, S. S. Chauhan, and D. S. Kalra. 1974. *Indian J Tub* 16:103.
4. Iyer, P. K. R. 1944. *Indian J Vet Sci* 10:271-275.
5. Mukhopadhaya, H. K., P. X. Antony, and R. M. Pillai. 2001. *Indian J Anim Hlth* 40:185-186.
6. Rathore, B. S. and N. P. Singh. 1968. *Indian J Anim Hlth* 8:85-87.
7. Tomar, S. S. and V. N. Tripathi. 1987. *Indian Vet J* 64:683-688.
8. Iyer, P. K. R. 1932. *Indian J Vet Sci* 11:41-48.
9. Nanda, P. N., and S. Karnail. 1944. *Indian J Vet Sci* 14:110-111.
10. Mohan, R. 1950. *Indian Vet J* 27:153-157.
11. Singh, G. 1951. Rep. I.C.A.R. Scheme for the investigation of tuberculosis and Johne's disease in animals, New Delhi.
12. Lall, J. M. 1969. *Vet Bull* 39:385-390.
13. Manisha, M., D. Hemant, G. D. Sharma, M. Mathura, and H. Dadhich. 2000. *Indian J Vet Pathol* 24:117-118.
14. Nanda, P. N., and S. Gopal. 1943 *Indian J Vet Sci* 13:70-74.
15. Singh, C. D. N. and P. B. Kuppuswamy. 1971. *Indian Vet J* 48:432-433.
16. Ajwani, G. A. and A. R. Venkataraman, 1932-1933. *Indian Vet J* 9:211.
17. Balasubramnian, N. N. M. S. Dewan, M. Mohammed, A. Sundararaj, and D. S. Reddy. 1990. *Indian Vet J* 67:259-260.
18. Jatkar. 1977. *Camel Disease in India*. Calcutta: Scientific Book Agency.
19. Datta, S. C. A. 1934-1935. *Indian Vet J* 11:93-98.
20. Dhanda, M. R., and J. M. Lall. 1959. *Indian Vet J* 36:467-472.
21. Rao Panduranga, P. and Venkatnarayanan. 1965. *Indian Vet J* 42:655-658.
22. Sadana, J. R. 1975. Ph.D. Thesis submitted to HAU, Hisar.
23. Katoch, R. C., S. Madhumeet, S. Verma, V. K. Gupta, and M. Sharma. 2004. *Indian Vet J* 81:216-217.
24. Rajkhowa, T. K. 2002. *Indian J Vet Pathol* 27:47.
25. Bhambhani, B. D. 1969. *Indian Vet J* 46:1023-1027.
26. Ahmad Niyaz, A. S., J. R. Khan, and M. A. Ganai. 1999. *Anim Reprod Sci* 57:15-21.

27. Rao Appaji, V. N., E. D. Rajaraman, and R. Manickam. 1995. *Indian Vet J* 72:523-525.
28. Mills, B. 1898-1899. *Ann Admn Rep Civil Vet Dept India*, 144.
29. Singh, G., G. Prasad, and B. R. SenGupta. 1956. *Indian Vet J* 32:330-335.
30. Singh, G. and B. R. SenGupta. 1957. *Indian Vet J* 34:183.
31. Nighot, P. K., O. P. Paliwal, and R. Kumar. 1996. *Indian J Vet Pathol* 20:23-26.
32. Nain, S. P. S. and R. K. Kaushik. 1985. *Indian J Anim Sci* 55:877-878.
33. Sharma, A. K., P. R. Vanamaya, O. P. Paliwal, T. P. Parai, and N. S. Parihar. 1987. *Indian Vet J* 64:711-712.
34. Soparkar, M. B. 1925. *Rep. Imperial Inst Vet Res Mukteswar*, 40-42.
35. Ahmad Niyaz, A. S., V. K. Batish, S. Grover, and R. C. Mittal. 1998. *Indian Vet J* 75:1034-1035.
36. Chandrasekharan, N. and R. Krishna. 1969. *Indian J Tub* 16:103.
37. Verma, R., A. K. Sharma, P. R. Vanamaya, P. N. Khana, I. H. Siddiqui, and B. R. Gupta. 1987. *8th Annual Conference of the Indian Association of Vety. Microbiol. Immunol. Inf. Dis. H.A.U.,* Hissar, 21-23 December, p. 68.
38. Chakraborty, A., B. Chaudhury, and D. K. Sarma. 1993. *Indian J Comp Microbiol Immunol Infect Dis* 18:147-152.
39. Verma, R., and S. K. Srivastava. 2001. Indian J Anim Sci 71:129-132.
40. Krishnaswamy, K. V. and K. R. Mani. 1983. *Indian J Publ Hlth* 27:60-63.

Chapter 18

Bovine Tuberculosis in Russia and the Former States of the Soviet Union

I. Pavlik, DVM, MVDr, CSc

Introduction

Data on bovine tuberculosis were analyzed from the available literature originating from the former Soviet Union, which has an area of 22,275, 858 km^2, with a total of 289.102 million inhabitants (in 2002), and where 74,437,315 head of cattle were kept in 2003. From the historical, political, demographic, and political view, this area can be divided as follows (Table 18.1): Baltic countries (Estonia, Latvia, and Lithuania) lying on 175,015 km^2, with 7.132 million inhabitants and 1,428,739 head of cattle; Russian Federation lying on 17,075,200 km^2, with 144.082 million inhabitants and with 43,000,000 head of cattle; and the remaining 11 former USSR countries (Armenia, Azerbaijan, Belarus, Georgia, Kazakhstan, Kyrgyzstan, Moldavia, Tajikistan, Turkmenistan, Ukraine, and Uzbekistan) lying on 5,025,643 km^2, with 137.888 million inhabitants and 30,008,576 head of cattle.

The above-mentioned 11 countries of the former USSR can be divided from the geographic, demographic, and political points of view, according to Ravilone et. al (1), into the following three groups: European countries (Belarus, Moldavia, and Ukraine), lying on 845,143 km^2, with 63.112 million inhabitants and 12,215,253 head of cattle; Central Asian countries (Kazakhstan, Kyrgyzstan, Tajikistan, Turkmenistan, and Uzbekistan), lying on 3,994,400 km^2, with 58.230 million inhabitants and 14,239,075 head of cattle; and Caucasian countries (Armenia, Azerbaijan, and Georgia), lying on 186,100 km^2, with 16.546 million inhabitants and 3,554,248 head of cattle.

Bovine Tuberculosis in Cattle in the Baltic Countries

On the basis of the official statistical OIE data over the period 1996–2003, all three Baltic countries (Estonia, Latvia, and Lithuania) can be considered to be free of bovine tuberculosis. The last outbreaks of bovine tuberculosis in Estonia, Latvia, and Lithuania were reported in 1986, 1989, and 2001, respectively (Table 18.1). In the human population, the epidemiological situation of lung tuberculosis in man is complicated predominantly by the incidence of *Mycobacterium tuberculosis* in

Table 18.1. Bovine tuberculosis in cattle in the former USSR

Geographic region	Country Area[a] (km²)	Population mil.[b]	No. of cattle[c]		Year[d] (year of the last reported occurrence of the disease)								Total
					1996[e]	1997[f]	1998[g]	1999[h]	2000[i]	2001[j]	2002[k]	2003[l]	
Baltic countries	Estonia 45,226	1.338	260,000	Outbreaks	1986	0	0	0	0	0	0	0	0
				Cases	0	0	0	0	0	0	0	0	0
	Latvia 64,589	2.329	389,639	Outbreaks	1989	0	0	0	0	0	0	0	0
				Cases	0	0	0	0	0	0	0	0	0
	Lithuania 65,200	3.465	779,100	Outbreaks	0	1	+?	1	+?	1	0	0	3
				Cases	0	17	NA	1	NA	1	0	0	19
Russia Federation	17,075,200	144.082	43,000,000	Outbreaks	712	593	186	140	145	78	71	87	2,012
				Cases	53,800	38,926	31,501	23,031	22,300	13,500	6,600	12,300	201,958
Former USSR countries	Armenia 29,800	3.072	514,244	Outbreaks	+	0	NA	NA	1	1	1	NA	3
				Cases	NA	0	NA	NA	32	48	16	NA	96
	Azerbaijan 86,600	8.297	1,934,422	Outbreaks	25	12	7	NA	0	0	+?	3	47
				Cases	249	381	33	NA	0	0	NA	9	672
	Belarus 207,600	9.940	3,924,100	Outbreaks	NA	52	13	NA	7	18	3	3	96
				Cases	NA	4,497	1,595	NA	711	803	285	166	8,057
	Georgia 69,700	5.177	1,105,582	Outbreaks	2	NA	NA	NA	3	3	3	2	13
				Cases	64	NA	NA	NA	10	3	28	8	125
	Kazakhstan 2,717,300	16.469	4,854,600	Outbreaks	NA	NA	NA	NA	NA	11	11	NA	22
				Cases	NA	NA	NA	NA	NA	1,090	1,079	NA	2,169
	Kyrgyzstan 198,500	5.067	988,016	Outbreaks	NA	NA	NA	1	1	NA	+	NA	2
				Cases	NA	NA	NA	400	80	33	NA	NA	513
	Moldavia 33,843	4.270	404,853	Outbreaks	1	0	2	1	+	0	0	0	4
				Cases	316	0	NA	NA	NA	0	0	0	479
	Tajikistan 143,100	6.195	1,131,459	Outbreaks	9	NA	7	2	NA	NA	6	1	25
				Cases	24	NA	70	15	NA	NA	25	232	366
	Turkmenistan 488,100	4.794	1,967,300	Outbreaks	1992	NA	NA	NA	0	NA	NA	NA	0
				Cases	0	NA	NA	NA	0	NA	NA	NA	0
	Ukraine 603,700	48.902	7,886,300	Outbreaks	139	144	100	67	55	69	29	27	630
				Cases	31,666	28,749	21,395	14,425	10,373	11,367	7,076	6,043	131,094
	Uzbekistan 447,400	25.705	5,297,700	Outbreaks	21	7	6	10	NA	NA	2	NA	46
				Cases	2,286	256	184	492	NA	NA	143	NA	3,361

aOfficial data from Index Mundi: http://www.indexmundi.com.

bOfficial WHO data from 2002: http://who.int.

cNo. of cattle in 2003 originated from OIE, 2004 (World Animal Health in 2003. Part 2, OIE, Paris), the data about the size of cattle population in Armenia, Kyrgyzstan, Moldavia, and Uzbekistan originated from OIE, 2003 (World Animal Health in 2002. Part 2, OIE, Paris) and data about the size of cattle population in Russia originated from FAO-OIE-WHO, 1997 (Animal Health Year Book 1995. Rome: FAO).

dNo. of outbreaks and infected cattle with bovine tuberculosis originated from official data from OIE.

eOutbreaks in 1996 originated from Handistatus: http://www.oie.int/hs2/help.asp.

f1997-2003 originated from OIE (1998-2004): OIE, 1998: World animal health in 1997. Part 2, OIE, Paris.

gOIE, 1999, World animal health in 1998. Part 2, OIE, Paris.

hOIE, 2000, World animal health in 1999. Part 2, OIE, Paris.

iOIE, 2001, World animal health in 2000. Part 2, OIE, Paris.

jOIE, 2002, World animal health in 2001. Part 2, OIE, Paris.

kOIE, 2003, World animal health in 2002. Part 2, OIE, Paris.

lOIE, 2004, World animal health in 2003. Part 2, OIE, Paris.

NA: No information available.

+: reported present or known to be present.

+?: serological evidence or isolation of the causal agent, but no clinical signs of disease.

175

middle-aged men of lower classes (2) and by the relatively frequent finding of multidrug-resistant (MDR) strains (3,4).

Bovine Tuberculosis in Cattle in the Russian Federation

A systematic control of bovine tuberculosis started in the Russian Federation in 1959, when the diagnostic methods were unified and an extensive examination of cattle by skin testing started. In 1950, 1.16% of the examined cattle were found to be positive, with great differences among the examined regions. Gradually, they managed, with the strong support of the government, to reduce positive cases to 0.08% of skin-tested animals by 1960. The increase of positive findings to bovine tuberculin, which appeared as a result of the failure of the sanitation program and a shortage of noninfected animals, reached 1.34% in 1964 and was resolved by an aggressive approach taken by all the responsible institutions, as follows (5):

1. All "isolation farms" were dissolved, and all animals positive to bovine tuberculin were immediately slaughtered.
2. In calves from dams positive for bovine tuberculin, feeding was finished, and then the animals were slaughtered at slaughterhouses (they were not further used for breeding).
3. The infected animals were, before dispatching to slaughterhouses, housed and provided with drinking water under safety conditions to prevent spreading *Mycobacterium bovis* in the environment.
4. In autumn, the infected farms were provided with equipment (special tractors, trucks, etc.) that enabled disinfection, or with manure composting to prevent spreading of the causative agent of bovine tuberculosis.
5. On farms where during winter animals infected with *M. bovis* were found, a 10–15-cm layer of soil was removed; the subsoil was then disinfected, based on a standard method, and was covered with noncontaminated soil.
6. On 38 farms with high incidence and prevalence of *M. bovis*, radical (stamping out) methods had been used for control of the infection, when about 10,000 healthy animals from noninfected regions of eastern and western Siberia were imported.

The above measures resulted in 1968 in drop of animals positive to bovine tuberculin to 0.77% of all skin-tested animals (5). Economic losses in some herds were extremely high, especially on farms where culling rate reached 56.7% (6).

Over the 8 years period of investigation (1996–2003), bovine tuberculosis was diagnosed in 2012 outbreaks, with 201,958 heads of cattle. Dating from 1996, a dramatic decrease was observed, from 712 recorded outbreaks then to 71 recorded outbreaks in 2002 (Table 18.1). At present, human tuberculosis in Russia is particularly complicated by the occurrence of MDR *M. tuberculosis* strains, which were recorded in the Ivanovo and Tomsk regions (7).

Complications at Allergenodiagnostics

In Latvia, nonspecific reactions to bovine tuberculin were observed during sanitation to get the herds from bovine tuberculosis. In 1963–1964, changes typical for tuberculosis were found in 41 (9.7%) of 425 slaughtered animals that reacted positively to bovine tuberculin, and isolated changes only in lymph nodes were found in 39 (9.2%) animals. Of the remaining 345 animals without pathological lesions, *Mycobacterium sp.* was isolated from lymph nodes in 32 of 81 animals selected at random. Using biological tests on guinea pigs, rabbits, and chickens, nonpathogenic bacteria were demonstrated in 20 animals, *M. bovis* in five, *Mycobacterium avium* in four, and *M. tuberculosis* in three (8).

Risk Factors Causing New Outbreaks of Bovine Tuberculosis in Cattle

Sanitation of cattle farms to eradicate bovine tuberculosis was, in the 1960s and 1970s, accelerated in all parts of the Russian Federation by the following procedures (9):

1. Clinically suspected animals that often did not react to the skin testing were systematically discarded to slaughterhouses or "isolation farms".
2. Extensive skin testing of all cattle, using bovine tuberculin, had been performed twice a year.
3. Test-positive animals were sent to the "isolation farms."
4. Only young cattle from tuberculosis-free farms had been purchased.
5. A minimal contact system of calf rearing with infected mothers and a minimal stay in the infected stable had been introduced.
6. On the infected farms, a system of antiepidemic measures including preventive management in livestock breeding, animal hygiene, manure processing, staff hygiene, and so on was introduced.

These procedures enabled us to control bovine tuberculosis on several farms within 3 years, and in the Vologodsk region, the 16.5% prevalence of bovine tuberculosis dropped to 0% in 1967. However, in the following decades new incidence of bovine tuberculosis in cattle was recorded on several farms, and anamnestic analysis of 17 outbreaks in cattle were performed (9). On two farms (11.8%) *M. bovis* had been introduced into a herd of purchased young breeding animals, on one farm (5.9%) *M. bovis* had been introduced by open herd turnover, and on 14 farms (82.3%) the infection appeared without being introduced to a herd ("spontaneous" outbreak). In these cases the reason might be infected animals kept in the time of existing outbreaks (a long incubation period), long-term persistence of the causative agent of bovine tuberculosis in the environment (insufficient disinfection), or the presence of latently infected animals in a herd.

While studying the significance of latently infected animals, lymph nodes without tuberculous pathological anatomic lesions from 170 animals reacting positively to bovine tuberculin were culture examined. *M. bovis* was isolated from 84 (49.4%) animals in a biological trial on guinea pigs. A subsequent study of the virulence of those isolates in guinea pigs and rabbits showed a decreased virulence compared to the isolates originating from cattle with tuberculous pathological lesions. As low positivity at skin testing (from 0.4% to 24.8%) was found in infected calves originating from farms with bovine tuberculosis, those calves represent a high risk for farms free from bovine tuberculosis. After the incubation period of 2–3 years, these animals can become a new source of *M. bovis* (9).

The source of *M. bovis* infection for animals can also be—in herds free from bovine tuberculosis—an infected person; on cattle farms, above all, the milkmaids, feeders, keepers, calf attendants, and herdsmen. The infection of the genitourinary system caused by *M. bovis,* with a lengthy course without clinical signs or excretion of *M. bovis* via urine, is considered to be the most dangerous. Such infected people, without hygienic awareness, can become a source of infection for cattle (10).

Bovine Tuberculosis in Humans in the Russian Federation

In the Soviet Union, among 2719 isolates from patients with tuberculosis (particularly the pulmonary form) *M. bovis* was isolated from 6.4% patients, predominantly children (11).

In the Kurgansk region, 88%–93% of inhabitants were examined by x-ray in the period 1973–1976 in village counties that were infected or free from bovine tuberculosis. It was found that in counties where no bovine tuberculosis was diagnosed in cattle, the morbidity rate in humans was 2.5-fold lower compared with that in counties with infected cattle farms. In the counties with *M. bovis*–infected cattle herds, 33.0%–54.6% of tuberculous patients came from farms with *M. bovis*–infected cattle. In contrast, significantly ($P < .05$) fewer patients came from farms with free herds. Concurrent with x-ray examination, in 14,000 inhabitants of the Kurgansk region, skin testing with a human tuberculin (2 TU *pro dosi*) had been carried out, and human tuberculin, simultaneous with bovine tuberculin (2 TU *pro dosi*), was applied to another 5100 persons during the above period of 4 years. In village counties with an occurrence of bovine tuberculosis in cattle, sensitivity to human tuberculin was found in persons of all age categories to be higher by 20%–25% ($P < .01$) when compared to the regions free from bovine tuberculosis in cattle. The level of human tuberculosis was in correlation with the level of *M. bovis* infection in cattle ($r = 0.85$). A sensitivity to bovine tuberculin 5.7 times higher was observed in workers on cattle farms who were infected with bovine tuberculosis, compared to workers on farms free from bovine tuberculosis (12).

Anamnestic Data about Humans Infected with Bovine Tuberculosis

Of isolates obtained from 1163 patients over the period 1974–1976, 197 (16.9%) were identified as *M. bovis*. The following conclusions were made from anamnestic data and laboratory examinations of the 197 patients (12).

First, a total of 184 (93.4%) patients suffered from lung tuberculosis. In 64.7% of these patients, the infiltrative to fibrous-cavernous process prevailed; in 66.0%, it was the destructive process, and in 13 (6.6%) patients, extrapulmonary tuberculosis was found. In 92 (46.7%) patients, tuberculosis was diagnosed for the first time, and in 105 (53.3%) patients, tuberculosis had previously been diagnosed (2–20 years ago). The patients were aged 17–70 years, with a significant prevalence of women who were working predominantly as milkmaids and cattle attendants on farms infected with bovine tuberculosis. The patients worked on cattle farms with bovine tuberculosis as attendants (45%), as machinery operators in agricultural co-operatives (21%), or as other workers in agriculture (15%); 10% were retired people or household women, and 9% came from the cities. The patients from the southern part of the above region were 3.4 times more often infected with *M. bovis* than were those from the northern part, which correlated with the level of cattle infection with the causative agent of bovine tuberculosis ($r = 0.76$). Finally, *M. bovis* was isolated in those patients from sputum, urine, punctures of the peripheral lymph nodes, and pleuropneumonial fluid.

In western Siberia, an incidence of tuberculosis was found to be 1.5 times higher in villagers than in city inhabitants. Epidemiological analysis of human tuberculosis in villages showed that the incidence of tuberculosis was 1.5–2.0 times higher in villagers possessing cattle infected with bovine tuberculosis than in those with noninfected cattle. Interestingly, this situation was found in regions with a prevailing agricultural production, as well as in regions with a prevailing industrial production (13).

The Most Important Risk Factors

One of the major causes of increased incidence of tuberculosis in humans was permanent occurrence of bovine tuberculosis in cattle on farms and the existence of the so-called "isolation farms." Cattle from the neighboring farms that were positive in the skin testing performed twice a year with bovine tuberculin, within sanitation, were gathered on the "isolation farm." Cattle on those farms were used (milked or calved). It was found that as early as 1981, all "isolation farms" were dissolved in this region, and the number of animals that tested positive to bovine tuberculosis had decreased during the past 5 years to 46.7%, and the number of outbreaks of bovine tuberculosis in cattle decreased to 40.0%. In spite of that, tuberculosis in workers on farms with bovine tuberculosis in cattle was diagnosed twice as frequently as in workers on noninfected cattle farms, and three times more frequently than in adults who did not work in agriculture. *M. bovis* was isolated in the Novosibirsk region in 7.2% of tuberculous patients, and in 9.5% of patients in the Omsk region. The frequency of tuberculosis in humans caused by *M. bovis* was two times higher in inhabitants of regions with an occurrence of bovine tuberculosis in cattle compared to those from regions free from bovine tuberculosis (13).

While studying the anamnestic data about tuberculous patients on farms with infective animals, a considerable sanitary–hygienic unawareness in those patients was found. Therefore, the causes of a higher incidence of tuberculosis in those farm workers could have been infection with *M. bovis* as well as the effect of the stressing environment massively contaminated with the agent of bovine tuberculosis. It was also found that in villages with farms on which bovine tuberculosis had been controlled, a more frequent x-ray diagnosis helped to control lung tuberculosis in humans. X-ray diagnosis was carried out once every 3 years for all inhabitants and twice a year for farm workers. Extrapulmonary tuberculosis was found by intradermal skin testing carried out in both children and adults (13).

Therapy of Bovine Tuberculosis in the Human Population

Monitoring of patients with tuberculosis caused by *M. bovis* shows that a progressive and torpid course of the infection had been observed, and the sensitivity of *M. bovis* isolates to antibiotics was monitored. Primary resistance was found in 17% of isolates, which was 2.2 times more frequent than in *M. tuberculosis* isolates. *M. bovis* isolates were resistant to first-line treatment. Therefore, antituberculosis drugs of the first line, together with Rifadin and ethambutol, were prescribed to those patients (12).

It was found that clinical signs in patients infected with *M. bovis* were more severe, and efficiency of therapy was lower, compared with the patients infected with *M. tuberculosis*, and mortality of patients infected with *M. bovis* was three times higher, healing of caverns was less frequent by 22.8%, and shedding of *M. bovis* could also be stopped 25.1% less frequently (12).

Bovine Tuberculosis in Other Animal Species than Cattle

Sheep and goats were considered to be greatly resistant to *M. bovis* or *M. tuberculosis* infections. In different regions of Kazakhstan 1728 sheep were examined by skin testing with bovine tuberculin, of which 17 (1.0%) animals tested positive, and of 772 examined goats, eight (1.0%) animals tested positive. In sheep originating from cattle farms where bovine tuberculosis had been diagnosed, prevalence of infection was two times higher. After slaughtering of 4960 sheep in different slaughterhouses of the region, tuberculous lesions were found in 429 (8.7%) animals. *M. bovis* was demonstrated in one sample only by cultivation of 440 samples of pathological material. After infection of guinea pigs with *M. bovis*, the agent was demonstrated in all samples. Study of the distribution of pathological lesions in 40 sheep revealed lung tuberculosis in 35 animals, with a tendency to exudation and a simultaneous infection of bronchi in 17 animals (epidemiological risk connected with *M. bovis* shedding). In addition to those findings, in three sheep with lung tuberculosis, caseous lesions were found in liver, which represents the risk of shedding the causative agent of bovine tuberculosis through bile into the intestinal tract. Therefore, sheep and goats had to be taken into consideration in the outbreaks of bovine tuberculosis in cattle while preparing the control measures (14).

In the tissues of 21 Maral deer with tuberculous lesions in their lungs, pulmonary lymph nodes, and submandibular, retropharyngeal, and mesenteric lymph nodes, *M. bovis* was demonstrated by culture in 17 animals. As different virulence levels were found in particular isolates that were tested on guinea pigs and rabbits, subcutaneous, oral, or contact infection with *M. tuberculosis* and *M. bovis* strains was carried out (15,16).

In Leningrad in the 1920s and 1930s, organ tuberculosis was detected by postmortem in 5.5% of 1089 dogs and in 3.5% of 1017 cats (17,18). Between 1960 and 1970, postmortems were performed in the same workplace in 1695 dogs, and organ tuberculosis was detected in one (0.06%) of them. Among 535 of dissected cats, organ tuberculosis was detected in four (0.74%) of them (18,19).

Occurrence of *M. bovis* in Milk and the Environment

The employees from farms of cattle infected with the causative agent of bovine tuberculosis, and the inhabitants of the regions with infected cattle, were exposed to various sources of *M. bovis*. Milk from infected cows was considered as the most common source. Among 164 pool samples of milk from cows kept in farms with the occurrence of bovine tuberculosis, *M. bovis* was isolated from five (3.1%) samples (12).

Farm workers (particularly milkmaids, cowmen, veterinarians, animal husbandry men, etc.) were exposed to *M. bovis* that was found in stables and the external environment of the infected cattle farms. *M. bovis* was detected in five (41.7%) of 12 samples of manure and in one (5.6%) of 18 scrapings of stable walls (12). In the soil of a pastureland, in the region of the Barabinska lowland, a strain of *M. bovis* was detected and was fully virulent for guinea pigs, surviving for 23 months (the entire period of investigation). Using experiments with guinea pigs, rabbits, and cattle fed with grass from naturally or artificially contaminated pastures, researchers have demonstrated the possibility of *M. bovis* transmission through grass. These conclusions were obtained by means of the following experiments (20).

In the region of the Barabinska lowland, *M. bovis* survival was investigated in the external environment of a pastureland in which spontaneously infected cattle grazed in the previous year. Since spring, the presence of *M. bovis* in soil (pH 7.5, containing 2.25% humus) was tested once a month by means of biological experiments in guinea pigs. Fully virulent *M. bovis* was detected even on the seventh to eighth months of investigation. Grass from that pastureland was mowed and fed to two guinea pigs and one rabbit. In one of the guinea pigs, tuberculous lesions caused by *M. bovis* were detected. With the aim of confirming this result, each of three young bulls was orally infected with 50 mg *M. bovis* culture. Over 3 months, feces from these animals was spread on a pastureland with an area of 1800 m^2. The following 3 months, fully virulent *M. bovis* was demonstrated to exist in the soil from the pastureland by means of the experiments in guinea pigs. Thereafter, one 10-month-old calf, noninfected with *M. bovis*, grazed on that pastureland for 55 days. Tuberculin test with bovine tuberculin and culture examination of urine and feces from that calf were positive on days 20, 40, and 52 after the beginning of grazing; after slaughter on day 55, tuberculous lesions were detected in the mesenteric lymph nodes. *M. bovis* was demonstrated by culture of bronchial, mediastinal, and mesenteric lymph nodes (20).

With the aim of testing these results, experiments investigating survival of *M. bovis* from cow organs with tuberculous lesions were conducted in three types of soil: A soil: deep columnar solonetz (pH 6.8, humus 7.36%); B soil: high columnar solonetz (pH 6.2, humus 16.34%); and C soil: soil crust solonetz (pH 9.5, humus 3.58%). Experimental areas of 20 × 20 cm were contaminated with 50 mg mycobacterial suspension in distilled water in the autumn (21 October 1969), and other areas were contaminated with 200 mg of mycobacterial suspension in distilled water in the spring (15 May 1970). Fifty grams of soil from the depth of 0–10 cm (soil contaminated in autumn) and 0–2 and 3–10 cm (soil contaminated in spring) from the areas contaminated with *M. bovis* was collected for laboratory examination (biological model in guinea pig and culture). In the soil infected in the autumn, which was monitored for 12 months, fully virulent *M. bovis* survived in soils A, B, and C for 9, 10, and 12 months, respectively. In the soil infected in the spring, monitored for 4 months, fully virulent *M. bovis* survived in soil A, B, and C for 2, 2, and 4 months, respectively, at the depth of 0–2 cm, and it survived at the depth of 3–10 cm during the entire 4 months (20).

In the pursuit to use a fully virulent strain of *M. bovis* for the contamination of the soil of type A (pH 6.8, humus 7.36%), blood from artificially infected calf was used; this was spread on an area of 0.5 m^2. It was confirmed by culture and in experiments with guinea pigs that fully virulent *M. bovis* survived after 6–12 and 19–23 months in the 0–2-cm layer. When mowed grass was fed to a guinea pig 7 months after contamination, organ tuberculosis caused by *M. bovis* developed in that animal (20).

Bovine Tuberculosis in Cattle in the 11 Remaining Countries of the Former USSR

On the basis of statistical data available among 11 former states of the USSR (Armenia, Azerbaijan, Belarus, Georgia, Kazakhstan, Kyrgyzstan, Moldavia, Tajikistan, Turkmenistan, Ukraine, and Uzbekistan), bovine tuberculosis was controlled in Turkmenistan; the last notification of the epicenter of tuberculosis was recorded in 1992. However, credibility of these facts is markedly decreased by the fact that during the monitored period of 1996–2003, it was only in 2000 that notification was received from that state that no fresh epicenter of bovine tuberculosis in cattle was detected. The OIE was not provided with any data in the remaining years (Table 18.1).

Tuberculosis in the Remaining Three European Countries

The European countries Belarus, Moldavia, and Ukraine lie on an area of 845,143 km^2, with 63.112 million inhabitants and 12,215,253 head of cattle (Table 18.1).

Bovine Tuberculosis in Cattle

Byelorussia

At the beginning of the attempts to put bovine tuberculosis in cattle farms under control, Byelorussia's economy suffered losses from the establishment of specific farms for the isolation of infected animals. However, as these farms for the isolation of the animals were not liquidated afterward, they became a source of infection for the animals from controlled farms, and since 1958, the prevalence of bovine tuberculosis increased. In 1964, among 599 farms infected with bovine tuberculosis, 162 of them had stables for the isolation of infected animals. Therefore, all these farms were liquidated, and before the end of 1966, all the animals from the farms for the isolation of infected animals had to be slaughtered in abattoirs. Sanitation of 769 cattle farms was thus accelerated during 1963–1966; 298 of them were sanitized in 1966. However, sources of *M. bovis* infection were still present in the sanitized farms, as 51 of the cattle farms were later that year diagnosed with *M. bovis* again (21).

The Ukraine

In 1970s, in the district of Odessa in the Ukraine, the efficiency of implemented methods of sanitation (two elimination methods and one radical method) was assessed in 25 herds of cattle infected with bovine tuberculosis. In all of the states, the infection was controlled for more than 10 years by (22), first, transfer of animals with a positive reaction to bovine tuberculin to farms for isolation of infected animals (eight cattle herds); second, culling of animals with a positive reaction to bovine tuberculin for slaughter (eight cattle herds); and third, replacement of all animals in the farm for healthy animals (nine cattle herds). Using these three methods, the following economic indices were detected:

1. Sanitation of infected herd lasted for 10.3 ± 1.6, 6.5 ± 1.3, and 3.2 ± 1.4 years, respectively.
2. Mortality in animals was 14.2 ± 8.4, 6.3 ± 4.0, and 6.1 ± 2.9, respectively.
3. Real economic losses in thousands of rubles were 665.1 ± 215.0, 151.6 ± 65.0, and 88.7 ± 10.0, respectively.
4. Losses per infected animal in rubles were 259.2 ± 130.0, and 87.3 ± 10.0, respectively.
5. Previous losses in thousands of Rubles were 74.5 ± 11.0, 504.4 ± 150.0, and 566.7 ± 176.0, respectively.
6. Recoverability per one expended ruble was 0.3, 5.8, and 21.8, respectively.

The limit of ill animals underlying the use of respective methods is 14.3% when the first method is used and 21.1% when the second method is used. It is suitable to use the third method, provided more than 21.1% animals in a herd are infected with bovine tuberculosis (it pays off when morbidity rate is 8.3%).

In 1970s, it was determined that different regions in the Ukraine (in the southern part of the country) had emerging bovine tuberculosis cases 3–4 years after sanitation in 76.7%–91.0% of farms. These cases were most often caused by inconsistent separated rearing of calves from infected animals: those animals were infected and they were anergents with repeated tuberculin testing with bovine tuberculin (23).

In the Ukraine, culture examination of organs from 148,973 head of cattle was performed in veterinary laboratories over 5 years (1984–1988); among these, mycobacteria were isolated from 7136 (4.79%) animals: *M. bovis* from 3606 (2.4%), *M. tuberculosis* from 30 (0.02%), *M. avium* subsp. *avium* from 125 (0.08%), and atypical mycobacteria from 3375 (2.27%). Among a total of 7136 isolates, 50.5% were species *M. bovis*, 0.4% *M. tuberculosis*, 1.8% *M. avium* subsp. *avium*, and

47.3% atypical mycobacteria. Those were members of 14 species: *Mycobacterium scrofulaceum, Mycobacterium gordonae, Mycobacterium intracellulare, Mycobacterium gastri, Mycobacterium nonchromogenicum, Mycobacterium xenopi, Mycobacterium terrae, Mycobacterium triviale, Mycobacterium smegmatis, Mycobacterium phlei, Mycobacterium fortuitum, Mycobacterium vaccae, Mycobacterium flavescens,* and *Mycobacterium chelonae* (24).

Tuberculosis in the Human Population

In addition to economic problems, an important factor in the causes of the increasing trends in incidence and prevalence of tuberculosis in people in Byelorussia is the increased radioactivity resulting from the nuclear power station breakdown in Chernobyl. The ^{137}Cs contaminated territory spanned over a 40,000 km^2 area, with radiation of more than 1 Cu/km^2. An increased incidence of tuberculosis in people was detected after the incident. The number of cases of caseous pneumonia of the tuberculous origin in other regions increased by only 31.8%, whereas in the affected territory, with higher radioactivity, it increased by 55.5% (25).

After the atomic power plant accident in Chernobyl, the people started to worry about radiation (radiophobia). Accordingly, the number of people examined by x-radiation for the presence of a tuberculous process decreased, which contributed to increased prevalence of tuberculosis in people. A decreasing trend in the incidence of tuberculosis in people in Byelorussia since 1993 has been recorded. In 1992, the total number of notified cases of human tuberculosis was 2414/100,000 inhabitants, and in 1997 it was 5832/100,000 inhabitants (26). Identical risks were detected in the Ukraine (27).

The prison houses became another risk factor for the spread of tuberculosis in people in Byelorussia. The incidence of tuberculosis in prisons in 1997 was 28.3 greater than that in the general population, which negatively affects the whole epidemiological situation (28). Tuberculosis of respiratory organs was studied in chronic alcoholics under the conditions of an industrial city in the Republic of Byelorussia after the Chernobyl atomic power plant accident. Respiratory tuberculosis was found to occur in chronic alcoholics more frequently than in those without chronic alcoholism. The disease ran relatively badly and in a destructive form. The efficiency of bacterial isolation was commonly therapeutically reduced in these patients, and long-term prognosis was under question. Controlled combined antituberculous and antialcoholic treatment should be performed in chronic alcoholics with tuberculosis (29).

Bovine Tuberculosis in the Human Population

A considerable risk factor for increased incidence and prevalence of bovine tuberculosis in people in rural regions is demographic development, where the population becomes older because the young people move to cities. In Byelorussia in 1984, for example, the proportion of people older than 50 years of age in the villages was 37.1%, whereas in the cities it was only 18.4% (30). Analysis of 77 cases of tuberculosis in villagers gives evidence of the successfulness of the sanitation program against tuberculosis in cattle and all measures adopted against the spread of the infection in the Ukraine during 1980–1982. Only *M. tuberculosis* was detected in the persons; 33% of them did not work in cattle farms and retired on a pension (31).

Tuberculosis in Five Central Asian Countries

Central Asian countries are represented by five states (Kazakhstan, Kyrgyzstan, Tajikistan, Turkmenistan, and Uzbekistan) lying on 3,994,400 km^2, with 58.230 million inhabitants and 14,239,075 head of cattle. The life in villages is particularly closely connected with cattle and other ruminants; those grazing on vast pasturelands are the most important sources of animal protein (Table 18.1).

Kazakhstan

In the 1990s, after the disintegration of the former Soviet Union and during transformation of industry and agriculture, in particular, the states in Central Asia found themselves in a considerably difficult situation. For example, in Kazakhstan, 4500 patients died of tuberculosis (mortality was increased by 50%), and about 11,000–12,000 inhabitants became infected with tuberculosis (increased by 11.1%). Although *M. bovis* infection in people may play an important role, particularly in villages with herds infected with bovine tuberculosis, the increasing prevalence and incidence of tuberculosis in people may be associated with (32) decreased quality of (lack of) protein, deteriorating economic conditions of the inhabitants, and decreasing amounts of finances spent for prevention of disease and treatment of patients.

In some districts the immune system of the inhabitants also decreased because of radioactivity coming from shooting ranges where experiments with underground atomic bombs were performed before 1979 (33).

The actual diets of children and adolescents also failed to provide their needs in nutrients, energy, vitamins, and gross and trace elements. The total calories of a daily diet failed to meet the energy requirements and were from 26.2% to 31.6% lower than the recommended doses. The level of total protein, fat, and carbohydrates were decreased by 13.7%–29.3%, 36.3%–47.5%, and 16.8%–25.1%, respectively. The diets contained vitamins A, B1, B2, PP, and C in small amounts, and there is a low intake of iron, phosphorus, magnesium, and occasionally potassium and calcium in all age groups. This all is a result of the inadequate intake of meat and meat products, milk, fish, eggs, vegetables, and fruits (34).

The incidence of tuberculosis was also markedly influenced by ethnic affiliation, as in Kazakhstan. According to the 1989 census, the basic ethnic groups in Kazakhstan were Kazakhs and Russians, who account for 40% of the whole population of the republic. A different risk of respiratory tuberculosis was revealed among them. The risk for tuberculosis in the Kazakh population was almost three times higher than that in the Russians—the Kazakh population accounted for 64% of the total tuberculosis morbidity (35).

Increased incidence of tuberculosis in alcoholics and drug-addicted persons represents a new problem. A study performed in cooperation with a narcological dispensary in Kazakhstan showed that persons suffering from active tuberculosis and alcoholism amounted to 11.2% of all the new cases registered in the tuberculosis dispensary and 5.9% of all the new cases registered in the narcological dispensary. Respectively, 2.5% of the persons registered in the narcological dispensary and 4.2% of the persons registered in the tuberculosis dispensary were subject to compulsory treatment. Among the new cases of drug addiction, the number of tuberculous patients amounted to 17.9%. A total of 1.6% of the patients with active tuberculosis registered in the tuberculosis dispensary (36).

Tajikistan

During the collapse of the Soviet Union in 1991, Tajikistan, one of the poorest Soviet Central Asian republics, was embroiled in a bloody civil war. Between 1991 and 1995, the gross domestic product declined 45%, and in 1996 more than 85% of the population was living below the poverty line. Per capita state expenditure on health care had dropped from US $300 in 1991 to less than US $1 in 1998, in a country where 5 kg of beef cost US $10 and a bar of soap US $1. This coincided with a downturn in vital health statistics (37). The 1992–1997 civil war in Tajikistan has taken its toll on the country's people, its economy, and its hospitals. The hospitals, which were once the centerpiece of the health care system, have been neglected for the past 10–15 years. Many were affected, and according to the World Health Organization, Tajikistan has one of the highest rates of maternal and infant mortality in the area (38).

Maternal mortality in Tajikistan increased from 41.8 per 100,000 live births in 1990 to 65.5 in 1997. During the Soviet period, patients with TB received paid leave from work and free TB treatment. In the crisis after 1991, however, the local 40-bed tuberculosis hospital in Badakhshan's capital, Khorog (population 20,000), was faced with a shortage of TB medicines. Drugs supplied by international organizations sustained the hospital for a short period, but soon the hospital was no longer able to provide patients with an effective treatment regimen of first-line antituberculous drugs such as isoniazid, rifampin, ethambutol, and pyrazinamide. This is consistent with national trends showing a dramatic increase in reported TB incidence, from 30/100,000 in 1995 to more than 250/100,000 in 1997 (39).

Uzbekistan and Turkmenistan

MDR tuberculosis has emerged as a major threat to tuberculosis control, particularly in the former Soviet Union. A cross-sectional survey of smear-positive tuberculosis patients was conducted in selected districts of Karakalpakstan (Uzbekistan) and Dashoguz (Turkmenistan). In Karakalpakstan, 14 (13%) of 106 new patients were infected with MDR-tuberculosis; 43 (40%) of 107 previously treated patients were similarly infected. The proportions for Dashoguz were 4% (4/105 patients) and 18% (18/98 patients), respectively (39).

In Turkmenistan, infection of children with *M. tuberculosis* in large families was 1.4 times higher than in small ones (61.6% and 44.7%, respectively), primary infection was 1.5 times higher (30.2% and 19.8%), and morbidity rate was 2.3 times higher: 22.7% in large and 9.8% in small families per 1000 people/years of observation (40).

Bovine Tuberculosis in the Human Population

In northern parts of Kazakhstan, during 1976–1980, expeditions were organized that diagnosed tuberculosis in the people and animals. Tuberculosis was diagnosed 3.6 times more frequently in the inhabitants of villages who were in contact with cattle infected with bovine tuberculosis compared to villagers who were not in contact with infected cattle. Examination of clinically healthy employees in farms with cattle infected with bovine tuberculosis (particularly milkers, milkmaids, feeders, and veterinarians) showed that their urine or vaginal lavage contained *M. bovis* detected by culture. During these expeditions, drawbacks in milk pasteurization and poor animal hygiene conditions were revealed; those increased the risk of *M. bovis* infection for humans (41).

In western parts of Kazakhstan, the relationship between human tuberculosis of people and tuberculosis in cattle was also investigated in the years 1977–1979. In families with occurrence of tuberculosis in people, three times higher occurrence of tuberculosis in cattle was recorded in comparison with cattle kept in families without tuberculosis (42).

A total of 6786 persons from different parts of Kazakhstan were bacteriologically tested between 1981 and 1986. Typing of mycobacterial isolates showed that only patients originating from southern Kazakhstan were infected with *M. tuberculosis*. In contrast, 89.0% of patients infected with *M. tuberculosis* and 11.0% of patients infected with *M. bovis* were detected in the western part of the country. Analysis of anamnestic data showed that they originated from agricultural farms situated farther from the cities and that most of them were farmers and machinery operators (43).

This epidemiological situation was confirmed by the following study conducted in children in the region of Koktava of Kazakhstan between 1985 and 1987. It was found that 70% of children suffering from tuberculosis originated from villages with a high incidence of bovine tuberculosis in cattle. Moreover, complicated forms of tuberculosis were diagnosed in almost 50% of these cases of children. Accordingly, between 1988 and 1990, 2150 children from villages with an occurrence of bovine tuberculosis in cattle were vaccinated twice a year with human tuberculin MANTU (2 TU *pro dosi*). A group of 1457 children without contact with infected cattle served as a control group. Antituberculosis treatment was started in 753 of children with the reaction: 366 children were primarily infected, 122 children had hyperreaction, and 265 children were earlier infected. After a 3-year study, primary infection of children was 2.8 times and local tuberculosis detection 6.4 times reduced because of early antituberculous therapy with isoniazid and ethambutol (44).

In the early 1980s, several cattle farms in Uzbekistan had workers suffering from tuberculosis. Examination with bovine tuberculin was performed, and culture examination of samples of feces, milk, external environment and tissues from animals with tuberculous lesions was conducted. By tuberculin testing, a four times higher positive rate was detected in the above farms, in comparison with farms with healthy workers. Among a total of 20 identified isolates, 12 isolates were *M. bovis*, six isolates were *M. tuberculosis*, one was a member of scotochromogenous, and one was nonfotochromogenous mycobacterial species. In the animals infected with *M. tuberculosis,* tuberculous lesions were detected in the following organs: pulmonary tissue and lymph nodes. Therefore, it was necessary to consider potential spread of *M. tuberculosis* in the farms with cattle infected with tuberculosis (45). Sensitization of cattle with *M. tuberculosis* was confirmed again at the end of the 1980s, when positive results were detected by tuberculin testing in only 0.1% of 694 examined animals from tuberculous-free owners of cattle herds and their families. In contrast, in cattle herds of owners and their families suffering from tuberculosis, 3.3% of 1216 examined animals were tested positive (46).

An expedition of experts into rural regions in Kazakhstan investigated the incidence of *M. bovis* isolates in patients from farms with cattle infected with bovine tuberculosis in the early 1960s. *M. bovis* was detected in one district in 12 (30.0%) and in another district in 21 (61.8%) patients suffering from lung tuberculosis (47). Ten years later, exposure of 52 workers to *M. bovis* was monitored in one farm with cattle infected with bovine tuberculosis by testing with human (MANTU) and bovine tuberculin (5 TU *pro dosi*). A positive reaction with bovine tuberculin was detected in all 52 workers, and a concurrent reaction with human tuberculin was found in seven of them. Reaction with only human tuberculin was not detected in any of the workers (48).

By the end of 1960s, among 721 isolates from tuberculous patients from villages, *M. bovis* was detected in 25.0% of them in northern Kazakhstan, and in only 9.5% patients from southern Kazakhstan, with a lower incidence of tuberculosis. In a further study (1975), the epidemiological situation improved a little, and from 626 isolates from people suffering from tuberculosis, *M. bovis* was detected in 23.8% of the patients from the northern part and in 8.9% of patients from the southern part. The sensitivity to streptomycin, isoniazid, para-amino-salicylic acid, and ethionamid was assessed by the disk method of 96 isolates of *M. bovis* from animals with bovine tuberculosis (48 isolates from cattle, 12 isolates from camels, 13 isolates from sheep, and 23 isolates from minks). Primary resistance was detected in 29 (30.2%) isolates: 19 (39.6%) from cattle, four (33.3%) from camels, three (23.1%) from sheep, and three (13.0%) isolates from minks (48). This primary resistance to antituberculotic agents was twice the level of the primary resistance of human isolates of *M. bovis* (49). These authors found primary resistance in 223 (14.6%) isolates of *M. tuberculosis* among the 1527 tested.

Localization of the process of tuberculosis in Kazakhstan was evaluated in the years 1967–1968 in the countrymen living near Alma-Ata in the mountain region and in the lowland. In the mountain region, pulmonary tuberculosis was detected in 71.9%, tuberculous lymphadenitis in 20.2%, tuberculosis of bones and joints in 5.2%, and eye tuberculosis in 2.7% of patients; in the lowland, pulmonary tuberculosis was detected in 70.2%, tuberculous lymphadenitis in 18.4%, tuberculosis of bones and joints in 6.6%, eye tuberculosis in 3.0%, and skin tuberculosis in 1.8% of patients. It follows from anamnestic data that the age of patients with tuberculous lymphadenitis ranged between 10 and 40 years, and all of them were in contact with cattle infected with bovine tuberculosis or patients infected with tuberculosis. Affected submandibular and cervical lymph nodes prevailed in both the regions. As more than 92% of inhabitants were Kazakhs, who drink only over-cooked milk, the possibility that they were infected with *M. bovis* from raw milk was doubtful. Despite that, *M. bovis* was isolated from the affected submandibular, cervical, parotid, and occasionally axillary lymph nodes from the majority of the patients who were in contact with cattle infected with bovine tuberculosis. It follows from anamnesis that 45% of patients with lymphadenitis worked in close proximity to the animals (veterinary technicians, shearers of sheep, milkmaids, etc.). Therefore, it was assumed that the main method of infection with *M. bovis* was percutaneous and small injuries. These assumptions were confirmed by different ways of infections performed in 120 guinea pigs and 29 rabbits with the isolates of *M. bovis* and *M. tuberculosis* (50).

More than a half of multidrug-resistant isolates originated from cattle and camels, and half of all the isolates were highly resistant to streptomycin (50 mg/ml) and isoniazid (25 mg/ml). Experimental infection of cattle with six resistant isolates of *M. bovis* from animals and six resistant isolates of *M. tuberculosis* from patients was induced with the aim of studying the stability of resistance of these isolates. During the experiment, strains identical with those used for infection were retrieved from nasal and oral cavities of all the animals (48).

In the northern part of Kazakhstan, 2562 urine samples from 1067 clinically healthy cowgirls and milkmaids from cattle farms were examined. The following mycobacterial isolates were obtained from 42 women: *M. bovis* from 18 (1.7%), *M. tuberculosis* from seven (0.7%), facultative pathogenic mycobacteria from 10 (1.0%), and saprophytic mycobacteria from seven (0.7%) women. In women with *M. tuberculosis* in their urine, cavernous tuberculosis of kidneys or infiltrative pulpitis of tuberculous etiology were diagnosed by subsequent examinations. Accordingly, it was recommended that we perform not only radiological examination of the lungs to diagnose potential pulmonary tuberculosis but also culture examination of urine for diagnosis of extrapulmonary tuberculosis in the "exposed workers in farms" with herds of cattle infected with bovine tuberculosis (48).

In addition to tuberculosis of the urinary tract, infection of genitals was detected in women in Kazakhstan, as follows: only 2.3% of all people with tuberculosis in the year 1973 were so affected; however, the percentage increased to 11.7% in 1980. All diseased women could be divided into three following groups, according to the clinical course (51): 18% patients had acute beginnings of the disease (high fever, severe pain in the lower abdomen, tympany (flatulence), discharge from genitals etc.), and among those, excretion of only *M. tuberculosis* was demonstrated in 16.0% patients; 74.8% patients had chronic torpid course of disease (subfebrility, less intense but long-lasting pain of the lower abdomen), and among those, excretion of mycobacteria from genitals was detected in 17.5% (36.8% isolates were identified as *M. bovis*); and 7.2% patients had other forms of genital diseases (fibromyom, ovarian cysts etc.), and tuberculomas in other organs were also detected in 52% of the women before the closing diagnosis was specified—they excreted mycobacteria in only 1.4% (however, *M. bovis* represented 25.0% isolates).

Ten years later (1986–1987), analysis of anamnestic data from 114 children suffering from tuberculosis was performed. It was found that the sources of the pathogen for 59 children were infected people: the source of infection was an ill parent (67.8% cases), brother or sister (11.8% cases), grandparent (10.2% cases), uncle or aunt (6.8%), or neighbors (3.4%). Epizootiological and epidemiological analyses revealed that 20.5% of children with the skin tuberculin reaction had been in contact with cattle infected with bovine tuberculosis. Identification of 42 isolates of the causative agent of tuberculosis from the environment gives evidence of the exposure of the children to the infection pressure: various subjects of hygiene 19.1%, kitchen table 14.3%, pillow 11.9%, blanket 9.5%, floor along the bed 11.9%, wall along the bed 7.1%, towel 7.1%, and door handle 2.4% (52).

Resistance of children to mycobacterial infection has been increasing since the Second World War as a result of obligatory vaccination with BCG. Despite that fact, vaccination was not performed at all in some cases (out of the way rural regions) or was not performed properly. Analysis of tuberculosis in children from Kazakhstan between 1978 and 1983 showed that the disease in many cases developed not only because the immune systems of children were weakened but also because vaccination with BCG was missing or performed inconsistently or because the revaccination commonly performed at the age of 11 years in children was missing (53).

In the early 1980s, analysis of anamnestic data from patients infected with *M. bovis* showed that 78.9% and 21.1% originated from villages and cities, respectively. Analysis of the origin of villagers with tuberculosis confirmed that *M. bovis* infection in 6.0% of patients in the parts of Uzbekistan where cotton was grown and in 11.6% of patients in the parts with cattle farms. Pulmonary tuberculosis and tuberculosis other than pulmonary was clinically diagnosed in patients infected with *M. bovis* in 63.0% and 37.0% of patients, respectively (45). The epidemiological situation did not change much at the end of the 1980s. From 2021 isolates from patients suffering from tuberculosis, *M. bovis* was diagnosed in 10.6%–18.3% of the patients from various districts of the country. The majority of the patients who worked in cattle farms suffered from pulmonary tuberculosis as follows: 47.3% had the fibrocavernous form, and 20.0% patients had the infiltration form (46). High contamination of the water and soil with pesticides used in plant production (particularly connected with cotton and fruit-tree cultivation) is connected with the emergence of the disease, as well as those factors that exert adverse effects on the immune system of people. The above statement was confirmed by the experiments conducted in 300 white mice fed with various doses of pesticides; their organs were more markedly affected after the infection with *M. tuberculosis,* and the mice died earlier (54).

Bovine Tuberculosis in Other Animals than Cattle in Kazakhstan

In Kazakhstan, in Alma-Ata, in the winter and spring of 1974, gross and culture examinations were performed in 105 stray dogs and two stray cats. Gross changes in the lungs (caseous necrosis demonstrated by histology) were detected in only one dog. Pathogenic mycobacteria were isolated by culture from two dogs (one *M. tuberculosis* and one *M. bovis* isolate), scotochromogenous mycobacteria in two dogs, and saprophytic mycobacteria in one dog. A total of 365 dogs were examined by testing using bovine (Strain Vinogradov) and human (Strain Akademia) tuberculins. From 269 dogs from tuberculosis-free families, 13 (4.8%) had a positive reaction as follows: eight (3.0%) dogs reacted with human tuberculin, two (0.7%) dogs with bovine tuberculin, and three (1.1%) dogs with both tuberculins concurrently. From 96 dogs from families with tuberculosis-infected people, 10 (10.4%) had a positive reaction as follows: seven (7.3%) dogs reacted with human tuberculin, one (1.0%) dog with bovine tuberculin, and two (2.1%) dogs with both tuberculins concurrently. The likely cause of the more frequent reaction to human tuberculin was the infection of dogs, particularly with *M. tuberculosis*, from infected people in the families. The results in 206 examined cats were similar: among a total of 115 examined cats in healthy families, six (5.2%) cats reacted, and among a total of 91 examined cats in families with tuberculosis-infected people, nine (9.9%) cats reacted (17).

In farms of cattle infected with bovine tuberculosis, *M. bovis* was likewise isolated from organs of extensively kept poultry; this had to be considered when measures were adopted with the aim of putting tuberculosis under control (42). Bovine tuberculosis was also detected in camels in Kazakhstan by allergological testing (from 285 camels, 15 gave a positive reaction with bovine tuberculin) and by gross examination. Accordingly, the risk of infection of people with *M. bovis* not only is represented by drinking raw cow milk but also is represented by drinking camel milk (47).

Bovine Tuberculosis in Three Caucasian Countries

Although the three Caucasian countries (Armenia, Azerbaijan, and Georgia) are situated in a geographically strategic position (oil and gas transport across their territory), the region was considerably politically and economically unstable after the collapse of the former USSR. Particularly because of the warfare of the early 1990s, the statistical data of the OIE concerning the incidence of bovine tuberculosis in cattle are missing (Table 18.1). Despite this, it is evident from the above partial data that bovine tuberculosis in cattle herds still occasionally occurs. It is difficult to obtain more data on the occurrence of bovine tuberculosis in cattle or other animal species in that region from literature available, particularly from databases such as PubMed (National Library of Medicine, Bethesda, MD) and the Web of Knowledge (ISI Thomson, Philadelphia, PA).

Bovine Tuberculosis in Cattle in Armenia

It follows from data given by Terovanesova (54) from Armenia that monitoring of bovine tuberculosis in this country in cattle began in 1948, particularly in dairy cattle herds. In the year 1950, when more than 160,000 head of cattle were examined, the positivity detected was 0.1%; because of the outbreak control, it was reduced to 0.02% of positive animals before 1957. However, because of inconsistent culling of animals reacting to bovine tuberculin from infected herds, bovine tuberculosis spread there similarly as in the Russian Federation, and the positivity detected in 1966 was 0.66%. After the analysis of 1.3 million tuberculin tests performed during 10 years, a markedly increased incidence of cattle that reacted to bovine tuberculin was found in August, in the summer, and minimum numbers were detected in December, in the winter. The occurrence of positive animals reacting to bovine tuberculin in the six spring and summer months (from May to October) was double that of the six autumn and winter months (November to April). That phenomenon was likely caused by the continental climate, which is characterized by hot summer months that cause heat stress in the animals and supports development of chronic forms of bovine tuberculosis.

Between 1952 and 1954, among 3489 animals with performed tuberculin tests, 181 (5.2%) reacted; the status of the condition of was assessed and was as follows: 32 animals were emaciated, 57 had an average level of body condition, and 92 animals were in good body condition. The lowest intensity of reactions was recorded in the group of emaciated animals in comparison with the group of animals in good body condition. It was also detected that the percentage of reacting animals was markedly elevated in the age group of 4–6 years, and it was the highest in the animals at the age of 8–10 years; that gives evidence about incidence of chronic forms of diseases in old animals (55).

Bovine Tuberculosis in Sheep in Armenia

Because cattle and sheep are kept together in farms, in 1949, incidence and the possibilities of diagnosis of bovine tuberculosis in three sheep herds kept together with cattle that were infected with bovine tuberculosis was investigated in mountain, submountain, and lowland regions. The most suitable site of tuberculin testing seemed to be above the knee fold or at the wool-free part of skin behind the anconeal joint. When tuberculin tests with bovine tuberculin were performed, the percentages of reacting animals from the mountain, submountain, and lowland regions were 2.05%, 1.57%, and 3.3%, respectively. Gross examination showed tuberculous lesions in the reacting animals in mesenteric lymph nodes (100% animals) and lungs (46% animals). Direct microscopy according to Ziehl-Neelsen staining revealed only occasional acid-fast rods in the tissue with tuberculous lesions, and by culture *M. bovis* was isolated. From the epizootiological aspect, excretion of *M. bovis* through feces on days 25–50 after their artificial infection was viewed as most important (55).

Tuberculosis in the Human Population in Three Caucasian Countries

In Caucasian countries, where underreporting and low case finding are recognized, case rates of tuberculosis in the human population have stabilized in Armenia, whereas in Azerbaijan and Georgia, there was a decrease from 1985 to 1990 (56). In 1994, the epidemiological situation in Armenia was very grave: the tuberculosis cases registered in this year were 19.6 per 100,000 inhabitants, which is 16.6% higher than the figure in 1993. Mortality rates in 1994 were 3.1 per 100,000 persons, and morbidity in males was 2.5 times higher than that in females. The greatest proportion of the first cases detected was in the age group of 25–34 years. Infiltrative tuberculosis with multiple decays and its acute course is prevalent in the pattern of tuberculosis morbidity. Activities in prophylactic measures have drastically declined because of the power crisis and grave socioeconomic conditions of the republic. Groups of migrants as potential carriers of undiagnosed tuberculosis forms were gaining a great significance among patients with tuberculosis (57). The staff of the organization Doctors without Borders also inform us about problems connected with the spread of the causative agent of tuberculosis with migrating people from this region (58).

The problem concerning the spread of tuberculosis in humans was not associated with the incidence of bovine tuberculosis in cattle during the last 10–15 years, but particularly with social and economic unrest in the society caused by various factors. In Armenia, an increased incidence of tuberculosis in people who lived in provisional conditions after the earthquake (and particularly children) was recorded in December 1988 (58,59). In Azerbaijan, a critical epidemiological situation concerning tuberculosis of people exists in the prison houses, with a high incidence and prevalence not only of tuberculosis but also of MDR strains (60–63). In Georgia, the epidemiological aspect of tuberculosis in humans is particularly threatening in its high prevalence in the immigrants who came to Tbilisi (the capital) from places affected by war (64). Another risk group are prisoners with a detected prevalence of smear- or culture-positive tuberculosis of 5995 per 100,000 prisoners ($n = 448$ cases among 7473 inmates). Of all the strains, 215 (77.9%) were resistant to at least one drug, and 37 (13.0%) were MDR (65).

At present, the only possibility is the establishment of directly-observed treatment, short-course. The effectiveness of that method in this sphere was successfully verified in an extensive pilot study performed in all three states (66).

Conclusions

Trends in HIV/AIDS associated with injecting drug use in the newly independent states in Eastern Europe (Belarus, Moldova, Russia, and Ukraine), and Kazakhstan in central Asia, were reviewed. Since 1995, there has been evidence of rapid HIV/AIDS spread in Belarus, Kazakhstan, Moldova, Russia, and Ukraine, with estimates indicating that between 50% and 90% of new HIV/AIDS infections occur among injecting drug users. At the same time, there have been rapid increases in the incidence of syphilis and declines in health and welfare status, including outbreaks of diphtheria, tuberculosis, and cholera. Findings emphasize the potential influence of the social and economic context in creating the "risk environments" conducive to HIV/AIDS and the epidemic spread. Key factors include rapid diffusions in injecting drug use; population migration and mixing; economic transition and decline; increasing unemployment and impoverishment; the growth of informal economies; modes of drug production, distribution, and consumption; declines in public health revenue and infrastructure; and political, ideological, and cultural transition (67).

The epidemiological relatedness of drug-resistant *M. tuberculosis* strains isolated in Germany in 1995 was evaluated by the standardized IS*6110* fingerprinting method. Altogether, 196 *M. tuberculosis* isolates from 167 patients were analyzed. A large degree of IS*6110* polymorphism was found, ranging from 1 to 20 copies. A total of 30 of the 167 isolates (approximately 18%) could be grouped in two fingerprint clusters, with a similarity of at least 78%. Approximately 60% of the patients of these two clusters were known to be immigrants from the former Soviet Union, and one patient is still living in Belarus (68).

Tuberculosis morbidity and mortality in the Moldova Republic has deteriorated since 1991. The percentage of advanced and rapidly progressive forms of the disease rose two- to threefold. Most of the patients are 21–50-year-old unemployed men living in poor financial and social conditions. Advanced and rapidly progressive tuberculosis forms are present clinically with multiple symptoms and destructions, high incidence of generalized dissemination, and involvement of the brain (69).

Acknowledgments

Partially supported by grant No. MZE 0002716201 of the Ministry of Agriculture of the Czech Republic. A. Maslanova and Z. Gregorova from VRI Brno are acknowledged for the literature and Maria Vass (Swinburne University of Technology, Victoria, Australia) for critical reading of the manuscript.

References

1. Ravilone, M. K., K. Esteves, A. Koshi, G. L. Rider, K. Stiblo, A. G. Khomenko. 1994. Trends in the field of tuberculous diseases in the Eastern Europe and former. *U. S.S.R. Probl. Tuberk.* 6:2-10.
2. Tekkel, M., M. Rahu, H. M. Loit, and A. Baburin. 2002. Risk factors for pulmonary tuberculosis in Estonia. *Int J Tuberc Lung Dis* 6:887-94.
3. Kruuner, A., S. E. Hoffner, H. Sillastu, M. Danilovits, K. Levina, S. B. Svenson, S. Ghebremichael, T. Koivula, and G. Kallenius. 2001. Spread of drug-resistant pulmonary tuberculosis in Estonia. *J Clin Microbiol* 39:3339-45.
4. Drobniewski, F. A., and Y. M. Balabanova. 2002. The diagnosis and management of multiple-drug-resistant-tuberculosis at the beginning of the new millennium. Review. *Int J Infect Dis* 6:S21-31.
5. Latyshev, A. S. 1969. Experience in bovine tuberculosis control. *Veterinariia* 45:37-38.
6. Latyshev, A. S., and I. J. Maslov. 1970. Hygienic measures on farms in relation to bovine tuberculosis (practical experience). *Veterinariia* 46:58-60.
7. Espinal, M. A., A. Laszlo, L. Simonsen, F. Boulahbal, S. J. Kim, A. Reniero, S. Hoffner, H. L. Rieder, N. Binkin, C. Dye, R. Williams, and M. C. Raviglione. 2001. Global trends in resistance to antituberculosis drugs. World Health Organization-

International Union against Tuberculosis and Lung Disease Working Group on Anti-Tuberculosis Drug Resistance Surveillance. *N Engl J Med* 344:1294-303.

8. Shtuikis, V. V., and V. V. Kublitskas. 1968. Nonspecific reactions to tuberculin in cattle. *Veterinariia* 45:33-34.

9. Kuzin, A. I. 1977. Latent course of tuberculosis. *Veterinariia* 7:47-50.

10. Ursov, I. G. 1976. Relationship between tuberculosis of farm animals and man. *Probl Tuberk* 3:10-14.

11. Tuzova, R. V. 1975. Interspecies circulation of mycobacteria. *Probl Tuberk* 7:66-70.

12. Shindler, E. M. 1979. Epidemiological importance of bovine tuberculosis for rural inhabitants. *Probl Tuberk* 1:12-15.

13. Kuzina, L. N. and S. A. Belichenko. 1984. Interrelations between human and bovine tuberculosis. *Probl Tuberk* 12:13-15.

14. Keldybajev, S., and K. A. Turkebajeva. 1969. The spread of tuberculosis by sheep and goats. *Veterinariia* 45:38.

15. Nikanorov, B. A. 1970. The role of *Mycobacterium tuberculosis* and *Mycobacterium avium* in epizootiology of Marals tuberculosis. *Veterinariia* 46:60-62.

16. Kapustin, L. A., and I. N. Nikitin. 1972. Economic loses caused by tuberculosis in maral deer. *Veterinariia* 48:43-45.

17. Gusev, A. A. 1935. *Proc Leningrad Vet Inst* 7:128-30.

18. Blagodarnyi I. A., and S. Basybekov. 1976. Tuberculosis in domestic animals and its relationship with human tuberculosis. *Probl Tuberk* 3:14-17.

19. Rotov, V. I., P. I. Kokyriev, and P. E. Savchenko. 1973. Tuberculosis in farm animals. Kiev, 381.

20. Kislenko, V. N. 1972. Survival of bovine tuberculosis mycobacteria in pasture soils. *Veterinariia* 48:48-51.

21. Kosko, F. A., M. A. Fishelevich, and P. K. Gulev. 1967. Controlling bovine brucellosis and tuberculosis. *Veterinariia* 144:46-48.

22. Kovanda, S. I., I. T. Nechval, E. I. Buriak, P. S. Sheverenko, and V. N. Vasilevskii. 1975. Effectiveness of different methods of eliminating tuberculosis from farms. *Veterinariia* 4:44-47.

23. Kovanda, S. I., and V. N. Vasilevskii. 1977. Tuberculosis morbidity in calves. *Veterinariia* 7:51-53.

24. Kassich I. I., V. A. Kochmarskii, A. I. Zavgorodnii, A. T. Borziak, N. V. Korotchenko, V. M. Manchenko, D. G. Kryzhanovskii, and M. I. Kozhushko. 1990. The interrelation of bovine and human tuberculosis. *Probl Tuberk* 6:23-26.

25. Surkova, L. K., and M. E. Shtilman. 1993. Characteristics of thanatogenesis and pathomorphology of tuberculosis in the Gomel region in relation to the Chernobyl AES accident. *Probl Tuberk* 2:20-24.

26. Takamura N., N. Kryshenko, V. Masyakin, H. Tamashiro, and S. Yamashita. 2000. Chernobyl-induced radiophobia and the incidence of tuberculosis. *Lancet* 356:257.

27. Dvoirin, M. S., P. P. Liabakh, L. A. Kharchenko, N. P. Androsova. 1990. Tuberculosis morbidity in the areas under strict radiation control. *Probl Tuberk* 11:12-14.

28. Krivonos, P. S., O. M. Kalechits, G. S. Avdeev, P. A. Zdanevich, V. N. Shamshur, V. K. Korban, and M. I. Snarov. 1999. Tuberculosis in penitentiaries of the Republic of Belarus. *Probl Tuberk* 6:8-10.

29. Shevchenko, A. A. 2001. Tuberculosis of the respiratory tract and chronic alcoholism. *Probl Tuberk* 8:6-8.

30. Lomako, M. N., and O. M. Kalechits. 1984. Improved methods of preventing tuberculosis and nonspecific lung diseases. *Probl Tuberk* 2:3-7.

31. Pilipchuk, N. S., and G. A. Borisenko. 1984. Tuberculosis among the rural population. *Probl Tuberk* 8:6-7.

32. Dzhunusbekov, A. D., Z. I. Khazhibaeva, and U. S. Dametov. 1997. Epidemiologic situation of tuberculosis in the Republic of Kazakhstan. *Probl Tuberk* 1:25-27.

33. Ivanova, E. S., I. I. Fisher, L. P. Fedorov, M. M. Utepkaliev, Z. A. Akpanov, G. T. Temresheva, and S. M. Polosukhin. 1991. Experience in joint activities of the Central Research Institute of Tuberculosis, USSR Ministry of Health, with therapeutic-preventive institutions of a Kazakhstan rural area. *Probl Tuberk* 11:27-30.

34. Bekbosynov, T. K., M. V. Baimagambetova, B. M. Myrzabieva, and R. Z. Kuandykova. 1991. Actual child and adolescent nutritional status in an epidemically unfavorable region of Kazakhstan. *Probl Tuberk* 12:37-39.

35. Khauadamova, G. T. 1991. The risk of tuberculosis in the principal ethnic groups of Kazakhstan. *Probl Tuberk* 4:22-24.

36. Khauadamova, G. T., V. A. Mingaliev, and K. O. Sharmagambetova. 1989. Incidence of alcoholism and drug addiction among patients with active tuberculosis. *Probl Tuberk* 10:7-10.

37. Keshavjee S. and M. C. Becerra. 2000. Disintegrating health services and resurgent tuberculosis in post-Soviet Tajikistan: an example of structural violence. *JAMA* 2839:1201.

38. Mashta, O. 2000. Building capacity for primary care in Tajikistan. *Lancet* 355:295.

39. Cox, H. S., J. D. Orozco, R. Male, S. Ruesch-Gerdes, D. Falzon, I. Small, D. Doshetov, Y. Kebede, and M. Aziz. 2004. Multidrug-resistant tuberculosis in central Asia. *Emerg Infect Dis* 10:865-72.

40. Murriev, A. 1990. Tuberculosis infection and morbidity in children of large and small families in relation to epidemic risks of tuberculosis foci. *Probl Tuberk* 9:21-24.

41. Kurmanbaev, K. K., R. A. Agzamova, V. F. Ipatkin, M. I. Blagodarnyi, and D. B. Balguzhinov. 1983. Experience in organizing specialist teams for the detection of tuberculosis cases in rural regions. *Probl Tuberk* 11:11-14.

42. Kurmanbaev, K. K., and I. A. Blagodarnyi. 1981. Interrelationship of human and animal tuberculosis. *Probl Tuberk* 5:6-8.

43. Krivtsova, A. E., and T. K. Bekbosynov. 1989. Bacteriological method of examination in the diagnosis of reactivation of the tuberculous process among contingents in ambulatory care group VII. *Probl Tuberk* 1:12-14.

44. Niiazbekova, K. Z., R. A. Arzamova, and E. T. Tleubergenov. 1991. Early detection of tuberculosis and its pharmacological prevention in children from the epizootologically unfavorable territories. *Probl Tuberk* 7:5-6.

45. Khamrakulov, R. S., A. B. Li, and Z. I. Ismailov. 1984. Examination of people and animals for tuberculosis and measures for its prevention. *Probl Tuberk* 3:12-14.

46. Ubaidullaev, A. M., R. A. Agzamov, E. A. Stoianovskii, R. S. Khamrakulov, and R. I. Zakharova. 1989. Role of comprehensive examination of the population in regard to tuberculosis in rural areas of Uzbekistan. *Probl Tuberk* 3:3-5.

47. Blagodarnyi, I. A., V. R. Levin, L. V. Koroteeva, B. S. Modelevskii, and D. M. Shapiro. 1965. Some problems concerning the epidemiology of tuberculosis in 1 of the Caspian lowland regions. *Probl Tuberk* 43:5-11.

48. Blagodarnyi, I. A., Z. Z. Bekmagambetova, L. I. Blonskaia, and E. V. Siderkina. 1975. Tuberculosis in stock breeders caused by *Mycobacterium bovis*. *Probl Tuberk* 10:72-75.

49. Krivtsova, A. E., and I. A. Blagodarnyi. 1974. Primary resistance of mycobacteria in Kazakhstan. *Probl Tuberk* 8:70-73.

50. Maskeev, K. M. 1970. Peripheral tuberculous lymphadenitis in rural regions of the Alma-Ata area. *Probl Tuberk* 483:10-15.

51. Bekbosynov, T. K. and A. E. Krivtsova. 1986. Role of the bacteriological examination method in the dispensary care of persons at increased risk for tuberculosis. *Probl Tuberk* 9:8-10.

52. Blagodarnyi, I. A., I. M. Blekhman, K. K. Alimbekova, B. S. Sergazin, and S. Z. Mynzhasarov. 1988. The value of an epidemiologic study in detecting sources of tuberculosis infection. *Probl Tuberk* 10:3-5.

53. Sakharova, E. A. and M. B. Bekezhanova. 1985. Children's groups with a high risk of developing tuberculosis. *Probl Tuberk* 1:12-14.

54. Kalankhodzhaev, A. A., R. A. Agzamov, R. S. Khamrakulov, E. S. Sodikov, and E. B. Morozko. 1983. Epidemiology of tuberculosis in various areas of Uzbekistan with diverse agricultural specialization. *Probl Tuberk* 11:7-11.

55. Terovanesova, O. G. 1967. Tuberculosis in animals and means of its eradication in the Armenian SSR. *Veterinariia* 447:51-52.

56. Raviglione, M. C., H. L. Rieder, K. Styblo, A. G. Khomenko, K. Esteves, and A. Kochi. 1994. Tuberculosis trends in Eastern Europe and the former USSR. *Tuber Lung Dis* 75:400-16.

57. Safrian, M. D., E. P. Stamboltsian, V. A. Avetisian, M. A. Sarkisian, L. T. Nikolaian, and N. R. Beglarian. 1997. Epidemiologic situation of tuberculosis in Armenia under the present condition. Review. *Probl Tuberk* 1:22-25.

58. Ivanova, E. S., N. S. Gvetadze, S. Kigan, and A. N. Nikiforov. 1996. Detection of pulmonary tuberculosis in migrants. *Probl Tuberk* 6:28-29.

59. Karapetian, E. T. and E. F. Markova. 1991. Pulmonary tuberculosis among the residents of the earthquake area in the Armenian SSR. *Probl Tuberk* 8:14-16.

60. Karapetian, E. T., E. F. Markova, and A. A. Gasparian. 1993. Development of tuberculosis in children and adolescents in extreme circumstances. *Probl Tuberk* 4:13-15.

61. Coninx, R., C. Mathieu, M. Debacker, F. Mirzoev, A. Ismaelov, R. de Haller, and D. R. Meddings. 1999. First-line tuberculosis therapy and drug-resistant *Mycobacterium tuberculosis* in prisons. *Lancet* 353:969-73.

62. Portaels F., L. Rigouts, and I. Bastian. 1999. Addressing multidrug-resistant tuberculosis in penitentiary hospitals and in the general population of the former Soviet Union. Review. *Int J Tuberc Lung Dis* 3:582-88.

63. Pfyffer, G. E., A. Strassle, T. van Gorkum, F. Portaels, L. Rigouts, C. Mathieu, F. Mirzoyev, H. Traore, and J. D. van Embden. 2001. Multidrug-resistant tuberculosis in prison inmates, Azerbaijan. *Emerg Infect Dis* 7:855-61.

64. Weinstock, D. M., O. Hahn, M. Wittkamp, K. A. Sepkowitz, G. Khechinashvili, and H. M. Blumberg. 2001. Risk for tuberculosis infection among internally displaced persons in the Republic of Georgia. *Int J Tuberc Lung Dis* 5:164-69.

65. Aerts, A., M. Habouzit, L. Mschiladze, N. Malakmadze, N. Sadradze, O. Menteshashvili, F. Portaels, and P. Sudre. 2000. Pulmonary tuberculosis in prisons of the ex-USSR state Georgia: results of a nation-wide prevalence survey among sentenced inmates. *Int J Tuberc Lung Dis* 4:1104-10.

66. Zalesky, R., F. Abdullajev, G. Khechinashvili, M. Safarian, T. Madaras, M. Grzemska, E. Englund, S. Dittmann, and M. Raviglione. 1999. Tuberculosis control in the Caucasus: successes and constraints in DOTS implementation. *Int J Tuberc Lung Dis* 3:394-401.

67. Rhodes, T., A. Ball, G. V. Stimson, Y. Kobyshcha, C. Fitch, V. Pokrovsky, M. Bezruchenko-Novachuk, D. Burrows, A. Renton, and L. Andrushchak. 1999. *HIV*

infection associated with drug injecting in the newly independent states, eastern Europe: the social and economic context of epidemics. *Addiction* 94:1323-36.

68. Niemann, S., S. Rusch-Gerdes, and E. Richter. 1997. IS*6110* fingerprinting of drug-resistant *Mycobacterium tuberculosis* strains isolated in Germany during 1995. *J Clin Microbiol* 35:3015-20.

69. Sain, D. O., G. G. Tsymbalar, L. P. Ryvniak, I. N. Khaidarly, N. N. Nalivaiko, and S. V. Pisarenko. 1999. Current characteristics of advanced and rapidly progressive forms of pulmonary tuberculosis. *Probl Tuberk* 1:27-29.

Chapter 19

Mycobacterium bovis in Africa

J. Zinsstag, DVM, PhD, R.R. Kazwala, DVM, PhD,
I. Cadmus, DVM, MVPH, and L. Ayanwale, DVM, MPH, PhD

Introduction

After HIV/AIDS, tuberculosis (TB) is responsible for the deaths of more people each year than any other single infectious disease, with more than 7 million new cases and 2 million deaths per year. Clinical disease caused by TB remains the largest attributable cause of death in HIV-infected individuals who are also infected with TB. TB is responsible for one-third of all deaths of HIV-infected individuals in Africa. In sub-Saharan Africa, where nearly 2 million tuberculosis cases occur each year, it is unknown what role cattle-derived *Mycobacterium bovis* plays in the rising epidemic of tuberculosis in Africa, fostered by HIV/AIDS. Studies in Malawi have shown that areas of high bovine tuberculosis prevalence are not necessarily matched by a concomitant high prevalence of tuberculosis in man. However, there is substantive evidence for significant transmission of *M. bovis* in pastoralist communities with close human-to-livestock contact (1).

In view of the considerable and continuing public health significance of *M. bovis* infection in humans, the World Health Organization convened a meeting on zoonotic tuberculosis in Geneva in November 1993 and elaborated a project protocol to investigate the zoonotic aspects of bovine tuberculosis (2). Despite the scarcity of information on *M. bovis* infection in Africa, there is sufficient evidence to indicate that it is widely distributed and is found at high prevalences in some animal populations. The public health threat of tuberculosis in Africa requires urgent investigation through collaborative veterinary/medical research programs (3). The available literature on *M. bovis* in Africa is focused on Bacille Calmette-Güerin (BCG) vaccination, public health, milk, livestock, game, or biological aspects, but very few reports mention isolation from humans and animals in the same setting. In addition, very little is known about the antibiotic resistance of *M. bovis* and mycobacteria in general in African countries. Ayele et al. (4) provides a comprehensive account of current knowledge on methods and geographical distribution of *M. bovis* in Africa. Among other reasons for the relatively little attention paid to *M. bovis* in Africa is the limited diagnostic capacity (3,4). In most countries, the diagnosis of tuberculosis relies on sputum microscopy alone. If strains are isolated, they are grown on media that are not suitable for *M. bovis*, and methods for molecular characterization are rarely available. Only very few veterinary mycobacteriology laboratories exist on the continent. Njanpop-Lafourcade et al. (5), for example, reported on molecular strain characterization by spoligotyping of *M. bovis* from North Cameroon, and similar strains were identified recently in Chad (6). In Tanzania, similar spoligotype patterns of *M. bovis* could be demonstrated in livestock and humans. At present, the variable number of tandem repeats method is being examined for its use in Africa and is further compared to microarray and the analysis of genomic deletions.

Although extensive pastoral systems may be less favorable for *M. bovis* transmission between animals than are intensive industrial systems, relatively high prevalences of tuberculin-positive animals were found in pastoral nomadic settings in Chad (7). Today, especially in peri-urban areas of larger cities, intensive dairy production is a livelihood for thousands of people, often migrating from remote rural areas. Cross breeding with exotic breeds is more and more widely practiced. Milk production systems are mostly informal/traditional, with little disease control in live animals and the milk (8). Milk is usually consumed after spontaneous fermentation, but raw milk consumption occurs frequently too, and isolation of *M. bovis* has been reported in raw milk (9). Cattle are the main host for bovine tuberculosis in Africa, but *M. bovis* was also isolated from small ruminants, camels, and many different wildlife species. Countries with endemic bovine tuberculosis implement various control efforts, but in most cases they are unable to compensate farmers for culled livestock. Attempts to protect cattle against tuberculosis by BCG vaccination in the 1970s had no success, but new trials are ongoing in Madagascar and are planned in Ethiopia.

Specific Country Reports

In this section, the tuberculosis situation in specific countries is reported. Reports are not available from all African countries, which reflects the need for further investigation. An overview on the reported occurrence of *M. bovis* is given in Table 19.1. More detailed information can also be obtained from the authors.

West and Central Africa

In West and Central Africa, bovine tuberculosis in humans seems to be specially prevalent among the nomadic Fulani tribe, who herd their cattle across the country borders of nations. They use milk, which they do not usually boil, from their cattle for food. Cross-border migration of livestock is allowed under the treaty of the Economic Community of West African States.

Nigeria

As in many African countries, not much work has been done on the national epidemiological study of TB in Nigeria. Reports on the prevalence of bovine tuberculosis in man and animals are few, local, and not often published. Most reports are from the few research scientists who demonstrated resourcefulness and determination in working with the pathogen, despite inadequate funding for research by the

Table 19.1. Bovine tuberculosis in cattle in 43 African countries, 1992–2001*

Country	1992	1993	1994	1995	1996	1997	1998	1999	2000	2001
Algeria	+	+	+	+	+	+	+	+	+	+
Angola	+	+	+	+	+	NR	+	NR	+	NR
Botswana	+	NR	000	1993	NR	NR	NR	NR	NR	NR
Burkina Faso	+	+	NR	+	+	+	+	+	+	NR
Cameroon	+	+	NR	NR	?	+	+	+	+	+
Cape Verde	NR	?	NR	NR	?	?	NR	1987	NR	NR
Central African Republic	?	?	+	+	+	+	NR	NR	NR	NR
Chad	+	+	+	+	—	+	+	NR	NR	NR
Comoros	?	?	NR	NR	NR	NR	000	NR	+	+
Ivory Coast	+	+	+	+	+	+	+	+	NR	NR
Democratic Republic Congo	NR	NR	NR	NR	NR	NR	NR	NR	NR	+
Egypt	+	+	+	+	+	+	+	+	+	+
Eritrea	+	+	+	NR	+	+	—	NR	NR	+
Ethiopia	NR	+	+	+	NR	—	NR	NR	NR	NR
Gabon	NR	NR	NR	+	NR	NR	NR	NR	NR	NR
Gambia	NR	NR	NR	NR	—	NR	NR	NR	NR	+
Ghana	+	+	+	+	+?	+	+	+	+	NR
Guinea	—	NR	—	—	+?	+	+	NR	+	+
Kenya	000	NR	NR	NR	+	+	NR	+	+	NR
Lesotho	—	NR	NR	NR	NR	NR	NR	+	+	+
Libya	+	?	+	+	NR	+	+	+	NR	+?
Madagascar	+	+	+	+	+	+	+	+	NR	NR
Malawi	+	+	NR	+	+	+	+	+	+	NR
Mali	+	NR	NR	NR	+	NR	NR	NR	+	NR
Mauritius	+	+	NR	NR	+	NR	+	+	NR	NR
Morocco	+	+	+	—	+	+	+	+	+	NR
Mozambique	1984	1984	+	NR	1995	1995	1995	1995	NR	NR
Namibia	+	+	+	+	+	1995	1995	1995	1995	1995
Niger	+	+	+	+	NR	+	+	NR	NR	+

Continues

Table 19.1. (Continued)

Country	1992	1993	1994	1995	1996	1997	1998	1999	2000	2001
Nigeria	+	+	+	NR	+	NR	NR	NR	NR	+
Reunion (FR)	+	NR	NR	NR	+	+	+	+	+	+
Sao Tome & Principe	NR	NR	NR	NR	NR	NR	NR	NR	NR	NR
Senegal	+	NR	NR	NR	—	—	—	NR	NR	NR
Seychelles	NR	NR	NR	NR	NR	NR	NR	NR	000	NR
South Africa	+	+	+	+	+	+	+	+	+	+
Sudan	+	NR	NR	NR	1992	1992	1992	1992	1992	1992
Swaziland	NR	+	NR	+	+?	+	+	NR		+
Tanzania	+	NR	NR	+	NR	+	+	NR	+?	+
Togo	+	NR	NR	+	NR	+	NR	NR	+	+
Tunisia	+	+	+	+	+	+	+	+	+	+
Uganda	+	+	+	+	+	+	+	+	+	+
Zambia	+	NR	—	+	—	+	+	NR	+	NR
Zimbabwe	NR	NR	NR	1990	1990	1990	1990	1990	1996	1996

*Data were extracted from the following sources: FAO-OIE-WHO Animal Health Yearbooks, Rome, Italy: OIE, 1992-1997, and OIE World Animal Health in 1997. Parts 1 and 2, Paris: OIE, 1998-2001.

NR: disease not reported; 000: never reported; 1987: year of last occurrence; ?: suspected but not confirmed; —: no information available; +?: serological evidence or isolation of causative agent, no clinical disease.

successive military governments of this country. In Nigerian hospitals, as in many African hospitals, all forms of pulmonary tuberculosis that are acid-fast-bacilli positive are considered as a single type of TB, even though patients suffering from *M. bovis* show no improvement in treatments. The application of direct smear microscopy as the only method of diagnosis of suspected cases of tuberculosis does not differentiate between species of the *M. tuberculosis* complex. The prevalence of bovine tuberculosis in cattle ranged between 3% and 9.6%, as reported by some workers through single intradermal tests conducted in some established farms and from abattoir samples (10). *M. bovis* has been isolated from test-positive cattle in nasal secretions and milk, abattoir granulomas, and human sputum and biopsies of lymph nodes of tuberculosis patients undergoing treatments at several large hospitals, including in Lagos, where over 6 million people live. There has not been any nationally coordinated study of TB either in cattle or human populations in Nigeria. Nigeria is the most populous country in Africa, and it has over 120 million people, with 13 million cattle and an unknown population of wildlife ruminants, which makes it a perfect opportunity for the easy transmission and spread of bovine type TB. The situation is further exacerbated by the advent of HIV/AIDS. The country has a test-and-slaughter policy for the eradication of TB in animals, but there is only a limited implementation. The increase of HIV/AIDS in Nigeria may have worsened infections of *M. bovis* in human patients who have also been infected with HIV/AIDS. The cumulative incidence of atypical mycobacteriosis isolated in a study of two Lagos hospitals over the 10-year period was between 21% and 26%. Analysis of the nature and frequency of the mycobacteria strains isolated over the period showed that infections with *M. tuberculosis* accounted for 74.7% of all the reported positive cases, followed by *Mycobacterium kansasii* (8.9%), *Mycobacterium bovis* (7.2%), *Mycobacterium fortuitum* (4.7%), *Mycobacterium avium* (4.0%), and *Mycobacterium Xenopi* (0.5%).

Cameroon

Between 1984 and 1986, abattoir records from Buyya showed a TB prevalence of 6% in cattle imported from Chad to Cameroon for slaughter. Human cases of bovine TB were estimated to be between 4% and 7%. Though the country imports local zebu cattle from Niger, Central African Republic, Chad, and Nigeria, France continues to be a major exporter of cattle to Cameroon. The first documented introduction of cattle to Cameroon was in 1913, when Charolais cattle were imported from Saone-et-Loire, France. In recent molecular epidemiologic studies of 75 *M. bovis* isolates obtained from Adamaoua and Northern Cameroon abattoir samples, European types of *M. bovis* were identified by molecular typing profiles (5). Although no definitive prevalence of TB in Cameroon could be estimated as a result of inadequate data from several other key provinces, the molecular typing studies show promise in their use for geographical mapping of *M. bovis* in Africa.

Ghana

Although Ghana continues to make dramatic progress in the reduction of tuberculosis in both human and livestock populations, the advent of HIV/AIDS in the country has led to the country's disproportionate share of bovine TB in man. In

1984 and 1985, the prevalence of human cases of tuberculosis was 3%. Between 1983 and 1986, single bovine caudal fold tests were conducted in several ranches in northern Ghana, using PPD (purified protein derivate) tuberculin imported from Weybridge, England; the TB prevalence obtained was between 0% and 2%. However, in a recent study on over 2860 animals, conducted in the major areas of cattle production, using standard single intradermal comparative cervical tests with PPD, the prevalence was between 10.8% and 19%. The specific prevalence data obtained are as follows: the area of Great Accra and Dangme established a 13.8% infection rate, 14.0% in Dodowa district, and 19.0% in the Ningo subdistrict. Prampram and Osudoku districts recorded 11.3% and 10.8% prevalence, respectively. Though the cattle owners and herdsmen in the communities often consume unpasteurized milk, the prevalence of bovine tuberculosis in human populations is not known.

Chad

Very little information, consisting mostly of unpublished reports, exists on the prevalence of *M. bovis* in Chadian livestock. Schelling et al. (7) found a prevalence of 17% using the *M. bovis* PPD tuberculin skin test. These *M. bovis* estimates are differentiated against *M. avium*, but it is not clear to what extent *M. farcinogenes* cross reacts. The quantification of *M. bovis* in livestock is thus even more important. Chad reported 949 cases of human tuberculosis, for a total population of nearly 7 million in 1996, and is suspected to have an incidence of tuberculosis ranging from 100 to 250 per 100,000. In this situation, we expect an incidence rate of *M. bovis*–derived tuberculosis of 4–25 per 100,000, depending on exposure to livestock and milk. Of the 1400 registered cases at the General Hospital in N'Djaména, 10% were smear positive after the Directly Observed Treatment Short Course (the World Health Organization–recommended control strategy). Bovine tuberculosis was one of the main causes for carcass condemnation at the largest slaughterhouse (Société Moderne des Abattoirs) in N'Djaména, Chad. During a prospective study from July to August 2002 at the slaughterhouse, meat inspectors condemned 727 of 10,000 cattle carcasses because of tuberculosis-like lesions. Microbiological examination of 201 lesions from 75 Mbororo zebu and 124 Arab zebu carcasses confirmed bovine tuberculosis by strain isolation. A significantly higher proportion of Mbororo than Arab carcasses were declared entirely unfit for consumption, in comparison to partial condemnation. *M. bovis* was more often cultured from specimens of Mbororo cattle than of Arab cattle. Spoligotyping of 56 M. bovis isolates showed a lack of the direct repeat in 30 of the isolates, as has been described for isolates from Cameroon (6).

Burkina Faso

In 1995, epidemiological studies of *M. bovis* in abattoir animals at Bobo-Dioulasso were reported. *M. bovis* was isolated from 38 of 100 granulomatous samples of suspicious lesions, and 1% were *M. tuberculosis* isolates (11).

Senegal and Gambia

In addition to zebus, there are important numbers of trypanotolerant N'Dama cattle in Gambia and Senegal. Although N'Dama cattle are comparatively resistant to parasitic diseases, it is not known to what extent they are susceptible to bovine tuberculosis infection. In a recent study by the International Trypanotolerance Centre in Gambia, very low prevalences of bovine tuberculosis were found. No record of bovine TB in humans is available.

Niger

In 1986 Niger had a population of 3,830,000 cattle. Between 1986 and 1994, over 1 million cattle that originated from Niger were documented as having been moved to the Shaki cattle market in Nigeria. An abattoir survey of 106 suspected TB granulomas conducted at Shaki slaughter establishments revealed 13% TB prevalence. Cultures where made from a few samples but could not be further characterized.

Eastern and Southern Africa

Bovine tuberculosis is known to be endemic in most of Eastern and Southern Africa (Table 19.1). In most countries, reports are sent to the OIE; however, there is a general scarcity of scientific publications regarding the occurrence of the diseases in most of the Eastern and Southern African region. The disease is found in various mammalian species ranging from domesticated animals to wildlife (9,12, 13). The mechanisms of disease transmission from these hosts to the human populations have also been subject to a number of studies in this region (14,15). Although *M. bovis* is a known pathogen to humans worldwide, little is known in this region because of the lack of diagnostic facilities to determine species of mycobacteria involved in human tuberculosis cases. This scenario has led to the underreporting of cases of *M. bovis* in humans (16). The lack of disease control measures allows for unrestricted progression of the disease and potential transmission to humans through consumption of raw milk, undercooked and sometimes raw blood and meat (as reported from Tanzania; 17), nonpasteurized milk and products from uninspected and informally (privately) slaughtered cattle, or directly through close animal-human contact. This currently unacknowledged risk to human health, locally, is of great concern to researchers in the Southern and Eastern African countries. The occurrence of *M. bovis* in humans, against the background of the soaring HIV/AIDS incidence in the region, implies that the risk of spillover of zoonotic tuberculosis to rural communities is rapidly increasing. Various researchers have reported on scientific evidence for acceleration of pathogen replication during coinfection of *M. tuberculosis* and HIV (18) and because of the close relationship among *M. tuberculosis* complex mycobacteria, the same can be assumed for *M. bovis*. At present, 50% of new TB cases can be attributed to HIV infection. For example, in the Hlabisa hospital, situated in the district where *M. bovis* is endemic, Hluhluwe-Umfolozi Park, in Kwazulu/Natal South Africa, is surrounded by more than 100,000 head of communal cattle, and the number of HIV-positive patients with tuberculosis increased from six in 1989 to 451 as early as in 1993 (19). Similarly, in Tanzania between 1991 and 1998, up to 44% of tuberculosis cases were coinfected with HIV (20).

South Africa

It is a well-established fact that domestic cattle act as a reservoir and maintenance species for bovine tuberculosis worldwide. Reports from South Africa indicate that African buffaloes (*Syncerus caffer*) are capable of maintaining *M. bovis* infection in self-sustaining ecosystems such as the Kruger National Park and Hluhluwe-Umfolozi Park in South Africa (21,22). Over time, this capability has not only led to uncontrolled spillover of infection to other wildlife species such as chacma baboon (*Papio ursinus*), lion (*Panthera leo*), cheetah (*Acinonyx jubatus*), kudu (*Tragelaphus strepsiceros*), and leopard (*Panthera pardus*) but also to contamination of the environment with *M. bovis* and its transmission to small mammals such as warthog, honey badger, and genet (13). Recently gathered data regarding *M. bovis* infection in a smaller game reserve in the Kwazulu/Natal Province of South Africa, which lacks buffalo, have strongly indicated that greater kudu might also possess maintenance host potential (21). Because the wildlife–livestock interface has essentially remained unchanged, it should be assumed that the same circumstances that originally led to the transmission of *M. bovis* from domestic cattle to wildlife would even allow for an easier transmission back to cattle, given the overwhelming amplification of the infection pressure in the wildlife population.

Surveys have been conducted to determine the bovine tuberculosis status of buffalo herds in the Kruger National Park. One study (23) used a new diagnostic approach, the gamma-interferon assay technique, to diagnose *M. bovis* in 608 adult buffaloes out of a total of 29 discreet herds. Postmortem specimens from gamma interferon assay–positive animals showed excellent correlation with the results of the antemortem gamma interferon test. The survey revealed that over and above the two positive herds that had been identified during a previous survey carried out in 1996, there were three additional but previously unidentified infected herds in the region north of the park. Using molecular biology techniques, a total of 12 cases of *M. tuberculosis* infection in eight different species were recorded in the National Zoological Gardens of South Africa in Pretoria (Tshwane). The genetic relatedness between seven of the *M. tuberculosis* isolates was determined by IS*6110* restriction fragment length polymorphism analysis. For the majority of isolates that were analyzed, a high degree of polymorphism indicated different sources of infection.

Evidence of *M. tuberculosis* transmission between animals is reported in two chimpanzees (*Pan troglodytes*) housed together from which samples were collected for analysis 29 months apart. Through its zoonotic character, the effects of an *M. bovis* epidemic in wildlife extend far beyond conservation aspects but have the potential to affect the wildlife–livestock–human interface. Transmission of *M. bovis* from cattle to humans is most likely to occur in resource poor rural communities whose livelihoods depend to a large extent on cattle farming.

Tanzania

Many of the recent studies carried out in Tanzania have centered on determining the involvement of *M. bovis* in the incidence of tuberculosis in the human population, particularly in communities involved in livestock keeping. Tuberculosis in man resulting from *M. bovis* generally occurs in the extrapulmonary form, and in particular, as cervical lymphadenitis. In Tanzania, the proportion of extrapulmonary TB among all forms of tuberculosis stands at around 16%. The major part of these cases has been recorded in the Arusha region in the north of Tanzania, where regional data indicate that up to 30% of total tuberculosis cases are the extrapulmonary form. In this region, the main ethnic groups comprise the Maasai Iraqws, and Barbaigs tribes, who form the majority of patients diagnosed as having extrapulmonary forms of tuberculosis. The predisposing factors for this condition in the aforementioned ethnic groups include the close contact between humans and cattle, as some of the groups keep their animals indoors, and the custom of drinking raw milk and blood.

In a more recent study, differences in local knowledge and practices that might influence tuberculosis control were assessed among 27 villages (16). In each village, a general and a livestock-keeping group were selected at random. The households were home visited, and 426 family members were interviewed. The finding from this study revealed that on average, 40% of respondents practiced habits that might expose them to both bovine and human tuberculosis. The Barbaig tribe had a significantly higher number of respondents ($P = .024$) who did not boil milk. Eating uncooked meat or meat products was practiced by 17.9% of all respondents. The habit was practiced more by the Iraqw ($P = .008$) and Barabaig ($P = .016$) tribes than by other tribes. The study also found about 75% of the respondents had a poor knowledge of tuberculosis.

In Tanzania, the increasing cases of extrapulmonary tuberculosis paralleled the increasing total cases of tuberculosis reported each year between 1983 and 2001. A positive correlation ($r = 0.67$) between the proportion of extrapulmonary tuberculosis and the cattle-to-human population ratio was found. In Tanzania, molecular epidemiology studies were conducted to ascertain the genetically relatedness of strains of *M. bovis* recovered from humans and those from cattle. In such work, it was shown that *M. bovis* from cattle has infected man or vice versa because the pTBN12 restriction fragment length polymorphism, IS*986* restriction fragment length polymorphism, and spoligotype patterns of some *M. bovis* from man were similar to those produced by *M. bovis* from cattle when these typing probes/techniques were assessed individually.

The genetic relatedness between these strains and those found in cattle ranged from as low as 43% to as high as 86% by pTBN12 restriction fragment length polymorphism typing, whereas with spoligotyping, these strains were genetically related to cattle strains by between 53% and 98%. These figures indicate that a clonal relationship might have existed in the past. In a mass DNA typing of strains from various parts of the world, it was found that strains of *M. bovis* with a higher copy number of IS*986* were those from wild animals, zoo animals, or humans without contact with cattle (24). In this study, two strains of *M. bovis* from patients residing in Usangu had 13 and 15 copies of IS*986*, respectively. There was no matching number among 18 cattle strains typed by this probe. It is possible that these strains came from people who might have acquired that infection from wildlife.

The increase in bovine tuberculosis could be associated to a certain extent with the following factors: declining living standards in villages, increased urban and peri-urban cattle keeping/raising, increased size and density of the urban population, improved detection, and most notably, emergence of the HIV/AIDS virus among people living in urban and peri-urban areas. Some of these factors have also been found to be confounding factors for the national effort toward the eradication of tuberculosis in the human population.

Uganda

In Uganda, bovine tuberculosis has been reported to be common among the long-horned Ankole cattle of western part of the country. Previous studies revealed a prevalence of 19.7% in pastoral cattle in that region. Abattoir slaughter reviews by the Ministry of Agriculture, Animal Industries, and Fisheries of the Government of Uganda, in 1990, based on gross pathological lesions, found 1.8% slaughter animals originating from eastern region (including Karamoja) to show generalized tuberculosis. Cattle raising/keeping in the Karamoja region is that of transhumance; this type of management is characterized by well-organized mobile herding groups, which traditionally move together under the leadership of kraals leaders in search of grazing and watering areas. The major animal species kept include short-horned zebu, cattle, sheep, goats, and few donkeys. Animals are not supplementally fed and receive little veterinary attention (25).

Although *M. bovis* transmission is reportedly low under such extensively managed systems, compared to intensive ones, documented risky practices that favor transmission, such as sharing of communal grazing and watering areas by livestock from different areas or herds, heavy fecal contamination of few stagnant water sources, and overcrowding in night enclosures, are routine and common in the transhumance system. In addition, long-distance migrations with large herds of greater than 35 cattle, and the formation and overcrowding in cattle camps during dry season, increase herd to herd contacts and create an ideal environment for transmission in this region.

According to James Oloya (personal communication), Uganda lacks a test-and-slaughter policy for test-positive animals. That, together with the culture of keeping animals in a pastoral farming system until they die of disease or old age, allows the infection to progress to advanced stages of clinical disease and long-term excretion of *M. bovis*. This ensures that the infection is maintained in herds within extensive grazing conditions.

The effect on human health of even a low prevalence of *M. bovis* infection may be severe in a system with intense level of contact between cattle and humans, as seen in pastoral groups in Karamoja District of Eastern Uganda. Notably, habits such as drinking raw milk mixed with cows' urine, consumption of raw meat, and close contact with cattle may be important risk factors for the spread of *M. bovis* from cattle to humans. No active *M. bovis* surveillance program exists in Uganda, and little is known about the magnitude of the problem of bovine tuberculosis in this farming system, despite the existence of risky practices mentioned.

Previous reports have documented the occurrence of bovine tuberculosis in the wildlife in warthogs and buffalo in the Ruwenzori National Park. As reported in South Africa, it is very likely that in Uganda cattle, *M. bovis* infection could spill over to wildlife, and vice versa (21), and pose a danger to human health.

Zambia

Many of the reports regarding bovine tuberculosis in Zambia have centered on infections in the wildlife, particularly in the free-living Kafue lechwe; *(Kobus leche kafuensis)*. In all those studies, the occurrence of *M. bovis* was confirmed in Lechwe found primarily in the Kafue River Valley. *M. bovis* has also been reported in other wildlife species such as bushbuck *(T. scriptus)*. In 1996, Cook and coworkers performed a cross-sectional survey on 176 randomly selected rural households in the Monze District of Zambia; 103 of these presented cattle for tuberculin testing. Of the 2226 cattle tested, 165 (7.4%) were positive reactors; 33% of herds contained positive animals. Risk of a positive reaction varied with an animal's age and body condition. Cattle in larger herds were more likely to give positive reactions. Ten households reported a human case of TB during the preceding 12 months; the herds or these households were 6 times more likely to have a tuberculin-positive animal than were herds in households without a reported human TB case.

References

1. Mposhy, M., C. Binemo-Madi, and B. Mudakikwa. 1983. Incidence de la tuberculose bovine sur la santé des populations du Nord-Kivu (Zaire) *Rev Elev Méd Vet Pays Trop* 36:15-18.
2. WHO. 1994. Zoonotic tuberculosis (*Mycobacterium bovis*): memorandum from a WHO meeting (with the participation of FAO). *Bull World Health Org* 72:851-57.
3. Daborn, C. J., J. M. Grange, and R. R. Kazwala. 1996 The bovine tuberculosis cycle—an African perspective. *Soc Appl Bacteriol Symp Ser* 25:27S-32S.
4. Ayele, W. Y., S. D. Neill, J. Zinsstag, M. G. Weiss, I. Pavlik. 2004. Bovine tuberculosis, an old disease but new threat to Africa. *Int J. Tuberc Lung Dis* 8:924-37.
5. Njanpop-Lafourcade, B. M., J. Inwald, A. Ostyn, B. Durand, S. Hughes, M. F. Thorel, G. Hewinson, and N. Haddad. 2001. Molecular typing of *Mycobacterium bovis* isolates from Cameroon. *J Clin Microbiol* 39:222-27.
6. Diguimbaye, C. 2004. La tuberculose humaine et animale au Tchad: Contribution à la mise en évidence et caractérisation des agents causaux et leur implication en santé publique. PhD Thesis, University of Basel, Switzerland.
7. Schelling, E., C. Diguimbaye, S. Daoud, D. M. Daugla, K. Bidjeh, M. Tanner, and J. Zinsstag. 2000a. Zoonoses in nomadic populations of Chad—Preliminary results obtained in humans and livestock. Proceedings of the 9th Conference of the International Society of Veterinary Epidemiology and Economics. Abstract 396.
8. Bonfoh, B., A. Wasem, A. N. Traoré, A. Fané, H. Spillmann, C. F. Simbe, I. O. Alfaroukh, Z. Farah, J. Nicolet, and J. Zinsstag. 2003. Microbiological quality of cow's milk taken at different intervals from the cow's udder to the selling point in Bamako (Mali). *Food Control* 14:495-500.
9. Kazwala, R. R., C. J. Daborn, L. J. Kusiluka, S. F. Jiwa, J. M. Sharp, and D. M. Kambarage. 1998. Isolation of Mycobacterium species from raw milk of pastoral cattle of the Southern Highlands of Tanzania. *Trop Anim Health Prod* 30:233-39.
10. Ayanwale, F. O., and D. Alonge. 1988. Bovine tuberculosis in Western Nigeria: An abattoir survey. *Zariya Vet* 3:62-65.

11. Delafosse, A., A. Traore, and B. Kone. 1995. [Isolation of pathogenic Mycobacterium strains in cattle slaughtered in the abattoir of Bobo-Dioulasso, Burkina Faso]. *Rev Elev Med Vet Pays Trop* 48:301-6.

12. Jiwa, S. F., R. R. Kazwala, A. A. Aboud, and W. J. Kalaye. 1997. Bovine tuberculosis in the Lake Victoria zone of Tanzania and its possible consequences for human health in the HIV/AIDS era. *Vet Res Commun* 21:533-39.

13. Alexander, K. A., E. Pleydell, M. C. Williams, E. P. Lane, J. F. C. Nyange, and A. L. Michel. 2002. *Mycobacterium tuberculosis*: an emerging disease of free-ranging wildlife. *Emerg Infect Dis* 8:598-601.

14. Kazwala, R. R., C. J. Daborn, J. M. Sharp, D. M. Kambarage, S. F. Jiwa, and N. A. Mbembati. 2001. Isolation of *Mycobacterium bovis* from human cases of cervical adenitis in Tanzania: a cause for concern? *Int J Tuberc Lung Dis* 5:87-91.

15. Weyer, K., P. B. Fourie, D. Durrheim, J. Lancaster, K. Haslov, and H. Bryden. 1999. *Mycobacterium bovis* as a zoonosis in the Kruger National Park, South Africa. *Int J Tuberc Lung Dis* 3:1113-19.

16. Mfinanga, S. G., O. Morkve, R. R. Kazwala, S. Cleaveland, J. M. Sharp, G. Shirima, and R. Nilsen. 2003. Tribal differences in perception of tuberculosis: a possible role in tuberculosis control in Arusha, Tanzania. *Int J Tuberc Lung Dis* 7:933-41.

17. Kazwala, R. R., et al. 2001. Risk factors associated with the occurrence of bovine tuberculosis in cattle in the Southern Highlands of Tanzania. *Vet Res Commun* 25:609-14.

18. Egwaga, S. M. 2003. The impact of HIV on transmission of tuberculosis in Tanzania. *Tuberculosis (Edinb)* 83:66-67.

19. Walker, A. R. P., B. F. Walker, and A. A. Wadee. 2003. The HIV/AIDS infection—the public health burden particularly in southern Africa. *South Afr J Epidemiol Infect* 18: 26-28.

20. Range, N., Y. A. Ipuge, R. J. O'Brien, S. M. Egwaga, S. G. Mfinanga, T. M. Chonde, Y. D. Mukadi, and M. W. Borgdorff. 2001. Trend in HIV prevalence among tuberculosis patients in Tanzania, 1991-1998. *Int J Tuberc Lung Dis* 5:405-12

21. Michel, A. L. 2002. Implications of tuberculosis in African wildlife and livestock. *Ann N Y Acad Sci* 969:251-55.

22. Keet, D. F., N. P. J. Kriek, M.-L. Penrith, A. L. Michel, and H. F. Huchzermeyer. 1996. Tuberculosis in buffaloes (*Syncerus caffer*) in the Kruger National Park: spread of the disease to other species. *Onderstepoort J Vet Res* 63:239-44.

23. Grobler, D. G., A. L. Michel, L. M. De Klerk, and R. G. Bengis. 2002. The gamma-interferon test: its usefulness in a bovine tuberculosis survey in African buffaloes (*Syncerus caffer*) in the Kruger National Park. *Onderstepoort J Vet Res* 69:221-27.

24. van Soolingen, D., P. E. de Haas, P. W. Hermans, P. M. Groenen, and J. D. van Embden. 1993. Comparison of various repetitive DNA elements as genetic markers for strain differentiation and epidemiology of *Mycobacterium tuberculosis*. *J Clin Microbiol* 31: 1987-95.

25. Karamoja-Data-Centre (2004) Sector Situational Analysis Available at: http://www. karamojadata.org/index.htm.

Chapter 20

Current Challenges to and Impacts on the U.S. National Bovine Tuberculosis Eradication Program: *Mycobacterium bovis* Outbreaks in Alternative Species and Surveillance Performance

M.J. Gilsdorf, DVM, MS, L. Judge, DVM, PhD, and E.D. Ebel, DVM, MS

Introduction

On May 1, 2007, the United States National Tuberculosis Eradication Program will be 90 years old. During this time, the program has made consistent adjustments to incorporate new scientific knowledge and changes in livestock marketing, management, and politics. The prevalence of *Mycobacterium bovis* (tuberculosis, or TB) infection in cattle has decreased from over 5% to less than 0.0001%. This declining prevalence has occurred within a dynamic population of cattle that has ranged from approximately 66 million to 100 million (1). The total cost of this effort has exceeded $5 billion in 2003 dollars. The international standard—established by the OIE (2)—for freedom from bovine tuberculosis is 0.2%. On the basis of analysis of reported prevalence in the United States, cattle prevalence has been less than 0.2% since before 1960. Nevertheless, since 1917, the U.S. program's goal has been to eradicate the disease from the country.

Current challenges to accomplishing the U.S. goal of eradication include infection of alternative species that can serve as reservoirs of infection for cattle, and the performance of routine surveillance activities to ensure adequate detection and reporting of infection. The existence of wild or captive reservoirs of TB infection within alternative species requires diversion of resources away from the focus on cattle. In addition, the declining incidence of TB infection in cattle within most of the United States, combined with the existing wildlife reservoir of infection in one state, places more importance on surveillance activities to detect infected cattle.

The challenges and effects of TB infection in alternative species and surveillance will be discussed separately. How the United States is working to overcome these challenges within its TB eradication program will also be discussed.

Alternative Species

Before 1994, outbreaks of *M. bovis* in alternative species within the United States occurred. These outbreaks were primarily limited to captive cervidae herds and to a wild, free-roaming population of deer located in northern Michigan. Infection within this free-roaming population was first reported in 1975. Because TB infection in alternative species has essentially been limited to cervidae, this discussion will be limited to this class of animals.

Captive Cervids

Few outbreaks of TB in cervids were reported in the United States before 1991. In 1991, a TB-affected elk herd was detected in the United States, and animal movements from that herd were responsible for an outbreak of TB in Canada. This incident lead to the incorporation of captive cervids into the U.S. national TB eradication program (3). Initially, the program's bovine standards were simply applied to cervids, but the standards have subsequently evolved in recognition of the differences between cattle and cervid industry management.

A total of 41 infected cervid herds have been discovered in the United States since 1991 (Fig. 20.1), but only four affected herds have been found since 2000. There were no TB-affected captive or farmed cervid herds found in 2000, 2001, or 2003, although three were found in 2002 and one was found in 2004. In contrast, a

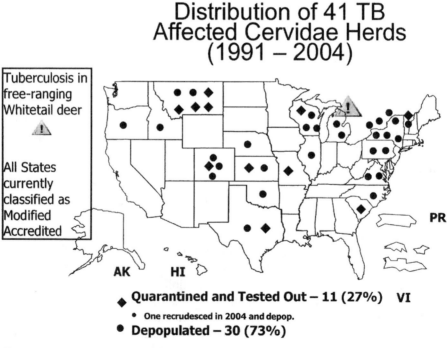

Figure 20.1.   Distribution of 41 tuberculosis-affected cervidae herds from 1991 to 2004.

total of 24 captive cervid herds were detected from January 1991 through December 1993. Therefore, these recent numbers indicate that the incidence of TB has been substantially reduced since captive cervids were included in the national program.

Of the 41 affected cervid herds, 30 were depopulated, and 11 were tested multiple times and qualified for release from quarantine. One of these 11 herds, which was an elk herd detected in 2004, was a recrudescence of a previous infection. This elk herd was initially found infected in 2001; was quarantined, tested, and released; and then was again found to be affected in 2004. The only infected animal found in that herd was an older bull that had repeatedly tested negative on annual single cervical skin tests. When that bull unexpectedly died, he was found to have extensive thoracic lesions during necropsy. The herd was subsequently depopulated.

There is continuing concern that the level of surveillance for TB in captive cervids may be inadequate. The passive slaughter surveillance system that constitutes a baseline monitoring tool for cattle is not appropriate for the captive cervid industry. Marketing of cervids for commercial slaughter is not yet routine in the United States. Several cervid herds are maintained primarily for recreational purposes or for the harvesting of antler velvet. Some cervid operations are managed for private hunting so that commercial slaughter is irrelevant. Therefore, developing a surveillance system based on slaughter is clearly inappropriate.

During 2004, a U.S. working group developed a surveillance plan for captive cervids that was presented to, and conditionally approved by, cervid industry leadership. This surveillance plan is integral to the TB eradication program's designation of individual state's TB status. It is a two-stage surveillance plan that stipulates the number of herds within a zone that must be sampled, as well as the number of animals to sample—within a specified time period—within each surveyed captive cervid herd. For a zone to move from a lower status (e.g., modified accredited) to a higher status (e.g., modified accredited advanced), it must statistically sample a greater share of the herds within the zone. This greater intensity of herd sampling increases confidence that the prevalence of affected herds within the zone is lower than a prescribed level. It is expected that this new surveillance system will be adopted into the national program standards for cervids sometime in 2005 or 2006.

Surveillance of cervids is primarily a result of animal testing in the United States. To assess the performance of animal testing, the national TB database was examined for the June 2003–June 2004 period. There were 29,230 single cervical tuberculin tests reportedly conducted on cervidae during this time period. There were 501 (1.7%) responders among these single cervical tuberculin tests. Testing was more common in the region east of the Mississippi River (69%) than west of that river (31%), but both regions reported similar fractions of responders. Comparative cervical testing for cervidae totaled 634 tests, with 93 (15%) suspects or reactors. A dramatic difference in the fraction of suspects or reactors in the east region (20%)—compared to the west (6%)—was primarily a result of fallow deer testing in a Michigan zoological park. These results indicate the need to examine the appropriateness of the comparative cervical scattergram for cervidae when applied to fallow deer and possibly other cervidae species. Therefore, the United States continues to strive for species validation of the comparative cervical test and gamma-interferon blood test in various cervid species (e.g., reindeer).

Free-Roaming Cervids

When the U.S. TB eradication program began in 1917, Michigan had a high prevalence level in its cattle population. Within Michigan, several high-prevalence counties were located in the northeastern (NE) part of the Lower Peninsula (LP). Nevertheless, whole-herd testing was effective in eliminating TB from the cattle population, and Michigan was granted TB-free status in 1979. This status was granted
despite finding a wild deer in 1975 in the NE part of the LP (Alcona County). At
this time, surveillance testing conducted on deer and cattle herds in close proximity to where this deer was found was negative. It was believed that TB could not be
maintained in a wildlife reservoir, and therefore this detection was determined to
be an isolated occurrence.

In 1993, a TB-infected cow was identified at slaughter and traced to a dairy
located in central Michigan (Isabella County); subsequent trace testing failed to
identify the source of this infection. In 1994, 19 years after the first infected deer
was disclosed, a second TB-infected deer was found in Alpena County. At that
time, the Michigan Department of Natural Resources began intensive surveillance
of wild deer based on hunter-killed samples. In 1995, several TB-infected deer
were found in this area of the state; subsequently, additional annual surveys of
hunter-killed deer began to discover an increasingly large number of infected wild
deer (Table 20.1). These findings prompted animal health officials to begin testing
cattle during 1995 in the area where these deer were discovered, and in June 1998,
the first TB-positive cattle herd was identified in the NE part of Michigan's LP. In
addition, a deer killed on a large privately owned (captive) deer facility was found
to be infected with *M. bovis* in October 1997.

During 1998 and 1999, three more cattle herds were discovered to be infected
in the NE part of the LP. As a result, Michigan's TB program status was reduced
from Accredited Free to Modified Accredited (MA) in June 2000. In addition,
Michigan established a quarantined area, to restrict cattle movement, that encom-
passed the area known to contain infected deer and cattle. Before June 2000, cat-

Table 20.1.   Tuberculosis testing in Michigan Wild Whitetail deer from 1995 to
2003

Surveillance Year	Number of Tuberculosis Positives	Total Number Tested
1975	1	1
1994	1	1
1995	27	814
1996	47	4,471
1997	73	3,705
1998	79	9,067
1999	58	19,501
2000	53	25,859
2001	60	24,278
2002	51	18,100
2003	32	17,257
Total	482	123,054

tle testing had focused on the NE part of the LP; statewide testing then began with a goal to test all cattle herds located in the state because of fears that the disease might spread over a larger area of the state. Ongoing testing in the NE part of the LP disclosed eight more TB-positive cattle herds during 2000. Also, because of the reduction in program status, the Pasteurized Milk Ordinance required that all dairy farms located in Michigan be tested for TB by June 2001.

During 2002, Michigan established three distinct zones (infected, surveillance, and disease-free). Each of these zones had testing requirements commensurate with the amount of risk of TB infection thought to exist in each zone and took the place of the state quarantine order. Concurrently with zoning, an agreement was signed between the State of Michigan and the U.S. Food and Drug Administration. This agreement allowed Michigan to implement a random-sampling plan, using whole-herd testing, as a substitute for the Pasteurized Milk Ordinance requirement to annually test all dairy herds in Michigan. The plan entails randomly sampling and testing approximately 1800 farms (proportionately distributed among beef and dairy herds) in the nonendemic area of Michigan every 2 years. A more targeted (risk-based) surveillance plan has been developed and is expected to be implemented over the next 3 years; it will replace the random selection of herds.

No infected cattle herds were found outside the TB-endemic area; therefore, Michigan applied for split-state status in August 2002. This status was subsequently granted in April 2004 and ended Michigan's zoning program while creating two TB program status zones in Michigan: the TB-endemic area remained at MA status, and the remainder of the state was upgraded to modified accredited advanced (MAA) status. The MA zone now includes the 11 counties in the NE portion of Michigan's LP plus the northern-most portions of two counties (Ogemaw and Iosco). This zone includes all cattle herds recently affected with TB. It also includes the locations where positive wildlife have been identified, except for one wild deer found in each of three contiguous counties to the MA zone.

As of 2004, a total of 33 cattle herds and one captive cervid herd in Michigan have been determined to be TB infected; this includes three herds that were found to be reinfected following depopulation and subsequent repopulation (two beef herds) or completion of a test-and-remove program (one dairy herd). It is believed that these herds were reinfected via contact with infected wildlife instead of recrudescence of infection remaining within the affected herd or the premises' environment. In addition to deer, several other species of wildlife have been found to be TB infected in Michigan, although the role these animals may play in disease transmission still remains unclear.

To discourage transmission among wild deer, feeding and baiting of deer is banned in seven counties of the NE portion of Michigan's LP. In addition, at the owners' request, the U.S. Department of Agriculture has been constructing fences surrounding feed storage areas on farms in the MA zone. These fences are expected to reduce contamination of feedstuffs consumed by cattle and thereby prevent transmission of TB from wildlife to cattle. Furthermore, risk mitigation strategies are now required for TB-accredited herds located in zones known to be endemic for TB in wildlife. These strategies focus on reducing contamination of stored feedstuffs by infected wildlife sources, restricting access of wildlife to areas where feed is presented to livestock, and reducing populations of wildlife in areas that are known to be infected with TB.

Wild deer numbers have been reduced in the MA zone through hunting. Furthermore, prevalence of TB in Michigan's wild deer has decreased from 5% to 1.4% (4) between 1997 and 2004. Although this trend is encouraging, the trend in the prevalence of affected cattle herds during this time period has remained relatively constant.

The establishment of different zones within Michigan is intended to prevent the establishment of new foci of TB in cattle and wildlife outside the MA zone. The primary function of zoning, however, is to restrict movement of cattle and require that only TB-negative cattle move from the MA zone to other parts of Michigan. Although movement of wildlife is less controlled than that of cattle, mitigation activities, such as the ban on feeding or baiting of deer within the MA zone, should reduce the likelihood of TB transmission to wildlife beyond the boundaries of the zone.

There are several factors that should be considered when assessing the importance of wildlife TB on the eradication of TB from cattle. These include costs to the farmers via increased testing requirements, movement restrictions, marketing restrictions, and other TB-preventive activities that reduce producer income. Other costs may include generally reduced value of livestock in TB-affected zones, reduced revenue from hunting in the area because hunters are concerned they might become infected from eating or touching infected deer, reduced revenue from businesses that rely on farmer and hunter purchases in the area, reduced tourism, and government costs for increased surveillance, testing, and continuing maintenance of quality control standards.

The economic consequences to Michigan cattle producers were briefly examined by Leefers et al. (4), who concluded that the total costs for Michigan's three agricultural industries—dairy, cow–calf operators, and cattle feeders—amounted to $35 million annually. Costs for wildlife management in Michigan are estimated by the amount spent on tuberculosis management and wildlife research activities by the Michigan Department of Natural Resources. These were estimated to be more than $2.5 million per year. Costs for the Michigan Department of Agriculture in tuberculosis management, outreach, and educational programs amounts to over $5 million per year (5). Michigan estimates that the state has spent $47 million in addressing TB infection in wildlife (6). These costs include maintaining an enlarged workforce to conduct testing, animal identification, record management, informing the public, and enforcing new TB movement restrictions.

Increased funding for surveillance and eradication is not the only challenge facing the national tuberculosis eradication efforts. The difficulties encountered with the detection of tuberculosis in wild white-tail deer and elk in Michigan has created a reservoir of disease in an animal species that is not under the authority of the state or federal animal health authorities. This had not been an issue in past tuberculosis eradication efforts in the United States. This is potentially a major program impediment because most of the other state and federal agencies do not have mandates that include disease control in animals. Therefore, there is sometimes reluctance from those agencies to become involved. In addition, their stakeholders often do not understand the importance of animal disease control and insist that those agencies require/implement wildlife management actions that are in direct conflict with sound, scientific disease management strategies.

Since 1998, this lack of authority for Animal Health Agencies in Michigan has been addressed through cooperation between the responsible state and federal agencies. To address the presence of TB in Michigan, the Michigan Department of Agriculture and the Michigan Department of Natural Resources formed a committee with the Department of Community Health, the U.S. Department of Agriculture/ Veterinary Services, and Michigan State University. The committee recommended that wildlife and livestock management activities, surveillance, public communication efforts, and additional research be conducted. The governor of Michigan identified actions that would be included in Michigan's tuberculosis eradication strategy, which included development of deer harvest quotas, development of methods to prevent livestock from being exposed, continued surveillance, and information dissemination. Michigan's wildlife strategy was a combination of wildlife disease surveys and deer management actions consisting of eliminating the feeding and baiting of deer and reducing the population in a special deer management area. After 1 year, there was an increase in the deer harvest of 38%. Michigan expanded its surveillance efforts to provide assurance to stakeholders that the disease was contained. However, in 2003, because of little improvement in the transmission of disease from wildlife for several years, Michigan formed an expert panel to recommend new strategies to address disease management in wildlife.

U.S. Department of Agriculture/Animal and Plant Health Inspection Service/ Veterinary Services has expended more than $12 million for tuberculosis eradication activities in Michigan since the outbreak of tuberculosis occurred in wild, free-roaming deer. Since 1997, more than $5 million per year in federal funds have been directed toward the Michigan eradication effort (5).

In 2000, a TB strategic plan was developed to identify the actions needed to complete the eradication of tuberculosis. This strategic plan was updated in 2004. The plan recommends increased eradication efforts and indemnity, increased surveillance, improved wildlife disease management strategies, risk mitigation, and increased information dissemination and education. The total costs of these measures are estimated to be over 33 million dollars.

Because the current amount of surveillance in wildlife is limited, the 2004 TB strategic plan (7) calls for an early, aggressive, and sustained management intervention to eradicate tuberculosis in wildlife. These interventions include expanded wildlife and livestock surveillance to define the scope of the problem and to monitor progress of eradication efforts, immediate cessation of activities that increase disease risks including supplemental feeding and baiting, population density reduction in specific locations to a level where tuberculosis is no longer maintained, and dissemination of information to involved stakeholders regarding risk factors associated with transmission of tuberculosis between wildlife and livestock. The estimated funding needed for these efforts is over 1 million dollars.

Because limited tools are available for eradicating tuberculosis from free-ranging wildlife, a better understanding of the epidemiology of tuberculosis in wildlife and livestock may identify additional or alternative eradication methods. In addition, the efficacy of current and future management actions must be continuously evaluated to identify the best strategies and methods for tuberculosis eradication. Therefore, research must be continued to identify key control points at which transmission among wild animals and transmission between wildlife and livestock can be precluded. It is estimated that another $500,000 is needed to fund these efforts.

The effect of TB in alternative species, and especially wildlife, is highlighted by the amount of resources already expended and the additional resources needed. Increased surveillance in both domestic animals and wildlife must be maintained as long as the disease remains in the domestic livestock or wildlife, which perpetuates program costs. The economic effect of these restrictions is difficult to measure. The discussion above provides an overview of the extent of the effects. However, successful completion of the TB eradication program relies on adequate surveillance, and TB in wildlife significantly affects how surveillance for TB will be conducted in the future.

Surveillance Performance

The surveillance challenges for captive cervids and the TB reservoir in Michigan's wild deer highlight the importance of surveillance to the national eradication effort. In addition to funds expended on eradication activities, the program has also had to increase surveillance in and around Michigan, which results in increased and prolonged surveillance costs as well as in maintaining and modifying surveillance standards to address continued infection in wildlife. For example, since the detection of TB in wildlife in Michigan, the amount of testing by state, federal, and accredited veterinarians has increased significantly. The number of cattle tested in Michigan each year before 1997 averaged 3000. In 1998 and 1999, there were more than 56,000 cattle, and in 2004 more than 124,000 cattle were tested (over 41,000 in the MA zone and over 86,000 in the MAA zone; 9).

To better understand the economic importance of TB surveillance on the program, because of continued potential for exposure to TB infection in livestock and wildlife, a description of the surveillance components of tuberculosis program is necessary.

In the early 1960s, TB surveillance in the United States converted from primarily individual animal testing to slaughter inspection. This transition was necessary because the prevalence of infection had become too low to rely on live animal testing for the purposes of proactively identifying infected cattle. Nevertheless, live animal testing using the caudal fold skin test remains an important tool for determining the status of cattle in interstate trade.

The application of the TB test is dependent on careful handling of the test reagent, accurate intradermal injection, and objective reading. Regulatory personnel, including accredited veterinarians, are responsible for ensuring that the testing is valid. In addition to Michigan, other U.S. states (e.g., Texas and California) are conducting thousands more tests than were needed before TB was again detected in their cattle populations. This has created several logistical problems, which include developing a more effective system to validate the surveillance testing.

Regardless of the system used, surveillance for TB is potentially biased if the application of the methods is invalid. For slaughter surveillance, each carcass must be carefully inspected for evidence of TB lesions. In the United States, the carcasses of all slaughtered cattle are required to be inspected in this manner. For skin testing, each injection site must be carefully palpated 72 hours postinjection, and any reaction—regardless of size—is considered a response. Responses are followed up with a more specific test—the comparative cervical test or the gamma interferon blood test—to classify a responder to the caudal fold test as a suspect or reactor. If slaughter inspectors are not attentive to evidence of TB, then the validity of that surveillance system is questionable. Similarly, if veterinarians who conduct skin testing do not report all responses, then the validity of that surveillance system is questionable.

On-Farm Surveillance

The TB eradication program relies on the competency of state, federal, and accredited veterinarians to correctly classify skin-test reactions and the competency of veterinarians and inspectors to correctly identify and submit lesions from slaughtered animals. Accredited veterinarians commonly conduct the caudal fold test on cattle for interstate movement. Because there is a wildlife reservoir in northern Michigan that has spread to cattle herds, there are hundreds of thousands more TB tests conducted each year for surveillance purposes. Because there is a greater potential for some animals to be exposed, there is a greater need to evaluate the performance of these veterinarians in a systematic and consistent manner. Therefore, one of the program changes needed in the U.S. Tuberculosis Eradication Program was to establish a performance standard.

The 2004 revised Tuberculosis Eradication Program's Uniform Methods and Rules includes a performance standard for conducting the caudal fold TB test. This performance standard provides veterinarians with the regulatory expectations and provides a quantitative tool for assessing compliance or noncompliance with these expectations. The concern regarding caudal fold TB testing is underreporting of reactions. If a veterinarian is rarely classifying a test as suspicious for TB, then it is possible that infected cattle are missed and that the eradication program is deficient.

In a completely noninfected population of cattle, the caudal-fold TB test is expected to result in a suspicious response in some predictable proportion of tested cattle. Test specificity (SPEC) measures the proportion of noninfected animals in a population that will be correctly classified as negative on a test. The quantity $1 - SPEC$ measures the proportion of false-positive results expected. For a low-prevalence disease like TB, the minimum observed proportion of suspicious responders in a population must be equal to, or greater than, the quantity $1 - SPEC$. If the population includes some infected cattle, then the observed proportion of suspicious responders could be greater than $1 - SPEC$, but in no case can it be less.

Assessments of the true specificity for the caudal fold TB test range from 90% to nearly 100%. For the purposes of this performance standard, it is expected that

99% of noninfected cattle should be classified as negative, and the remaining 1% of noninfected cattle should be classified as responders to the caudal fold test. Given this expectation, there remains the quantitative assessment of performance by individual veterinarians.

According to the performance standard, each caudal fold test a veterinarian conducts has a 1% probability of being positive. The expected number of positive results in *n* tests is predicted by the binomial distribution. This distribution implies that there should be at least one positive test among, for example, 300 tests. The purpose of the performance standard is to verify that a veterinarian is classifying tests at prevalence above or equal to 1%. Nevertheless, the performance standard must account for the random variability inherent in the binomial distribution.

The caudal fold TB test performance standard should result in consistent application of this test. In turn, this performance standard should improve detection of remaining infected cattle in the United States. Having a performance standard should also assist the United States in withstanding scrutiny of its national TB surveillance effort. The standard also allows evaluation of other countries' performance of this test.

The benefits of this standard—in terms of disease detection and validation of testing—far outweigh the costs incurred because of an increase in reported false-positive cattle. False-positive cattle are not a result of the standard, but a biologic phenomenon inherent in the skin testing. If responses are arbitrarily classified by the veterinarian conducting the test, then a responder could be a false-positive animal or a true-positive animal. The cost avoided by not classifying the false-positive animal as a responder is likely much less than the cost of allowing a true-positive animal to remain unreported.

Slaughter Surveillance

As long as the potential for TB infection exists in a country, the importance of maintaining surveillance at slaughter is magnified. The presence of TB in alternative species, such as wildlife in Michigan, affects the Tuberculosis Eradication Program by prolonging the time period that each carcass must be examined. In conducting surveillance at slaughter, every carcass is required to be inspected for TB. This results in maintaining a significantly increased number of veterinary inspectors until after the disease has been eradicated from the country. Therefore, the expected number of lesions submitted from slaughtered animals for testing also increases. Because slaughter inspection for TB is so critical to the eradication of TB from the United States, a system of validating proper numbers of samples to be collected at slaughter was developed.

If we know the number of cattle slaughtered annually, then the threshold of infection that we can detect via slaughter surveillance can be determined. Yet, inspection must be thorough to detect TB in carcasses. There is much pathology that grossly resembles TB lesions. If carcass inspection is valid, then granulomas must occasionally be submitted, even in the absence of infection. If submissions from a slaughter plant are occurring with sufficient frequency, then it is concluded that monitoring activities are valid.

In the past, the frequency of granuloma submissions by slaughter establishments has been highly variable. From year to year, the frequency of granuloma submissions per plant has ranged from zero per 10,000 carcasses processed to greater than 30 per 10,000 carcasses processed. This variability raises concerns about the validity of slaughter surveillance in the United States.

Similar to the caudal fold TB test, slaughter inspection for TB should have some fraction of false-positive carcasses. These are carcasses with lesions that resemble TB but that are distinguished by histopathology or culture (or polymerase chain reaction assay) as not being caused by TB. Among the population of cattle carcasses processed in the United States with any type of gross lesion, there is a subpopulation of carcasses with lesions that are called granulomatous. For example, there is some percentage of actinomycosis, actinobacillosis, coccidiomycosis, and malignant lymphoma lesions that grossly resemble TB.

During 2003, there were 5078 submissions from slaughter establishments to the National Veterinary Service Laboratories and the State of California Veterinary Diagnostic Laboratories for suspicion of TB (Fig. 20.2). The largest percentage of these lesions were classified as ACTI—meaning either actinobacillosis or actinomycosis. ACTI is a condition that the U.S. Department of Agriculture's Food Safety Inspection Service (FSIS) specifically keeps track of in their Animal Disease Reporting System database. Other histopathology categories, such as pyogranuloma, are not specifically identified in this FSIS database. Instead, these other conditions may fall within other FSIS categories such as pneumonia, abscess pyemia, or miscellaneous inflammation.

FSIS reports the number of carcasses that are restricted because they have evidence of ACTI. Most of the time, these restrictions simply involve trimming out the affected part, although a small number of ACTI-affected carcasses are condemned.

However, because ACTI is a common histopathologic diagnosis for TB, and it can be linked to the FSIS database, this condition is used to establish a minimum

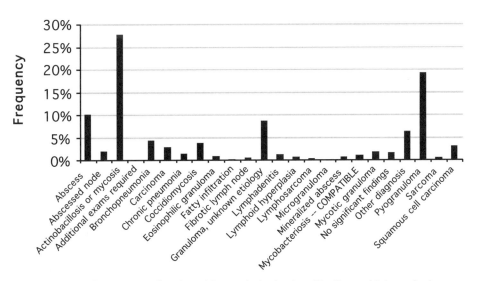

Figure 20.2. Frequency of various histopathologic classifications of tuberculosis submissions in 2003.

Table 20.2.   Summary of ACTI-affected carcasses in FSIS-inspected slaughter plants during 2003

Region	Number Slaughtered	Number of ACTI-Affected Carcasses	Fraction Affected
United States	6,057,653	57,024	0.94%
Eastern United States	2,969,802	11,137	0.38%
Western United States	3,087,851	45,887	1.49%
Northern United States	4,296,066	36,478	0.85%
Southern United States	1,761,587	20,546	1.17%

submission frequency standard for suspicious TB lesions by slaughter establishments. The minimum submission frequency standard is defined as $S = P \times f$, where S is the fraction of carcasses with TB-suspicious lesions slaughtered in an establishment, P is a prevalence of ACTI-affected carcasses, and f is the fraction of ACTI-affected carcasses whose lesions resemble TB.

To establish a standard that all slaughter establishments can meet, the lowest regional prevalence of ACTI-affected carcasses (0.38%) is chosen as the value for P. The number of ACTI-affected carcasses reported by FSIS in 2003 was evaluated for the east and west regions of Veterinary Services, as well as for the north and south regions of the United States. There was little difference in the prevalence of ACTI-affected carcasses between the north and south regions, but there was a much lower prevalence in the eastern United States when compared to the west. Nevertheless, ACTI was reported at perceptible levels regardless of region (Fig. 20.2 and Table 20.2).

To estimate the fraction of ACTI-affected carcasses whose lesions resemble TB, data from the 40 largest cow–bull slaughter establishments were examined. Regardless of regional location of the slaughter establishment, there was a concentration of slaughter establishments that submitted fewer than 5 TB samples for every 10,000 carcasses processed (Fig. 20.3). Nevertheless, there were 13 plants that submitted samples at substantially higher frequencies. Based on experience, it is recognized that these plants are staffed with veterinarians committed to TB surveillance.

The relationship between the number of TB samples with histopathologic diagnoses of ACTI and the number of carcasses reported as being ACTI affected indicates that plants committed to TB surveillance are likely submitting lesions from ACTI-affected carcasses because those lesions look like TB (Fig. 20.4). A proportional trend in this relationship is noted for the top 12 submitting slaughter establishments, but no such trend is evident among the other 27 slaughter establishments. One establishment among the top submitting plants was considered an outlier because personnel changes at the plant—which contributed to an improvement in TB submission frequency—occurred late in 2003.

Using data from the top 12 submitting slaughter establishments, the fraction of ACTI-affected carcasses whose lesions resemble TB (f) is estimated as 14%. From the top 12 submitting slaughter establishments, there were 3213 TB submissions from more than 2 million adult cattle slaughtered in 2003. Following histopathology,

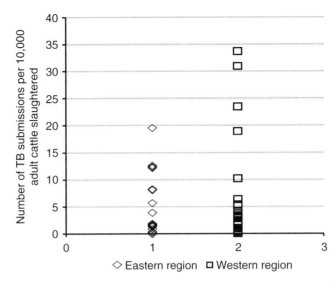

Figure 20.3. A comparison of adult cattle tuberculosis submission rates from the 40 largest eastern and western region slaughter facilities for 2003.

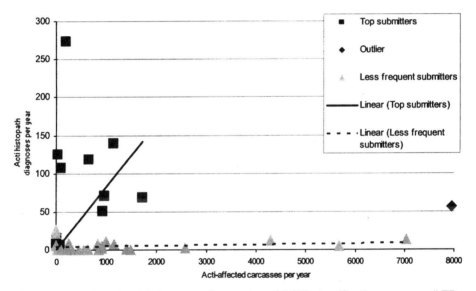

Figure 20.4. Relationship between the number of ACTI classifications among all TB submissions and the number of ACTI-affected carcasses for the 40 largest adult cattle slaughter plants in financial year 2003. There were 12 slaughter plants identified as frequent tuberculosis submitters (Top Submitters), 27 slaughter plants identified as less frequent submitters, and one plant identified as an outlier.

990 (31%) of these 3213 TB submissions were diagnosed as ACTI. According to FSIS data, there were 5919 carcasses reported as being ACTI affected from these top 12 slaughter establishments in 2003. Assuming the TB submissions that were later diagnosed as ACTI contribute to the total number of ACTI-affected carcasses

from these plants, the fraction of ACTI-affected carcasses whose lesions resemble TB equals

$$14\% = \frac{990}{990 + 5919}$$

Based on this analysis, it is concluded that slaughter establishments should be submitting samples suspected of TB at a frequency of 0.05% (= $P \times f$ = 0.38% × 14%). This equates to one submission per 2000 carcasses processed. Failure to meet this standard indicates that the inspection of carcasses for TB may be inadequate. Inadequate inspection of carcasses could delay the successful eradication of TB in the United States.

The benefits of this slaughter surveillance standard are similar to those mentioned for the caudal fold TB testing performance standard. Because slaughter surveillance is a very important element of the U.S. TB program, the benefits are magnified. If TB-infected cattle are routinely missed because slaughter inspection is inadequate, then the cost to the eradication program is large.

This increase in sampling and testing represents another increased cost to the program. In addition, laboratories must have increased staffing and resources to handle the increase in sample submission. In the 2004 TB strategic plan, it is estimated that an additional $5.6 million is needed annually to meet the increased surveillance cost.

Summary

In summary, TB in wildlife costs citizens an estimated $35 million in lost revenue each year. Wildlife TB has cost the national TB eradication effort at least $30 million since 1994 in surveillance, eradication activities, and research efforts alone. Wildlife TB will continue to require adequate funding to prevent its spread and to make progress toward its eradication. Significant efforts are needed to prevent the disease from spreading to other areas through wildlife movement and livestock movements. The tuberculosis strategic plan has identified more than $10.5 million in resources to adequately address this situation in wildlife. Research is being conducted to find improved management techniques, effective vaccines, or better tests to incorporate into the program. More resources are needed in this area. However, even with adequate resources, disease management authorities must also be in place through interagency cooperation and collaboration to adequately eliminate this disease from the country in all species.

The persistence of TB in cattle, as well as captive and wild cervids, highlights the importance of surveillance to detect TB infection. To ensure that data coming from the existing surveillance systems is accurate, the performance of testing and inspection needs standardization. The national TB eradication program's methods and rules now incorporate such standards.

The finding of TB infection in wild deer has had a significant effect on the tuberculosis eradication efforts in livestock in that area and on the entire eradication program. Until the exposure of domestic livestock to TB-infected wildlife can be effectively prevented, the outbreak of TB in the white-tail deer and elk will continue to have a significant effect on the eradication of bovine tuberculosis in the United States.

References

1. US Department of Agriculture, Animal and Plant Health Inspection Service, Veterinary Services.
2. OIE World Organization for Animal Health, Health Standards, Chapter 2.3.3, Article 2.3.3.1, bovine tuberculosis, 2003.
3. Essey, M. A., and J. S., VanTiem. 1995. *Mycobacterium bovis* Infection in Animals and Humans, 1st edition. Ames: Iowa State University Press, 152.
4. Leefers, L., J. Ferris, D. Propst. 1997. Economic Consequences Associated with Bovine Tuberculosis in Northeastern Michigan, Report to the State of Michigan Commission of Agriculture.
5. US Department of Agriculture, Animal and Plant Health Inspection Service, Veterinary Services.
6. Bridget, P. 2003. Michigan Tuberculosis TB Eradication Project, Michigan Department of Community Health, December.
7. US Department of Agriculture, Animal and Plant Health Inspection Service. 2004. Veterinary Services Tuberculosis Strategic Plan.

Chapter 21

Effect of Bovine Tuberculosis in Wildlife on a National Eradication Program—Canada

M.A. Koller-Jones, DVM, C. Turcotte, DVM, PhD,
C. Lutze-Wallace, and O. Surujballi, PhD

Canada's Bovine Tuberculosis Eradication Program: Cattle

In 1897, only 5 years after Robert Koch discovered the bacterium responsible for tuberculosis, Canada was one of the first countries in the world to commence a program to deal with the disease by offering testing to livestock owners free of charge. In 1907, a national meat inspection system was implemented, which provided reliable statistics on the incidence of tuberculosis in slaughter animals and permitted the tracing of diseased livestock to their farm of origin. This, in turn, provided the impetus for the development of programs aimed first at control and then the complete eradication of the disease in cattle. The initial voluntary program of testing herds and removing animals with a positive reaction to the tuberculin test was replaced in 1923 with a mandatory farm-to-farm whole-herd testing program. During the first nationwide testing campaign, which lasted until 1961, the rate of test-positive animals was reduced from more than 4% of cattle tested to approximately 0.1%.

Between 1961 and 1978, the mandatory on-farm testing program continued through a second, third, and fourth complete test of all cattle herds in Canada, using an eradication strategy of repeated herd testing and the removal, to slaughter, of test-positive animals only. However, the rate of skin test–positive animals remained at approximately 0.1%, and the number of infected herds detected each year stabilized. In 1979, a comprehensive review, including an economic analysis, was conducted to identify the obstacles to successful completion of Canada's bovine tuberculosis eradication program (Management Consulting Services, 1979).

The review resulted in several significant changes to the eradication program beginning in 1980: first, disease surveillance was shifted from on-farm herd testing to slaughterhouse monitoring through the submission of any granulomatous lesions found during routine postmortem inspection to the laboratory for microscopic (histopathology) and microbiological (culture) examination; second, detailed epidemiological investigations were instituted to identify all possible sources of infection whenever *M. bovis* was confirmed; and third, disease eradication required the destruction of all susceptible animals found by the epidemiological investigation to have been exposed to *M. bovis*—those present on the infected farm as well as those previously removed (trace-out animals). Although other eradication options were considered, the computer simulation model used in the economic analysis determined that the whole-herd destruction option yielded the best benefit/cost ratio.

The implementation of these program enhancements was followed by a steady decline in the number of infected cattle herds found in Canada each year. In 2005, bovine tuberculosis has been eradicated from cattle herds in all regions of the country, except for a small area around Riding Mountain National Park in the province of Manitoba. During the preceding 5 years (2000–2004), bovine tuberculosis was found in six cattle herds in Canada, five of which were located in, or associated with, the Riding Mountain area. The situation in the Riding Mountain area, the only region in Canada where bovine tuberculosis continues to be present in livestock, is discussed later in this chapter.

Canada's Bovine Tuberculosis Eradication Program: Farmed Bison and Cervids

Ventures into the commercial farming of game animals in Canada began in the early 1980s, expanding from a handful of enterprises to several thousand herds over the next two decades. The emergence of this farming sector occurred as Canada was nearing the complete eradication of bovine tuberculosis in traditional livestock. Game farms, which in Canada raise primarily bison, elk, red deer, white-tailed deer, mule deer, and fallow deer, were identified as potential reservoirs of *M. bovis* that, if left unexamined, could result in the recurrence of bovine tuberculosis in traditional livestock and humans, as well as serve as an avenue by which the disease could spread to, and become established in, free-roaming wildlife.

In 1989, Canada's bovine tuberculosis eradication program was expanded to include farmed bison, farmed cervids, and other captive ungulate species. The disease was made notifiable in all species of animals, and disease surveillance was achieved through on-farm testing of those species considered to be suitable for tuberculin skin testing: bison and other Bovidae using the caudal fold site and Cervidae using the midcervical site. Disease eradication methods were identical to those in place for cattle: a detailed epidemiological investigation to identify all possible sources of infection and the destruction of all susceptible animals found by the investigation to have been exposed to *M. bovis*.

During the first 11 years of the expanded eradication program (1989 through 1999), bovine tuberculosis was found on 40 game farms in five of Canada's 10 provinces. Nineteen of these infected herds were associated with the importation of one or more shipments of infected farmed elk from the United States into Alberta during the mid- to late 1980s, before the implementation of stricter import controls (Essey and Koller, 1994). During the next 5 years (2000–2004), bovine tuberculosis was found on a single game farm in Canada—a bison herd in Alberta in 2001.

In 2005, bovine tuberculosis has been eradicated from farmed bison and farmed cervids in all regions of the country.

Elements of Canada's Bovine Tuberculosis Eradication Program

The Canadian bovine tuberculosis eradication program has three major elements: disease surveillance, disease eradication, and disease reservoir management. The collective results of these three elements are reflected in the fourth aspect of the program—area status classification. The program also includes provisions for the payment of compensation.

Disease Surveillance

Bovine tuberculosis is a federally notifiable disease in Canada in all species and in all regions. Active surveillance is directed at three livestock sectors: cattle, farmed bison, and farmed cervids. It consists of routine slaughterhouse inspections, the submission of tuberculous-like lesions for laboratory examination, and the tracing and investigation of the herd of origin of all lesions suspected or confirmed to be caused by *M. bovis* infection. This slaughter monitoring program is augmented by periodic on-farm testing targeted at livestock sectors with insufficient slaughter volumes to support slaughter monitoring as the sole method of surveillance (farmed cervids), and regions in Canada where the risk of *M. bovis* being present in, or introduced into, livestock herds warrants more aggressive surveillance (i.e., the area around Riding Mountain National Park in Manitoba). Passive surveillance relies on Canada's extensive veterinary infrastructure, encompasses all species, and consists of routine postmortem examination by private veterinary practitioners and diagnostic laboratories, as well as tuberculin testing of animals for other reasons, such as export, entry into an artificial insemination center, or change of ownership. The tuberculin tests used in on-farm testing include the caudal fold test to screen cattle and farmed bison, the midcervical test to screen farmed cervids, and the comparative cervical test to evaluate cattle, bison, or farmed cervids that react to the screening test. An interferon-gamma assay (Bovigam) was added to the program in 2003 for use in cattle and farmed bison that react to the screening test. Animals suspected of being infected with bovine tuberculosis are destroyed for detailed necropsy and confirmatory laboratory testing of their tissues. If *M. bovis* is isolated, disease eradication activities are initiated.

Disease Eradication

The response to confirmed cases of bovine tuberculosis in farm animals involves measures to eliminate the infection from the premises (quarantine, destruction of all susceptible exposed animals, cleaning and disinfection, vacant period, and monitoring of the restocked herd); identify any spread of *M. bovis* from the infected premises, and eliminate it (tracing and destruction of exposed trace-out animals); and prevent future spread of the infection (trace-back and investigate all possible sources of the infection).

Disease Reservoir Management

Two reservoirs of bovine tuberculosis, both in free-roaming ruminants, have been identified in Canada. Their presence has resulted in the development and implementation of risk-management measures to prevent the spread of the disease from these reservoirs to Canadian livestock herds. Bovine tuberculosis is endemic in free-roaming herds of approximately 3000 wood bison in and around Wood Buffalo National Park in northwestern Canada. Because of their distance from agricultural enterprises, the diseased bison currently pose a very low risk to livestock herds. Bovine tuberculosis is also present in wild Cervidae (approximately 2000 elk and white-tailed deer) in and around Riding Mountain National Park in southern Manitoba. Unlike the situation in northern Alberta, this reservoir is believed to be the source of bovine tuberculosis for five of the six infected cattle herds found in Canada between 2000 and 2005. The effect of the presence of these wildlife reservoirs is discussed later in this chapter.

Area Certification and Movement Control

Federal legislation sets out criteria that must be satisfied for a region (area) in Canada to be classified as officially free from bovine tuberculosis. These criteria meet or exceed those set out by the World Organization for Animal Health (OIE). Criteria for two other levels of tuberculosis certification—tuberculosis-accredited-advanced (very low prevalence) and tuberculosis-accredited (low prevalence)—are prescribed. The legislation also requires that certain livestock—cattle and farmed bison moved from a region of lower status to one of higher status, and cervids moved between any premises—are accompanied by a permit issued by the federal veterinary authority. In 2005, cattle and farmed bison in all regions of Canada, except those in the eradication area around Riding Mountain National Park, have been classified as officially tuberculosis free. The Riding Mountain eradication area is classified as tuberculosis-accredited-advanced, and a permit is required for cattle and farmed bison leaving this area. In 2005, farmed cervids in all regions of Canada were classified as being officially tuberculosis free.

Compensation

Federal legislation provides for the payment of compensation for animals that are destroyed under eradication programs in the amount of the market value of the animal up to a prescribed maximum amount, as well as reasonable disposal costs. The level of compensation endeavors to strike a balance between encouraging the early reporting of suspected disease by animal owners and veterinarians to facilitate effective control of outbreaks, providing assistance to owners in replacing their animals, and ensuring that disease does not become profitable.

Wood Buffalo National Park

By the 1890s, the once enormous herds of plains bison in North America had been reduced to a handful of herds held in private ownership. In Canada, a morphologically distinct subspecies, wood bison, was reduced to a few animals surviving in a small area of woods and small prairies in northwestern Canada. Early in the last century, the Canadian government established Buffalo Park in central Alberta and stocked it with a herd of purchased plains bison. In 1922, Wood Buffalo National Park was established to protect the surviving wood bison. At 44,800 square kilometers in an area that straddles the boundary between the province of Alberta and the Northwest Territories, it remains Canada's largest national park. By 1923, the plains bison in Buffalo Park had become too numerous for their range to support. Attempts to cull the herd by slaughtering older animals caused a public outcry (and revealed the presence of bovine tuberculosis). Faced with the need to reduce the population, more than 6000 plains bison were transported to Wood Buffalo National Park between 1925 and 1928, introducing bovine tuberculosis and resulting in the interbreeding of the two subspecies (Northern Diseased Bison Environmental Assessment Panel, 1990).

Bovine tuberculosis is endemic (estimated prevalence of 49%) in the free-roaming bison herds in and around Wood Buffalo National Park (Joly and Messier, 2001). A risk assessment conducted in 1998 concluded that these herds pose their greatest threat to adjacent disease-free wild bison herds (Animal and Plant Health Risk Assessment Network, 1998). As they remain sufficiently geographically isolated from areas of livestock-rearing operations, the diseased bison represent a very low risk to bison farming operations located to the south and west of the park, and to cattle farms, which occur further south. However, as drought conditions in the south, the growth of economic enterprises such as oil and ecotourism in the north, and climate change contribute to the northward expansion of human habitation and agricultural activities, the risk of spread of bovine tuberculosis from the diseased herds to disease-free populations can be expected to increase.

In response to the findings of the risk assessment, a number of measures were instituted to minimize the risk of the bovine tuberculosis spreading to healthy free-roaming bison herds, farmed bison, or cattle. These measures include a bison containment plan operated by the provincial and territorial governments and designed to prevent diseased bison from leaving their current range. This is achieved through the creation of no-bison buffer zones around the herds, the killing of stray bison that enter these zones, expanded hunting opportunities in areas outside the park, and restrictions on the grazing of livestock on public lands in northern Alberta.

As a result of the spatial separation that exists between the diseased free-roaming bison herds and livestock herds and the containment measures that have been instituted, no cases of spread of bovine tuberculosis to farmed animals have been detected. Despite the disease not having spread to livestock, the presence of this wildlife reservoir has significant economic implications for Canada. First are the ongoing costs to governments and livestock operations of maintaining aggressive active surveillance programs in both the livestock and wildlife populations. The appropriateness of these surveillance strategies must be constantly reviewed and enhanced to ensure they incorporate the best available science and technology. Efforts are underway to develop a suitable fluorescent polarization assay as a screening test for bovine tuberculosis that would permit the screening of cattle and farmed bison at auction markets and other assembly points in Alberta and neighboring provinces—something currently not feasible using the tuberculin screening test, which requires animals to be held for 72 hours. Governments incur ongoing costs to operate, monitor, and enhance, as needed, the various containment measures in place to maintain adequate spatial separation between the diseased free-roaming bison herds and livestock operations, as well as healthy wildlife.

Also of economic significance are the restrictions that have been placed on the development and expansion of livestock enterprises in the northern part of Alberta as a result of the presence of diseased bison in and around the park. As these ongoing costs and lost economic opportunities continue to mount, governments may, at some time in the future, have the public support and the financial resources to embark on a program to eradicate bovine tuberculosis from wildlife in the Wood Buffalo National Park area.

Riding Mountain National Park

Throughout much of the last century, cases of bovine tuberculosis were reported in free-roaming elk and deer in Canada and the United States: elk in Alberta (1942) and Manitoba (1992); white-tailed deer in New York (1934 and 1963), Ontario (1962), and Michigan (1975 and 1997); axis deer in Hawaii (1974); and mule deer in Alberta (1942) and Montana (1995) (Schmitt et al., 1997). The vast majority of these findings were geographically associated with infected livestock herds, and when no further cases were found in wildlife following the eradication of the disease from livestock, the risk that bovine tuberculosis could establish and maintain itself in free-ranging Cervidae populations in North America in the absence of diseased livestock appeared to be very small. Protecting the health of free-roaming wildlife became another motive for eradicating the disease from livestock. Unfortunately, findings in Michigan in the late 1990s and soon thereafter in Manitoba dispelled this commonly held belief.

Riding Mountain National Park is, by Canadian standards, a very small park, covering just under 3000 square kilometers and extending only 115 km from east to west and 60 km from north to south. Established in 1929, it represents a transition zone between the prairies and the northern Boreal Plains and is dominated by the Manitoba Escarpment, which rises up to 475 m above the surrounding, largely flat, landscape. Described as an island of wilderness in a sea of agriculture, the park is home to approximately 2000 wild elk and a similar number of moose. White-tailed deer are found near the perimeter of the park and in the surrounding agricultural area, which is predominated by cereal crops, pasture, and hay production (Brook and McLachlan, 2004). Not permitted inside the park, big-game hunting is a significant recreational and economic activity in areas immediately outside the park. Until the late 1960s, when management of the park shifted from resource and recreational use to protection of the ecology, cattle owners in the area pastured their livestock in the park during the summer months.

In contrast to the history of Wood Buffalo National Park, precisely how or when bovine tuberculosis became established in the wild elk and deer population in and around Riding Mountain National Park is unknown. The earliest documented finding of *M. bovis* in wildlife in the park was in 1978, when it was confirmed in two wolf pups (Carbyn, 1982). It is not known whether this infection originated from diseased livestock or wildlife carcasses, as bovine tuberculosis was still present in Manitoba cattle herds. No further wildlife cases were reported until 1992, when *M. bovis* was confirmed in a wild elk harvested during a special hunt conducted near the southwest boundary of the park (Lees et al., 2003). This hunt was prompted by an outbreak of bovine tuberculosis involving six cattle herds in the area in 1990–1991. In keeping with the belief at the time, this elk was seen as another case of self-limiting transmission from livestock to wildlife that would resolve itself once the disease was eradicated from livestock herds in the area.

Five years later, in 1997, bovine tuberculosis was confirmed in a cattle herd located in the vicinity of the 1990 outbreak that had been tested several times, with negative results, following that outbreak. By this time, findings in Michigan were beginning to indicate that free-roaming Cervidae populations could indeed sustain bovine tuberculosis and, furthermore, could spread the disease to surrounding livestock herds. In late 1997, an ongoing comprehensive wildlife survey was implemented in the Riding Mountain area, resulting in the confirmation of *M. bovis* infection in a total of 26 elk and six white-tailed deer from 1998 to 2005. During the same period, five infected cattle herds (one in 2001, three in 2003, and one in 2004) were found in Manitoba, all located in (four) or originating from (one) the area immediately around the park. The investigation of these herds indicated that, in each case, the most likely source of the infection was diseased wild elk or deer, indicating that free-roaming elk and deer in and around the park were maintaining bovine tuberculosis and could serve as a source of the disease for surrounding livestock herds.

Isolates of *M. bovis* obtained from 11 infected cattle herds detected in the vicinity of the park, and one infected cattle herd (2004) that originated from the vicinity of the park and was moved to another part of Manitoba before the implementation of movement controls in 2003, as well as all wildlife isolates of *M. bovis* (elk and deer) obtained during the period 1992–2003, have been characterized by spoligotyping. These isolates were found to be predominantly of a single strain type, with minor deviation only at oligonucleotide 12 in 9% of the isolates examined (Lutze-Wallace et al., 2005). The uniqueness of the molecular characteristics of this strain support the epidemiological finding that wild elk and deer are the most likely source of the outbreaks of bovine tuberculosis found in livestock in the Riding Mountain area in recent years.

Managing Bovine Tuberculosis in Wildlife in the Riding Mountain Area

In response to the findings of bovine tuberculosis in livestock and wildlife in the Riding Mountain area, the federal and provincial veterinary and wildlife authorities established a multiagency working group to develop and implement a management strategy with the objectives of determining the prevalence and distribution of bovine tuberculosis in wildlife in the Riding Mountain ecosystem, preventing the spread of the infection to livestock herds, and eliminating the disease from wild Cervidae populations in the area. This strategy operates alongside the Canadian bovine tuberculosis eradication program, which is responsible for disease surveillance, eradication, and certification activities in farmed animals.

Prevalence and Distribution

On the basis of the results of hunter–harvest surveys conducted outside the park from 1997 to 2005 and a capture-test-removal program carried out inside the park from 2003 to 2005, the prevalence of bovine tuberculosis in the free-roaming elk population in the Riding Mountain area is estimated to be between 1% and 5%. Although *M. bovis* was confirmed in six white-tailed deer between 2001 and 2005, sampling data has not permitted an estimation of disease prevalence in this species. To 2005, active sampling of other species of wild Cervidae (moose, mule deer) and other wild mammals in the Riding Mountain area has failed to detect *M. bovis* infection. Bovine tuberculosis in wild elk and deer does not appear to be evenly distributed in the Riding Mountain ecosystem, with the vast majority of positive cases occurring in or outside the western third of the park. To 2005, all confirmed wildlife cases have been found inside the park or within 10 km of the park boundary, with sampling at further distances yielding negative results.

Preventing Spread to Livestock

The investigations of the infected cattle herds found in the vicinity of the park have concluded that the most likely source of the infection was feed or water contaminated by diseased wild elk or deer. During the winter months, wild elk and deer may be observed gathering at, and feeding on, livestock feedstuffs (primarily hay) that are stored outdoors or that have been placed out for feeding of livestock. Wild elk or deer are rarely observed in close proximity to cattle at any time of year, and transmission of the disease under summer pasture conditions is not believed to play a significant role in the epidemiology of bovine tuberculosis in the Riding Mountain ecosystem. Given these considerations, key elements of the wildlife management strategy are measures implemented to establish spatial or temporal separation between wild Cervidae and livestock. These include installation of barrier fences around feed storage areas and cattle feeding yards to prevent elk or deer from accessing and possibly contaminating these areas; limitations on crop insurance for hay left in the field through the winter to encourage its removal to secure storage areas; improvements to the habitat in the park, such as prescribed burning, to encourage animals to remain in the park and reduce visits to farms where barrier fencing is not in place; and management of elk and deer populations through increased hunting opportunities outside the park to numerically reduce the elk and deer in the area.

Eliminating Disease from Wild Cervidae

The measures described above to prevent the spread of bovine tuberculosis from wild elk and deer to surrounding livestock herds also contribute to eliminating the disease from the wildlife population itself. The fencing of feed storage sites and cattle yards and the prompt removal of harvested hay from the fields reduce the incentives and opportunities for elk or deer to gather in groups and come into close contact with one another, thereby reducing animal-to-animal spread among wild Cervidae. The habitat improvements that encourage animals to remain in the park also permit wider dispersal of the animals, contributing to fewer opportunities for wildlife-to-wildlife spread in the park. The reductions in population size achieved by increased hunting opportunities for wild elk and deer and an additional measure that prohibits the feeding or baiting wild elk or deer for hunting or other reasons also reduce contacts between wildlife that could spread disease. From 2002 to 2005, approximately 500 elk were captured in the park, identified with a radio collar for recapture if needed, and tested for bovine tuberculosis, using blood tests (lymphocyte stimulation test and fluorescent polarization assay). Elk found to have a positive or suspicious test result were recaptured (132), humanely killed, and subjected to a detailed necropsy and tissue collection for confirmatory laboratory testing. *M. bovis* infection was confirmed in 15 of these elk. Although its primary objective has been to determine the prevalence and distribution of bovine tuberculosis in the park, this capture-test-removal program also contributes to the elimination of infected animals from the free-roaming population.

The costs of carrying out the bovine tuberculosis management strategy in wildlife in the Riding Mountain area are largely borne by the federal and provincial public treasuries at an estimated cost of $1,500,000 (Canadian funds) annually. Although hunting and tourism contribute to the local economy in the Riding Mountain area, albeit not to the same extent as in the Upper Peninsula in Michigan, the presence of bovine tuberculosis in wild Cervidae, and the measures implemented in response to it, have had a negligible economic effect on nonagricultural enterprises. The program is widely supported by residents, landowners, and businesses in the area.

Eradicating Bovine Tuberculosis from Livestock in the Riding Mountain Area

In the mid-1990s, Canada was nearing the complete eradication of bovine tuberculosis from livestock, including game-farmed species, and looking forward to maintaining this enviable status through ongoing slaughter inspection monitoring, appropriate import controls, and maintenance of the spatial separation between livestock and diseased bison in the Wood Buffalo National Park area. Instead, as the new century dawned, the findings in the Riding Mountain area required that the bovine tuberculosis eradication program be ramped up instead of wound down.

Using provisions contained in federal legislation, a special eradication area was established around the park. The eradication area encompasses approximately 50,000 breeding cattle on 650 farms, representing approximately 10% of the cattle herds in the province of Manitoba and 1% of cattle herds in Canada. For ease of administration and because the hunting zones reflect the range of wild elk in the area, the boundaries of the eradication area mirror those of the two provincial hunting zones surrounding the park. To 2005, all findings of bovine tuberculosis in cattle and wildlife in the Riding Mountain area have occurred within the eradication area boundaries. Following an initial test of all livestock herds in the eradication area during the period from 2000 to 2003, these herds have continued to undergo periodic retesting at intervals of 12–36 months, with the appropriate interval for any given herd determined by the previous year's findings (in wildlife and livestock) in the area where the farm is located. To confirm that cattle herds in the regions outside but adjacent to the eradication area continue to be free from bovine tuberculosis, these herds are also tested from time to time. Periodic on-farm testing of livestock herds in the Riding Mountain area is expected to continue for as long as the threat of spread of infection from wild elk and deer is believed to be present.

Under the surveillance program, 20,000–40,000 head of livestock are tested each year, 450–900 of which undergo ancillary testing by interferon-gamma assay or comparative cervical test, and 20–40 of these are slaughtered for confirmatory tissue testing. Any herd in which *M. bovis* is confirmed is subjected to the disease eradication measures previously described in this chapter.

The findings of bovine tuberculosis in cattle herds in the Riding Mountain area have resulted in the downgrading of the area's tuberculosis status. Although the rest of the Manitoba and other Canadian provinces are certified as officially free from bovine tuberculosis, the eradication area around the park is classified as tuberculosis-accredited-advanced. As a consequence, the owners of cattle, farmed bison, and farmed cervids located in the eradication area require a permit from the federal veterinary authority before removing animals from the area. In addition to these restrictions on domestic movements, cattle going to the United States from anywhere in Manitoba require a negative tuberculin test before export, unlike cattle from the rest of Canada.

The costs of carrying out disease surveillance and eradication activities for bovine tuberculosis in livestock and administering and monitoring livestock movement controls in the Riding Mountain area are largely borne by the federal public treasury, at an estimated annual cost of $1,000,000 (Canadian funds), with an additional estimated cost of $300,000 for every infected cattle herd found. These costs include on-farm testing of livestock herds and compensation for any animals slaughtered for confirmatory tissue testing, issuing movement permits to owners and conducting herd inventory audits, and the investigation of infected premises, including the payment of compensation for animals slaughtered to eradicate the infection.

Although livestock owners support the disease surveillance, control, and eradication measures implemented in response to the presence of bovine tuberculosis in wild elk and deer in the Riding Mountain area and its apparent spread to surrounding livestock herds, these measures have significant economic implications for livestock owners and related industries. Owners are responsible for providing suitable animal handling facilities and the labor to gather their animals for testing, as well as any costs related to injuries their animals sustain during testing, including abortions, and any damage to their property, and for the costs associated with obtaining movement permits and keeping the required records. Owners of herds under

1

precautionary quarantine while suspicious findings are investigated incur costs/losses resulting from restricted marketing opportunities for their cattle. If *M. bovis* is confirmed, the herd owner faces uncompensated costs/losses associated with lost production, a longer quarantine period, cleaning and disinfection, and restocking. When animals of superior genetic value are required to be slaughtered, in addition to lost genetics, the compensation payable is often significantly less than the animals' market value. Owners also face the possibility that their animals will be discounted or rejected by the marketplace because they originate from the Riding Mountain area. The cost of tuberculin testing cattle being exported to the United States from Manitoba is another cost borne by the owners.

Conclusion

After almost 100 years of effort and financial investment by Canadian taxpayers and livestock owners, all livestock herds in Canada, except those in a small area of Manitoba surrounding Riding Mountain National Park, are now officially free from bovine tuberculosis. This hard-won status has many positive effects. It provides public health benefits, improves the productivity of livestock operations, contributes to the international marketing of Canadian animals and animal products, and protects free-roaming wildlife. Having reached this point, Canada has been faced with two wildlife reservoirs that threaten to reintroduce the disease into livestock herds. This has required the federal and provincial veterinary and wildlife authorities to implement aggressive and sustained measures to protect what has been achieved and complete the eradication campaign. The costs incurred by the public treasury to carry out these disease surveillance, containment, and eradication activities in livestock and wildlife, and the costs and losses incurred by livestock owners as a result of these measures, represent the most visible economic effect of the presence of bovine tuberculosis in the free-roaming bison of Wood Buffalo National Park and the free-roaming elk and deer of Riding Mountain National Park. Less visible, but perhaps even more significant, are the lost opportunities for economic growth and prosperity in the livestock sector and other enterprises when this serious zoonotic disease is present in a wildlife reservoir. In Canada, the cost of doing nothing is greater than the cost of acting.

References

Brook, R. K., and S. M. McLachlan. Elk-Agriculture Interactions in the Greater Riding Mountain. Available at: www.thegreenpages.ca/tb/documents/reports/brook_dec2003 interim_report.pdf. Interim report January 2004. Last accessed 17 March 2005.

Carbyn, L. N. 1982. Incidence of disease and its potential role in the population dynamics of wolves in Riding Mountain National Park, Manitoba. *In* F. Harrington and P. Paquet (eds.), Wolves of the World: Perspectives of Behaviour, Ecology and Conservation. Park Ridge, NJ: Noyes Publications, 106-116.

Essey, M. A. and M. A. Koller. 1994. Status of bovine tuberculosis in North America. *Vet Microbiol* 40:15-22.

Joly, D. O., and F. Messier. 2001. Limiting effects of bovine brucellosis and tuberculosis on wood bison within Wood Buffalo National Park. Final Report, March 2001. University of Saskatchewan, Saskatoon, Saskatchewan.

Lees, V. W., S. Copeland, and P. Rousseau. 2003. Bovine tuberculosis in elk (*Cervus elaphus manitobensis*) near Riding Mountain National Park, Manitoba from 1992 to 2002. *Can Vet J* 44:830-31.

Lutze-Wallace, C., C. Turcotte, M. Sabourin, G. Berlie-Surujballi, Y. Barbeau, D. Watchorn, and J. Bell. 2005. Spoligotyping of *Mycobacterium bovis* isolates found in Manitoba. *Can J Vet Res* 69:143-45.

Management Consulting Services. 1979. Evaluation of Alternative Tuberculosis Programs by Benefit/Cost Analysis, Volume I Technical Report, Volume II Summary Report. Ottawa: Agriculture Canada.

Northern Diseased Bison Environmental Assessment Panel. 1990. Northern Disease Bison: Report of the Environmental Assessment Panel. Ottawa: Minister of Supplies and Services Canada (Cat. EN 106-16/1990).

Schmitt, S. M., S. D. Fitzgerald, T. M. Cooley, C. S. Bruning-Fann, L. Sullivan, D. Berry, T. Carlson, R. B. Minnis, J. B. Payeur, and J. Sikarskle. 1997. Bovine tuberculosis in free-ranging white-tailed deer from Michigan. *J Wildl Dis* 33:749-58.

Chapter 22

Bovine Tuberculosis Program in South Africa: The Impact of *M. bovis*-infected Wild Species

N. Kriek, DVM, PhD

Introduction

There is little doubt that in recorded history, tuberculosis is one of the oldest known diseases of humans and animals. For many years before the introduction of pasteurization of milk, and the active control of the disease in livestock on an international basis, infection with *Mycobacterium bovis*, the cause of the disease in cattle and other animals, was a significant zoonotic disease, particularly at times of war and in communities of the lower socioeconomic strata. Thus, in the United Kingdom during the 1930s, 50,000 people (of which 2500 died) contracted bovine tuberculosis; at present, because of control measures, it is estimated that only 1% of cases (about 40 a year) are caused by bovine tuberculosis (Anonymous, 2000). Similar data are available for other European countries (Pavlik et al., 2003)

Internationally, bovine tuberculosis is a controlled disease of animals primarily because of its zoonotic potential. However, the importance of zoonotic bovine tuberculosis because of the control of the disease in developed countries paled into what certain (many) authorities consider to be insignificant. It is at present often implied that *M. bovis* is of no importance from the point of view of human infection and disease, even when considered against the risk posed by the rampant spread of HIV/AIDS and other debilitating diseases in humans on the African continent (particularly in South Africa) and elsewhere in the world.

Current Shifts in Paradigm

However, there is increasing evidence that zoonotic *M. bovis* infections may be much more important than generally considered. A survey along the United States–Mexico border revealed that 10.8% of all cases of tuberculosis in children there were caused by *M. bovis* infection, and that 33.9% of 180 positive cultures from individual patients proved to be *M. bovis* (Danker and Davis, 2000). Similarly, in

Ethiopia, of 29 cases of tuberculosis, 17.1% were caused by *M. bovis* infection (Dawit Kidane et al., 2004).

The importance of zoonoses because of HIV infections worldwide is increasingly stressed. Articles outlining the risks have appeared regularly in publications of the World Health Organization (Anonymous, 1994; Cosivi, et al, 1994), FAO (Pasquali, 2004) and in other scientific publications (Wedlock, 2002). Confirmation of the occurrence of such infections and the predisposing role played by HIV-1 infection has been published detailing a series of such cases in Arusha, Tanzania (Mfinanga, et al, 2004). Furthermore, transmission of *M. bovis* from patient to patient with advanced HIV-1 infection (Guerrero, 1997; Samper et al, 1997) and from patients to HIV-negative hospital staff (Bernad, et al, 2003) has been documented.

Increasingly, opinions are expressed that emphasize the growing concern about the role of zoonotic *M. bovis* infections in the developed and developing world (Ayele et al., 2004). In many instances, few such infections have been recorded over the last number of decades, but in others, there is increasing evidence that the infection may be of greater significance than assumed (Ayele et al., 2004). Data pertaining to these issues are particularly inferior in poorer countries, where resources to diagnose the cause of tuberculous infections accurately even in humans are inadequate and the cause of infection is merely recorded as "mycobacterial infection." The knowledge about the role of *M. bovis* in many of these countries, and even in the developed world, remains unclear and speculative.

In terms of newly emerging diseases, a number of contributing factors play a significant role in their future development: a rapid increase in the movement of people, environmental change, expansion of the human population, destruction of animal habitats, and changes in animal husbandry and production technologies (Thiermann, 2004). The ability to recognize and rapidly deal with new or newly emerging diseases is important when seen against the role that these diseases play in the current process of globalization and protection of markets. The appearance of a new disease, or even a new epidemiological event of a known pathogen, is likely to result in a much more severe effect on international trade (Thiermann, 2004).

Current Realities in South Africa

In South Africa, there are also differences of opinion about the significance of the infection dependent on whether the proponents' biases are toward conservation, control, or eradication of the disease in domestic stock, or the relevance of the infection as a zoonosis, as expressed currently by members of the medical profession in South Africa and in the developed world.

The general opinion in medical circles in South Africa is that *M. bovis* infection as a cause of tuberculosis is of negligible significance as a zoonotic disease. Furthermore, in terms of conservation, in the agenda of a recent scientific meeting in the Kruger National Park, one of the senior conservationists in the Park expressed the following opinion in a paper (Mills, 2005): The essence of the argument revolves around hypothetical effects of the infection on wildlife without considering the likely risks posed by sustained high levels of the infection in increasing number of animals of different species in the Kruger National Park to the surrounding commercial and communal cattle and subsistence farmers living in those areas. This attitude also does not consider the wider implications of the effect of sustained foci of the infection in wildlife maintenance hosts within the park and elsewhere on the future control of the disease in South Africa and its neighbors.

The changes that have taken place about the perceived status of *M. bovis* infection in South Africa over 10–20 years are interesting, if not alarming. At the beginning of the 1990s the prevalence of bovine tuberculosis in commercial cattle was assessed to be less than 0.01% (Anonymous, 1990–2003). At that time too, the infection in wildlife was considered to be an oddity and of historical importance. The disease in greater kudu *(Tragelaphus strepsiceros)* that was prevalent in the Eastern Province of South Africa during the course of the 1930s was deemed to have largely disappeared because of the decline in prevalence of domestic stock resulting from eradication programs instituted by the South African government. The current trends reveal a very different perspective: the number of outbreaks of tuberculosis in commercial and communal stock has increased (Table 22.1), and the extent of the disease in wildlife is increasing exponentially. Increasing numbers of wildlife species are becoming infected, and there are strong indications that greater kudu also act as maintenance hosts (Bengis, Cooper, unpublished data, 2004). Kudu appear to have been the source of an *M. bovis* infection in the Spioenkop reserve in KwaZulu-Natal in a group of tuberculosis-free African buffaloes. The control of tuberculosis is less than adequate because of limitations in human and financial resources. Recent outbreaks in livestock and wildlife will have to prompt a rethink of policies and execution of control and eradication programs.

The increasing levels of infection in an increasing number of species (currently 12) in the park and surrounding areas should also be seen against the current development of transfrontier conservation areas in the Southern African Development Community. These so-called Peace Parks have as their main objective reducing poverty by promoting sustainable biodiversity, increased ecotourism, job creation, wealth creation and the improvement of the economy of the countries involved in the development of these parks. The fact of the matter is that tuberculosis of domestic and wild animals, because of its potential as a zoonosis, is one of the major impediments to progress with the establishment of the transfrontier parks, particularly in southern Africa.

The eventual consequence for South Africa of the unbridled increase of tuberculosis in wildlife, and the current increase in reinfection of herds that have been clean for extended periods, may have severe adverse effects. Future eradication strategies will have to contend with sustained foci of infection—many perhaps unknown—in wildlife, and with the cost of increased numbers of outbreaks of the disease in previously TB-free herds and the increasing importance of the disease becoming visible as a zoonosis, particularly in the poor rural areas of the country, where subsistence farming is practiced.

Further increases in outbreaks of the disease in domestic stock will most likely have serious negative effects on future trade in livestock and their products nation-

Table 22.1. Multiannual disease status (South Africa): tuberculosis

Year and Species	Number		
	Outbreaks	Cases	Deaths
2003			
Cattle	17	394	1
Buffaloes	2	103	1
2002			
Cattle	4	123	0
Buffaloes	2	2	1
2001			
Cattle	1	33	0
Buffaloes	0	0	0
2000			
Cattle	10	174	0
Buffaloes	0	0	0
1999			
Cattle	6	80	0
Buffaloes	0	0	0
1998			
Cattle	11	162	1
Buffaloes	1	?	?
1997			
Cattle	8	20	0
Buffaloes	4	18	13
1996			
Cattle	5	8	2
Buffaloes	0	0	0

ally, regionally, and internationally. In addition, the cost of managing the infections in an increasing number of wildlife species in the various national and provincial parks, game ranches, and breeding establishments should be taken into account. The effect on value of scarce species; the likelihood of illegal trade in rare, disease-free wildlife species; the inability to diagnose the infection in various species (also endangered species), and the levels of risk taken in trading in these species have not been assessed and factored into the future cost of the presence of the disease to the country.

The real threat of *M. bovis* infection in South Africa is unknown in many respects, and although it is clear that it will have some negative effect on the economy of the country, its extent has not been contemplated. Given the current international trade agreements and the international control of animal diseases, the zoonotic potential of the infection, its expected effect on the sustainability of biodiversity, the sustainability of the ecotourism trade, and the cooperation between countries in the region, there should be some concern. All these factors should be considered when assessing the future effect of the infection in livestock, and particularly in wildlife in which there are now established host species that will sustain the infection in the country long beyond its likely eradication, should it not have been present in those species (Michel, 2002).

In a country with many problems, the one caused by *M. bovis* cannot be minimized or ignored for the sake of convenience or because of a lack of appreciating
its likely role in negatively affecting the economy of the country. The country's
future ability to trade regionally and internationally, and maintain the health of its
citizens, is dependent on addressing these problems as a matter of urgency.

References

Anonymous. 1990–2003. Annual and monthly disease prevalence reports of the Department
of Agriculture, Republic of South Africa.

Anonymous. 1994. Zoonotic tuberculosis (*Mycobacterium bovis*): memorandum from a
WHO meeting. *Bull World Health Org* 72:851-57.

Anonymous. 2000. MAFF Fact Sheet. TB in cattle: protecting human health. Available at:
http://www.defra.gov.uk/animalh/tb/publications/index.htm.

Ayele, W. Y., S. D. Neill, J. Zinsstag, M. B. Weiss, and I. Pavlik. 2004. Bovine tuberculosis: an old disease but a new threat to Africa. *Int J Tuberculosis Lung Dis* 8:924-37.

Bernad, S., M. J. Hernández Navarette, J. I. Martín Sánchez, E. V. Martínez Sánchez, and
J. L. Arribas Llorente. 2003. Occupational exposure to multiresistant *Mycobacterium
bovis* at a hospital in Zaragoza, Spain. *Rev Espanõla Salud Pub* 77:201-209.

Cosivi, O., J. M. Grange, C. J. Daborn, M. C. Raviglioni, T. Fujikura, D. Cousins, R. A.
Robinson, H. F. K. A. Huchzermeyer, I. de Kantor, and F.-X. Meslin. 1994. Zoonotic
tuberculosis due to *Mycobacterium bovis* in developing countries. Available at:
http://www.cdc.gov/ncidod/eid/vol4no1/adobe/cosivi.pdf.

Dankner, W. M., and C. E. Davis. 2000. M*ycobacterium bovis* as a significant cause of tuberculosis in children residing along the United States–Mexico border in the Baja
California region. *Pediatrics* 105:E79

Kidane D., J. O. Olobo, A. Habte, Y. Negesse, A. Aseffa, G. Abate, M. A. Yassin, K. Bereda,
M. Harboe. 2004. Identification of the causative organism of tuberculous lymphadenitis
in Ethiopia by PCR. *Ethiopian Med J* 42:15-22.

Guerrero, A., J. Cobo, J. Fortun, E. Navas, C. Quereda, A. Asensio, J. Canon, J. Blazquez,
and E. Gomez-Mampaso. 1997. Nosocomial transmission of *Mycobacterium bovis*
resistant to 11 drugs in people with advanced HIV-1 infection. *Lancet*: 350:1738-42

Mfinanga, S. G. M., O. Morkve, R. R. Kazwala, S. Cleaveland, M. J. Sharp, J. Kunda, and
R. Nilsen. 2004. Mycobacterial adenitis: role of *Mycobacterium bovis*, non-tuberculous
mycobacteria, HIV infection, and risk factors in Arusha, Tanzania. *East African Med J*
81:171-78.

Michel, A. 2002. Implications of tuberculosis in African wildlife and livestock. *Ann N Y
Acad Sci* 969:251-55.

Mills, M. G. L. 2005. TB in Kruger: wildlife crisis or red herring? Scientific Services, South
African National Parks.

Pasquali, P. 2004. HIV infections and zoonoses. Available at: http://www.fao.org/docrep/
007/y5516e/y5516e00.htm.

Pavlik, I., W. Y. Ayele, M. Havelkova, M. Svejnochova, V. Katalinic-Jankovic, and M.
Zolnir-Dovc. 2003. *Mycobacterium bovis* in human population in four Central European
countries during 1990-1999. *Vet Med* 48:90-98

Samper, S., C. Martin, A. Pinedo, A. Rivero, J. Blazquez, F. Baquero, D. van Sooligen, and
J. van Embden. 1997. Transmission between HIV-infected patients of multidrug-resistant tuberculosis caused by *Mycobacterium bovis*. *AIDS* 11:1237-42

Thiermann, A. 2004. Emerging diseases and implications for global trade. *Rev Sci Tech Off Int Epiz* 23:701-708.

Wedlock, D. N., M. A. Skinner, G. W. de Lisle, B. M. Buddle. 2002. Control of *Mycobacterium bovis* infections and the risk of human populations. *Microbes Infect* 4:471-80.

Chapter 23

Bovine Tuberculosis in China

D. Zhao, PhD, C.D. Wu, PhD, and Z. Ning, MS

Bovine tuberculosis continues to be a threat to cattle industry and human health in China even after many years of prevention and a treatment campaign. This disease occurs sporadically among cattle populations, especially in rural areas, and thus represents a serious problem to human health.

A number of investigations on the prevalence of bovine tuberculosis were carried out during 1997–2003 in some regions of China. Results of these investigations are presented in Table 23.1.

Bovine tuberculosis is also a source of human infection. An investigation conducted in 1979 involving 1,338,080 people from 888 sites of 29 provinces showed that 13.0% of people were positive to the purified protein derivative (PPD) test. Another investigation carried out in 1984–1985 demonstrated that 4.2% of human tuberculosis cases were caused by *Mycobacterium bovis*.

Prevention of tuberculosis has been made a priority to improve human health. A series of regulations and laws has been issued by the Chinese government and legislature to control animal infectious diseases, including bovine tuberculosis, such as Regulations of Animal Quarantine (1981), Guidelines of PPD Operation (1988), Regulations of Veterinary Surveillance (1990), Prevention and Control of Infectious Diseases in Domestic Animals (1997), and so on. These legislative documents provide guidelines for diagnosis, quarantine, isolation, treatment, and slaughter of bovine tuberculosis cases, disinfection of animal facilities, depopulation and repopu-

Table 23.1. Prevalence of bovine tuberculosis in some regions of China

Region	Year	No. Cattle	No. Cattle Positive (%)
Anhui	2000	238	39 (16.38)
Fujian	1997	230	16 (6.96)
Gansu	2001	123	9 (7.32)
Guangdong	1997	58733	41 (0.07)
Guangxi	1998	1531	192 (12.54)
Jilin	1997	17479	228 (1.30)
Shanghai	2001	8979	221 (2.46)
Xinjiang	1997–2000	45606	199 (0.44)
Zhejiang	2001	6841	6 (0.09)

lation of cattle herds, coordination for prevention campaign, and disbursement for economic loss.

Diagnosis of bovine tuberculosis relies on three methods, including the bacteriological method—*Mycobacterium bovis* cultivation and coloration check-up, immunological method—PPD and ELISA, and molecular biological method—polymerase chain reaction, probe of nucleic acid, and atlas of DNA. These methods have been developed and applied by following international standards. The PPD test that is recommended by OIE is used in case investigation, and bacteriological and molecular biological techniques are used as complementary tools for accurate diagnosis.

Regular examination of cattle herds by the PPD test has been adopted to monitor the status of bovine tuberculosis. The number of animals subject to examination varies depending on the usage of herds. The percentage subject to examination is 100% for dairy and breeding herds, 10% for feedlot herds, and 5% for other herds. All animals from a herd in which suspicious cases are identified should be examined individually, and results should be confirmed by bacteriological and molecular biological methods. If any animals are suspected to have bovine tuberculosis, local veterinarians must report the cases to higher authorities for further examination and confirmation.

Chapter 24
Mycobacterium bovis Infections in Cattle in Germany

R. Weiss, DVM, PhD

Tuberculosis caused by *Mycobacterium bovis* was widespread in the German cattle population during the first half of the 20th century. Between 1920 and 1950, infection rates can be estimated at about 60% of the cattle herds and at 30% of all bovines. A sanitation scheme according to Ostertag, initiated at the beginning of the 20th century and based on the registration and eradication of cattle with open tuberculosis of the lungs, udder, uterus, or intestines, did not lead to a decline of the infection rates. Instead, an increase of cows with tuberculosis at slaughter from 20.1% in 1908 to 37.0% in 1935, and a major field trial in 1939, yielding prevalence rates of 31% and 63% of infected animals and herds, respectively, demonstrated the insufficiency of the program and resulted in its stop.

After World War II, the incidence of bovine tuberculosis was extremely high—over 60% of the cattle were infected—and a new, at first voluntary, bovine tuberculosis control program, supported governmentally, started in 1952. It was based on the eradication system developed by Bang that had been applied in Denmark successfully. In particular, it comprised the use of the tuberculin test as the most relevant method for identifying *M. bovis*–infected cattle, as well as the experience that all cattle reacting tuberculin positive sooner or later would start to shed the agent and, thus, were expected to become a possible source of infection. The most important measures consisted of periodical tuberculinization of all cattle above 6 weeks of age, separation and in-time slaughtering of animals reacting positive, removal of calves from reacting mothers immediately after birth, certification of herds as "admittedly tuberculosis-free herd" after a twofold tuberculin test control of all cattle of a farm with negative results, and so on. Farmers were supported by governmental subsidies like tuberculinization at reduced or no charge, and by economic stimuli (i.e., higher prices for milk and meat from animals of tuberculosis-free herds, as well as trading facilities).

This kind of sanitation resulted in a strong decline of tuberculosis in German cattle between 1952 and 1961 and, vice versa, in an enormous increase to 99.7% of herds registered to be tuberculosis free. After 1970, the number of infected farms continued to decrease to <0.01% in 1982, and since 1997, Germany has had a tuberculosis-free status, with fewer than 10 outbreaks per year (Fig. 24.1).

Periodical use of tuberculin tests, meat inspection at the abattoir, and identification of diseased animals, as well as of suspected cases, were the main methods for controlling the tuberculosis situation in German cattle. However, the frequency of tuberculinization was adjusted to the decrease of positive rates. Until 1963, periodical herd tests were performed once per year; until 1972, they were performed once every 2 years; and until 1997, they were performed once every 3 years. Now, Germany is controlling for tuberculous cattle routinely by meat inspection only. Cattle suspected for or showing tuberculous lesions are traced back to their original herd, and tuberculin testing of the herd usually follows.

Herds No.

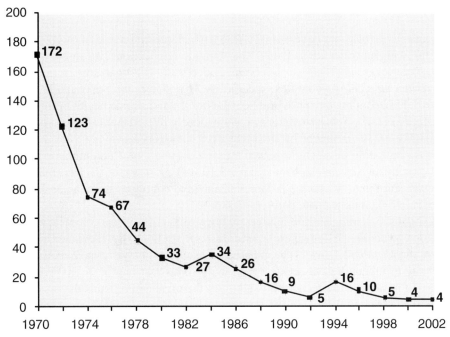

Figure 24.1. Bovine tuberculosis outbreaks per year in Germany between 1970 and 2002.

Chapter 25
Tuberculosis in Captive Exotic Animals

G. West, DVM

Mycobacterial diseases have historically been a significant cause of morbidity and mortality in zoo collections (1–12). The zoonotic implications of captive wild animals with tuberculosis are an important concern (2–4). Organisms in the *Mycobacterium tuberculosis* complex, specifically *Mycobacterium bovis* and *M. tuberculosis*, have continued to pose problems for human and animal health in zoological institutions (1–9). These two organisms are closely related and infect a broad host range (5). *M. bovis* has been identified as a pathogen in a wide variety of zoo species, including clinically diseased carnivores, ungulates, nonhuman primates, and recently an African elephant (1,3,6,7,8,10–13). *M. tuberculosis* has emerged as a significant threat to captive Asian elephants and continues to be a considerable threat to nonhuman primate colonies (2,4,6–9).

Diagnostic testing and obtaining a clinical diagnosis in captive wild animals continue to challenge zoo veterinarians (14–29). Traditionally, the diagnosis of *M. bovis* and *M. tuberculosis* has been based on results of delayed-type hypersensitivity tests to tuberculins injected intradermally. This test has been challenging to interpret in many zoo species, and culture of the organism remains the only definitive diagnostic test.

This chapter discusses clinical and pathological findings in zoo animals with tuberculosis, as well as diagnostic testing and control strategies. The focus will be on *M. tuberculosis* complex, specifically *M. bovis* and *M. tuberculosis*, including ungulates, elephants, and nonhuman primates.

Clinical Findings

Clinical signs of tuberculosis in zoo animals are often minimal until the disease is in the advanced stages (1,3,9,10,12,14). Zoo animals may show progressive lethargy, weight loss, and respiratory disease. Clinically affected animals may die suddenly or die during diagnostic evaluations requiring anesthesia (3). Zoo species may not show clinical signs and may just be found dead with disseminated disease (14). Complete physical examination is essential, and advanced disease may be detected with radiography, the finding of lymphadenopathy, or detection of pulmonary lesions. However, in one report macaques evaluated with radiography, gastric and tracheal washes, and skin testing found that the skin test was the most sensitive diagnostic test (6).

Ungulates, which include exotic ruminants, rhinoceros, elephant, hippopotamus, camelids, and tapir, have various clinical signs. These signs may range from chronic respiratory disease with weight loss to sudden death. A white rhinoceros infected with *M. bovis* showed a productive cough and purulent nasal discharge and progressive deterioration (3). Camels may only exhibit chronic weight loss as a primary clinical sign (17).

Large ungulates often do not show clinical signs, and tuberculosis is diagnosed at necropsy (3,12,18). Elephants may show chronic weight loss and intermittent ventral edema, but this species often has extensive pulmonary disease without clinical signs of respiratory disease. A black rhinoceros was culture positive for *M. tuberculosis* after multiple gastric washes and was found dead during treatment; *M. tuberculosis* was also isolated from pulmonary lesions at necropsy (19).

Nonhuman primates may have minimal clinical signs until the disease is advanced. Occasionally, clinical signs of respiratory disease or debilitation may be observed, but often a definitive antemortem diagnosis is elusive. Intradermal skin testing is the most commonly used diagnostic test and has been a relatively sensitive test (6–8). One species that is an exception to this is the orangutan. Orangutans have a greater sensitivity to tuberculin than other primate species. Exposure to nonpathogenic mycobacteria has resulted in false-positive or nonspecific responses in orangutans (15,16).

Pathology

Gross lesions can be very extensive in captive exotic animals with chronic disease. Many organ systems can be involved in the disease process. An oryx in a U.S. zoo had granulomas in the lungs, liver, uterus, and lymph nodes (20,21). *Mycobacterium* sp. was also isolated from this animal's mammary gland fluid (20,21). Unfortunately, progressive disease in zoo animals may only be apparent when extensive tuberculous lesions are seen at necropsy.

These lesions typically have yellowish, caseous necrotic areas in nodules of firm, white, fibrous tissue. Tubercles may not be grossly discrete lesions and can become diffuse in tissues. Miliary patterns may be seen in disseminated disease in species such as nonhuman primates (6,8,16,22). Cavitation and calcification or caseocalcification may occur in lesions. This has been seen in advanced pulmonary disease in many species.

Tubercles are granulomatous lesions with a caseous, necrotic center bordered by epithelioid cells, some of which may form multinucleated giant cells (Fig. 25.1). In addition, there is an accumulation of lymphocytes, granulocytes, and encapsulation of fibrous connective tissue. There may also be considerable variation of the formation of lesions in nondomestic species. Tubercles may not always be consistently formed, and multinucleated giant cells may not always be present. In camels, gross sarcomatoid lesions are seen, and solid pyogranulomas with few giant cells are often observed in histologic sections (17).

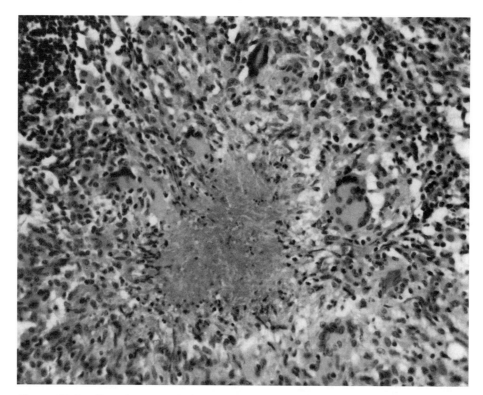

Figure 25.1. Granulomatous lesion with necrosis in a monkey tissue; multinucleated giant cells, epithelioid cells, and other inflammatory cells are present. *Mycobacterium bovis* was isolated.

Nonhuman primates may have extensive pulmonary tubercles with caseous cavitation and lymphadenopathy of bronchial lymph nodes. Fulminate tuberculosis may also be exhibited as miliary lesions in primates. Tubercle lesions in primates have been described as having few Langhan's cells or multinucleated cells. Also, classic tuberculosis in primates has traditionally not had extensive calcification and fibrosis. In addition, nonhuman primate colonies may be infected with both *M. bovis* or with *M. tuberculosis* with similar lesions (6,7).

Nondomestic ruminants will typically have lesions similar to those of domestic bovidae (Fig. 25.2). Granulomatous lesions of the lung, pleura, thoracic cavity, and lymph nodes of the head, neck, and pleural cavity are often seen in bovids. Kudu are a species of bovid that develop severe, progressive disease and potentially shed large numbers of organisms (10,24,25). Wild kudu often have abscessed and draining parotid, mandibular, and cervical lymph nodes that may be easily visible from a distance (23). In addition, kudu may have severe disseminated disease that involves several organ systems (10). Cervids often have retropharyngeal lymph node involvement, as well as involvement of the pulmonary tissue and pleural cavity (22–25). Microscopically, there are large amounts of central necrosis and liquefaction of granulomas (Fig. 25.3).

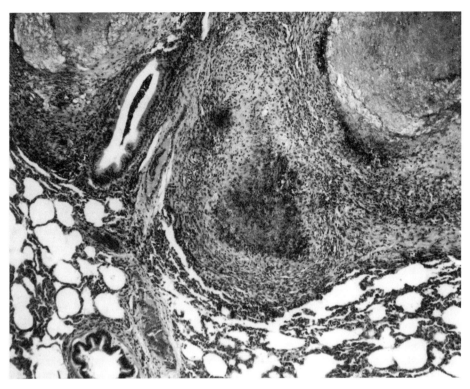

Figure 25.2.   Section of lung of a bison granuloma with caseous necrosis and mineralization. *Mycobacterium bovis* was isolated.

Elephants with *M. tuberculosis* primarily have lesions in the lung and thoracic lymph nodes. Granulomatous lesions of the trachea have also been observed. Elephants with chronic disease may die with few premonitory signs and have severe caseocalcareous lesions with cavitation. In elephants, large coalescing pulmonary abscesses form, and other thoracic sites may have firm granulomatous nodules (12,16).

Diagnosis and Control

The diagnosis of tuberculosis in ungulates and other captive wild animals has been based on the intradermal skin test. In ungulates other than elephants, the intradermal skin test is the preferred method of testing. However, in large ungulates such as hippopotamus, rhinoceros, and tapir, interpretation of skin-test responses can be a challenge (18). Factors such as dose, location of testing, and nonspecific responses can complicate the skin test. Evaluation of biopsy of skin-test sites may help distinguish positive from negative reactions. Biopsy to evaluate the delayed hypersensitivity site can be used in conjunction with ELISA. Biopsies of comparative antigen testing sites can also be very helpful in distinguishing nonspecific responses

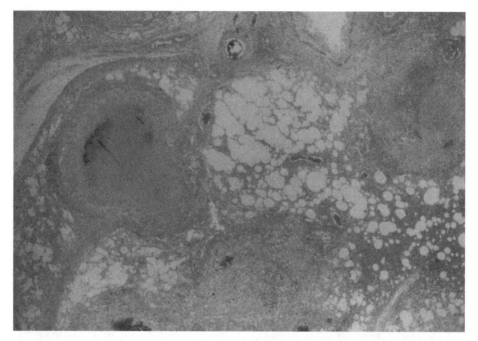

Figure 25.3. Photomicrograph of lung of an elk from which *Mycobacterium bovis* was isolated. Note multiple granulomas, some caseation necrosis and mineralization. One granuloma is adjacent to a bronchiole.

(18). Nonspecific reactions are often observed in camelids, and skin test results can be variable. The axillary site is currently the preferred site of skin testing in camelids. However, one study emphasized the need to further evaluate the skin test in llamas and its effect on serodiagnosis (30).

Domestic cattle are typically skin tested with 0.1 mL or 5000 TU intradermally in the caudal tail fold (34). Cervids are typically tested with a single cervical test of 5000 TU intradermally in the cervical region. This test is interpreted at 72 hours postinjection. An ancillary test used to help diagnose infected animals and possibly decrease handling in difficult species is the gamma-interferon test. Presumably, gamma-interferon will be increased with the cell-mediated response to infection with mycobacterial organisms. Results of the gamma-interferon are comparable to those obtained with intradermal tests in some domestic cattle (31,32). However, additional investigations are needed to validate the test in cervids and other captive wild animals (31,32).

Elephants, however, have frequent false-positive and false-negative skin tests when correlated with culture results. At present, the most reliable testing method for elephants is a trunk wash. Sterile saline is instilled into the nostrils and trunk of an elephant, and respiratory secretions are lavaged or washed out. This material is then submitted for mycobacterial culture. Three samples on different days are collected. Food and water should be withheld for 2 hours beforehand, to alleviate dilution or contamination that may occur. Also, if elephants can be trained to have a forced exhalation during a wash, this would yield a better laboratory sample.

In addition, elephants have been diagnosed with tuberculosis after sneezing out purulent exudate from their trunks. Exudate sampled off an enclosure floor had large numbers of acid-fast organisms present, and *M. tuberculosis* was cultured. Ancillary testing to help characterize clinical disease in elephants includes a nucleic acid amplification test and a serum ELISA test (9,26,27,33). The amplification test uses transcription-mediated amplification to replicate RNA from *M. tuberculosis*. This test has very good sensitivity for detecting *M. tuberculosis* in elephant trunk wash samples. The serum ELISA uses multiple antigens to screen elephants for tuberculosis (26). This test shows promise for detecting clinically affected animals. However, there is still concern about sensitivity. Cross-reactions may also be a problem, as many nonpathogenic mycobacteria have been cultured from elephant trunk washes. However, certain antigens used in the ELISA have shown good specificity when tested in culture-positive animals (26,27).

Intradermal skin testing is the screening test of choice in nonhuman primates and may be more sensitive than other diagnostic tests (4). Nonhuman primates show an attenuated response to tuberculin and require up to 10,000 times as many antigen units as humans. Thus, human tuberculin is not appropriate for testing nonhuman primates.

Orangutans are an exception to reliable skin testing results in nonhuman primates (15). Orangutans have increased sensitivity to tuberculins compared to other nonhuman primates. A comprehensive study of orangutans was conducted comparing gastric lavage, serum enzyme-linked immunosorbent assays, skin testing, thoracic radiographs, and physical examinations (15). Orangutans appeared to be sensitized to nonpathogenic mycobacteria and have false-positive skin-test responses. Standard tuberculin testing in primates uses the eyelid and abdomen for intradermal skin testing. Quarantine and multiple skin testing should be conducted in nonhuman primate additions to any collection. An anergic response or false negative may occur in primates with advanced tuberculosis, animals exposed to immunosuppressive viruses, or those receiving antituberculosis drug therapy (7,28).

Additional testing in nonhuman primates has included ELISA testing, gamma-interferon testing for antigen 85 protein, chest radiographs, and tracheal or gastric washes (29). Some of these tests may be useful as adjuncts to the skin test to help obtain a clinical diagnosis. Cross-reactions with nonpathogenic mycobacteria may give erroneous results on some tests. In a colony of macaques, the most accurate diagnostic test was the tuberculin skin test (6).

Culture remains the gold standard for diagnosis, and postmortem samples are often confirmatory of a diagnosis of tuberculosis. Polymerase chain reaction detection of mycobacterial organisms in formalin-fixed tissues may also be used to help establish a diagnosis in culture-negative animals (33). Restriction fragment length polymorphism is also useful in detecting the relatedness of organisms that may be infecting multiple species in a zoo (34). This will help determine whether one strain has infected multiple animals and may be very useful in epidemiological investigations when involving humans (2–4,9).

Treatment for tuberculosis in animals is controversial and of unknown effectiveness. Bongos were administered antituberculosis drugs in food and water, and acceptable serum levels of the drug were achieved (13). Similar treatment has been used in Arabian oryx to attempt to release disease-free animals. Although treatment greatly reduced tuberculous lesions in oryx, the organism was still recovered at necropsy (20).

Elephants with tuberculosis were initially treated with isoniazid (INH) alone. *M. tuberculosis* in certain individual elephants was resistant to INH; therefore, multiple-drug treatment with pyrazinamide rifampin (RIF) was administered. Elephants had poor oral acceptance of INH, so the drug was then administered transrectally as a liquid suppository (Fig. 25.4). INH is water soluble and well absorbed when administered in the rectum of infected animals. Pyrazinamide was also absorbed transrectally, and good serum levels were obtained. Adequate serum RIF levels were not achieved with transrectal administration. Oral administration of RIF was used to get acceptable serum levels of the drug. RIF was more palatable, and elephants accepted it in food or were trained for oral administration. Doses of antituberculosis therapy had to be intermittently titrated on the basis of serum drug levels and side effects seen in treated elephants. In general, initial doses were based on human studies. Serum drug levels were monitored to be sure that adequate levels were maintained. INH doses often had to be decreased because of toxic side effects such as anorexia, lethargy, leukopenia, and increased liver enzymes.

Camels treated with INH showed severe bone marrow suppression, leukopenia, and death resulting from the toxicity of this drug (17). Nonhuman primates in infected colonies have been prophylactically treated with INH, but treatment is not always effective in preventing disease, and multiple drug regimen may be needed (7,8). In addition, prophylactic treatment may complicate diagnostic testing. Animals on prophylactic treatment with INH may revert to a negative skin test and

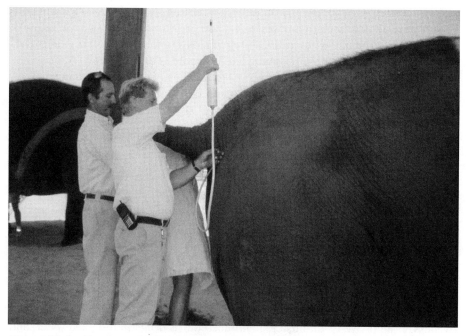

Figure 25.4.   Transrectal administration of isonicotinic acid hydrazid in an elephant.

still have disseminated tuberculosis at necropsy (6–8). Therefore, INH prophylaxis of an animal in a colony in which tuberculosis has been diagnosed cannot be recommended. Multiple drug therapy has been more effective in treating infected animals. If this is undertaken for valuable animals, they should be isolated and treated for prolonged periods of up to a year or more. Poor acceptance of drugs is another factor that can affect the success of treatment.

Mycobacterium bovis Bacille Calmette-Güerin (BCG) vaccine has been evaluated in nonhuman primates (35). This vaccine would likely be of limited value in a colony, where massive numbers of bacilli would likely overwhelm an immune response. The effects of stress on animals in these colonies are also a complicating factor to diagnostic testing, and stress may influence immune responses. Moreover, BCG vaccination could complicate interpretation of the intradermal skin test. Animals vaccinated with BCG may always respond to a skin test. Also, animals that have been vaccinated but become infected may not respond to the skin test because of immunosuppression (35).

It is important to emphasize that animal additions to a collection should be made only from tuberculosis-free populations. Animals of unknown status should be held under quarantine for 90–120 days, and appropriate retests should be conducted before animals are added to a collection. Only caretakers who are negative on the tuberculous skin tests conducted annually should be in contact with the animals.

References

1. Morris, P., C. Thoen, and A. Legendre. 1996. Pulmonary tuberculosis in an African lion (*Panthera leo*). *J Zoo Wildl Med* 27: 392-6.
2. Oh, P., R. Granich, J. Scott, B. Sun, M. Joseph, et al. 2002. Human exposure following *Mycobacterium tuberculosis* infection of multiple animal species in a metropolitan zoo. *Emerg Infect Dis* 8:1290-93.
3. Stetter, M., S. Mikota, A. Gutter, E. Monterroso, J. Dalovisio, C. Degraw, and T. Farley. 1995. Epizootic of *Mycobacterium bovis* in a zoologic park. *J Am Vet Med Assoc* 207: 1618-21.
4. Michalak, K., C. Austin, S. Diesel, et al. 1998. *Mycobacterium tuberculosis* infection as a zoonotic disease: transmission between humans and elephants. *Emerg Infect Dis* 4:2883-87.
5. Thoen, C. O. and R. G. Barletta, 2004. Mycobacterium. *In* C. L. Gyles, J. F. Prescott, J. G. Songer, and C. O. Thoen (ed.), Pathogenesis of Bacterial Infections in Animals. Ames, IA: Blackwell Publishing, 69-76.
6. Jannssen, D., M. Anderson, S. Abildgaard, and S. Silverman. 1989. Tuberculosis in newly imported Tibetan macaques (*Macaca thibetans*). *J Zoo Wildl Med* 20:315-21.
7. Dillehay, D. and M. Huerkamp. 1990. Tuberculosis in a tuberculin-negative rheus monkey (*Macaca mulatta*) on chemoprophylaxsis. *J Zoo Wildl Med* 21: 480-84.
8. Silberman, M. 1978. Tuberculosis in a band of imported hamadryas baboons. *In* R. Montali (ed.), Mycobacterial Infections of Zoo Animals. Washington, DC: Smithsonian Institution Press. p. 161-162.
9. Mikota, S., L. Peddie, J. Peddie, R. Isaza, F. Dunker, G. West, et al. 2001. Epidemiology and diagnosis of *Mycobacterium tuberculosis* in captive Asian elephants (*Elephas maximus*). *J Zoo Wildl Med* 32:1-16.

10. Himes, E. M., D. B. LyVere, C. O. Thoen, M. A. Essey, J. L. Lebel, and C. F. Freiheit. 1976. Tuberculosis in greater kudu. *J Am Vet Med Assoc* 169:930-1.
11. Silberman, M. 1978. Epidemiology of tuberculosis outbreak in a Sitatunga antelope housed at a municipal zoo. *In R.* Montali (ed.), Mycobacterial Infections of Zoo Animals. Washington, DC: Smithsonian Institution Press, 193-94.
12. Montali, R. 2001. *Mycobacterium bovis* in an African elephant (*Loxodonta africana*). Proceedings of the International Elephant and Rhinoceros Research Symposium. Vienna, Austria.
13. Auclair, B., S. Mikota, C. Peloquin, R. Aguilar, and J. Maslow. 2002. Population pharmokinetics of antituberculosis drugs and treatment of *Mycobacterium bovis* infection in bongo antelope (*Tragelaphus eurycerus isaaci*). *J Zoo Wildl Med* 33:193-203.
14. Himes, E., D. Luchsinger, J. Jarnagin, C. Thoen, H. Hood, and D. Ferrin. 1980. Tuberculosis in fennec foxes. *J Am Vet Med Assoc* 177: 825-6.
15. Calle, P., C. Thoen, and M. Roskop. 1989. Tuberculin skin test responses, mycobacteriologic examinations of gastric lavage, and serum enzyme-linked immunosorbent assays in orangutans (*Pongo pygmaeus*). *J Zoo Wildl Med* 20:307-14.
16. Montali, R., S. Mikota, and L. Cheng. 2001. *Mycobacterium tuberculosis* in zoo and wildlife species. *Rev Sci Tech* 20:291-303.
17. Bush, M., R. Montali, L. Phillips, and P. Holobaugh. 1990. Bovine tuberculosis in a bactrian camel herd: clinical, therapeutic and pathologic findings. *J Zoo Wildl Med* 21: 171-179.
18. Mann, P., M. Bush, D. Jannssen, E. Frank, and R. Montali. 1981. Clincopathological correlations of tuberculosis in large zoo mammals. *J Am Vet Med Assoc* 179:1123-9.
19. Barbiers, R. 1994. *Mycobacterium tuberculosis* in a black rhinoceros (*Diceros bicornis*). Proceedings of the American Association of Zoo Veterinarians, Pittsburgh, PA. 171-172.
20. Rietkerk, F., F. Griffin, B. Wood, S. Mubarak, E. Delima, O. Badri, N. Lindsay, and D. Williamson. 1993. Treatment of bovine tuberculosis in an Arabian oryx (*Oryx leucoryx*). *J Zoo Wildl Med* 24:323-27.
21. Lomme, J. R., C. O. Thoen, E. M. Himes, J. W. Vincent, and R. E. King. 1976. *Mycobacterium tuberculosis* infection in two East African oryxes. *J Am Vet Med Assoc* 169:912-14.
22. Hadley, R., C. Sauter-Louis, I. Lugton, R. Jackson, P. Durr, and J. Wilesmith. 2001. Mycobacterial diseases. *In* Infectious Diseases of Wild Mammals, 3rd ed. Ames: Iowa State University Press, 340-41.
23. Thoen, C. O., W. J. Quinn, L. D. Miller, L. D. Stackhouse, B. F. Newcomb, and J. M. Ferrrel. 1992. *Mycobacterium bovis* infection in North American Elk (*Cervus elephus*). *J Vet Diagn Investn* 4:423-427.
24. De Lisle, G., C. Mackintosh, and R. Bengis. 2001. *Mycobacterium bovis* in free-living and captive wildlife, including farmed deer. *Rev Sci Technol* 20:86-111.
25. Rapley, W., O. Kelton, N. Scollard, K. Mehren, and L. Trillo. 1978. Diagnosis and control of tuberculosis during the establishment of a modern zoo. *In R.* Montali (ed.), Mycobacterial Infections of Zoo Animals. Washington, DC: Smithsonian Institution Press, 163-172.
26. Thoen, C. O., K. Mills, and M. P. Hopkins. 1980. Enzyme- linked protein A: an enzyme-linked immunosorbent assay reagent for detecting antibodies in tuberculous exotic animals. *Am J Vet Res* 40:833-35.
27. Larsen, R., M. Salman, S. Mikota, R. Isaza, R. Montali, and J. Triantis. 2000. Evaluation of a multiple-antigen enzyme-linked immunosorbent assay for detection of *Mycobacterium tuberculosis* infection in captive elephants. *J Zoo Wild Med* 31:291-302.

28. Good, R., and N. McCarroll. 1978. BCG vaccination in rhesus monkeys: study of skin hypersensitivity and duration of protective immunity. *In* R. Montali (ed.), Mycobacterial Infections of Zoo Animals. Washington, DC: Smithsonian Institution Press, 115-22.

29. Kilbourn, A., H. Godfrey, R. Cook, et al. 2001. Serum antigen 85 levels in adjunct testing for active mycobacterial infections in orangutans. *J Wild Dis* 37:65-71.

30. Stevens, J. B., C. O. Thoen, E. B. Rohonezy, et al. 1998. The immunological response of llamas (*Lama glama*) following experimental infection with *Mycobacterium bovis*. *Can J Vet Res* 62:102-9.

31. Wood, P. R., L. A. Corner, J. S. Rothel, et al. 1991. Field comparison of the interferon-gamma assay and the intradermal tuberculin test for the diagnosis of bovine tuberculosis. *Aust Vet J* 68:286-90.

32. Whipple, D. L., C. A. Bolin, A. J. Davis, et al. 1995. Comparison of the sensitivity of the caudal fold skin test and a commercial gamma-interferon assay for diagnosis of bovine tuberculosis. *Am J Vet Res* 56:415-19.

33. Miller, J. W., A. L. Jenny, and J. B. Payeur. 2002. Polymerase chain reaction detection of *Mycobacterium tuberculosis* complex and *Mycobacterium avium* complex organisms in formalin-fixed tissues from culture negative ruminants. *Vet Microbiol* 87:15-23.

34. Kaneene, J. B. and C. O. Thoen. 2004. Tuberculosis. *J Am Vet Assoc* 224:685-91.

35. Janicki, B. W., R. C. Good, P. Minden, L. F. Affronti, and W. F. Hymes. 1973. Immune responses in rhesus monkeys after Bacillus Calmette-Guerin vaccination and aerosol challenge with *Mycobacterium tuberculosis*. *Am Rev Respir Dis* 107: 359-66.

Chapter 26

Tuberculosis in Fur Seals and Sea Lions Caused by *Myocbacterium pinnipedii*

D. Cousins, PhD

Tuberculosis in pinnipeds was first diagnosed after causing significant disease in a captive colony of seals in a marine park Western Australia in 1986 (1). The disease affected both the New Zealand fur seal (*Arctocephalus forsteri*) and the Australian sea lion (*Neophoca cinerea*). The zoonotic risk of tuberculosis in seals was demonstrated when a seal trainer who had worked with the affected seals in the zoological park was diagnosed with tuberculosis caused by the same strain in 1988 (2). In subsequent years, tuberculosis was diagnosed in an Australian fur seal (*Arctocephalus pusillus doriferus*) in Tasmania (3); in captive Southern sea lions (*Otaria flavescens*) in Uruguay (4); and in the South American fur seal (*Arctocephalus australis*), Southern sea lion, and Sub Antarctic fur seal (*Arctocephalus tropicalis*) in Argentina (5,6); in captive South American fur seals in the United Kingdom (7); and in New Zealand fur seal and New Zealand sea lion (*Phocarctos hookeri*) in New Zealand (8; Duignan, personal communication, 1998). Although *M. bovis* was originally implicated as the cause of the tuberculosis in pinnipeds (1,4,8), slight differences noted in pathogenicity and phenotypic characteristics and basic molecular typing indicated divergence from the classic *M. bovis*, and the organism was labeled the "seal bacillus" (9,10). Genomic deletion studies indicate that these organisms evolved from the classic human pathogen *M. tuberculosis* and diverged to form a separate evolutionary branch, along with *M. microti* and *M. africaunum* (11,12). These findings, along with comprehensive molecular characterization of a collection of 37 seal-related isolates originating from six species of pinniped, human, and other animal species from five countries, has resulted in the organism causing tuberculosis in seals being accepted as a new species within the *M. tuberculosis* complex; namely, *M. pinnipedii* sp. nov. (7). So far, tuberculosis has been only reported in pinniped species that originate from the southern hemisphere. To the author's knowledge, there has been only one anecdotal report of tuberculosis caused by *M. bovis* in a seal originating from the northern hemisphere (Thoen, personal communication, 1996), and it is unknown whether the disease is a serious risk to seal species that populate the oceans north of the equator. *M. pinnipedii* is known to be pathogenic in guinea pigs and rabbits, and the apparent incidental infection of a human, bovine, Brazilian tapir, llama, Chilean pudu, and Western lowland gorilla indicates the species may have a wide host range. The remainder of this chapter describes in detail the disease aspects and taxonomic characteristics of *M. pinnipedii* and discusses the potential origin of the species and its implications.

Disease in Pinnipeds

M. pinnipedii is capable of causing serious disease in several species of seal and fur seals that inhabit the southern hemisphere. So far, *M. pinnipedii* has been isolated from four species of fur seal and two species of sea lion. In addition, tuberculosis has been diagnosed in a New Zealand sea lion histologically (Table 26.1).

M. pinnipedii is also known to be pathogenic in other species, as well as capable of infecting humans, cattle, laboratory guinea pigs and rabbits, Brazilian tapir (*Tapirus terrestris*), llama (*Lama glama*), Chilean pudu (*Pudu pudu*), and Western Lowland gorilla (*Gorilla gorilla gorilla*; Table 26.2.). Apart from the laboratory animals that were infected for pathogenicity studies, the other cases have all evolved as a result of transmission from infected seals.

Clearly *M. pinnipedii* has the potential to have a wide host range similar to that of *M. bovis* (7). In seals, the strain predominantly causes granulomatous lesions in the peripheral lymph nodes, lungs, pleura, spleen, and peritoneum (Fig. 26.1).

Cases with pulmonary, liver, and mesenteric node involvement, a case with pulmonary lesions and meningitis, and a case with lesions confined to the liver have

Table 26.1.   Species and origin of pinnipeds recorded with tuberculosis from various countries from 1985 to 2004

Species	Common Name	Country of Origin	Wild	Year Captive	Recorded
Arctocephalus australis	South American fur seal	Argentina	14	0	1989–2000
		United Kingdom	0	6	1996–1998
		Uruguay	5	0	1997–2004
Arctocephalus forsteri	New Zealand fur seal	Australia	1	2	1986–1995
		New Zealand	3	0	1997–1998
Arctocephalus pusillus doriferus	Australian fur seal	Australia	1	0	1992
Arctocephalus tropicalis	Sub antarctic fur seal	Argentina	1	0	1996
Neophoca cinerea	Australian sea lion	Australia	2	4	1985–1992
Otaria flavescens (byronia)	Southern sea lion	Argentina	2	6	1987–2003
		Uruguay	2	5	1987–2004
Phocarctos hookeri	New Zealand sea lion	New Zealand	3	0	2001–2004
Total			34	23	1985–2004

Table 26.2.   Other species naturally infected with *M. pinnipedii* or known to be susceptible to infection from artificial infection or pathogenicity studies

Species	Common name	Origin	Situation	Number	Year
Homo sapiens	Human	Australia	Seal trainer	1	1988
Bos taurus	Bovine	New Zealand	Farmed near coast	1	1991
Tapirus terrestris	Brazilian tapir	United Kingdom	Zoo enclosure adjacent to infected seals	1	1996
—	Laboratory guinea pig	Australia	Pathogenicity testing	2	1986
—	Laboratory rabbit	Australia	Pathogenicity testing	2	1986
Lama glama	Llama	United Kingdom	Zoo enclosure adjacent to infected seals	1	—
Gorilla gorilla gorilla	Western Lowland gorilla	United Kingdom	Zoo enclosure adjacent to infected seals	2	—

been described, as well as cases of disseminated disease with lesions in mesenteric nodes, kidney, spleen, and liver. Mycobacteria have been recovered from the lung and associated lymph nodes and from mesenteric lymph nodes and liver. Histologically, the reaction is often characterized by proliferation of spindle cells, sometimes resulting in a sarcomatous appearance, particularly in serosa and lymph

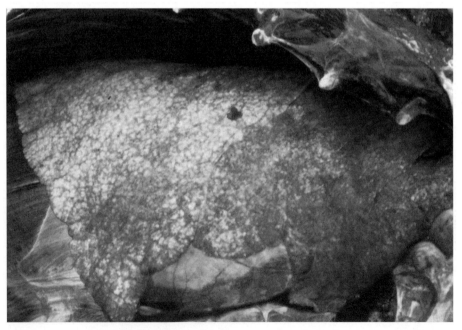

Figure 26.1.   Adult female New Zealand sea lion with diffuse miliary granulomas throughout the right lung.

nodes. Typical necrogranulomas and pyogranulomas are common in the lungs, but the presence of mineralization and multinucleate giant cells is variable (Figs. 26.2 and 26.3). The presence of acid-fast bacilli in lesions also varies from large numbers of organisms to none detectable (Fig. 26.4). As with other members of the *M. tuberculosis* complex, aerosols are considered to be the primary route of transmission,

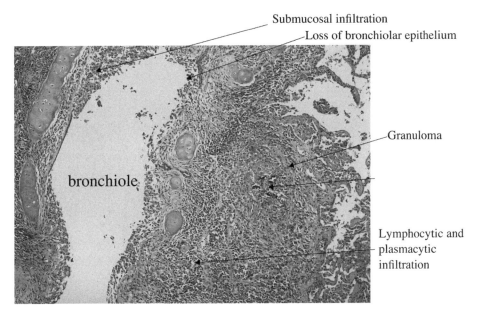

Figure 26.2.　New Zealand sea lion lung (×10, hematoxylin and eosin).

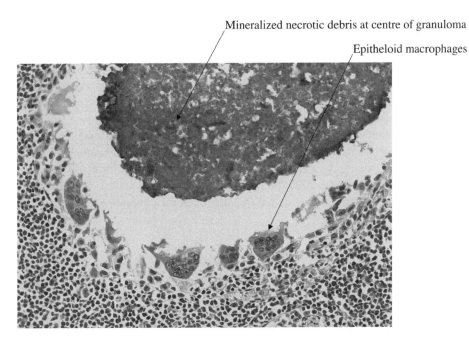

Figure 26.3.　New Zealand sea lion, bronchial lymph node (×40, H&E stain).

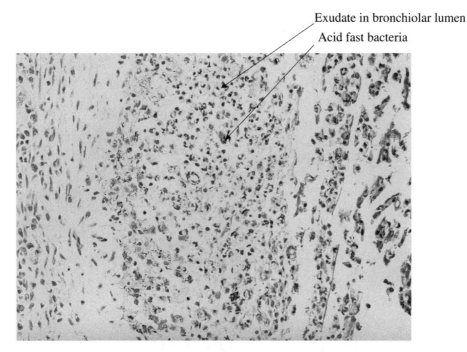

Exudate in bronchiolar lumen

Acid fast bacteria

Figure 26.4.   New Zealand sea lion bronchiole (×40, Ziehl Neelsen stain).

although mesenteric lymph node and hepatic infection in some animals also indicates that an alimentary route is possible.

Phenotypic Characterization of *M. pinnipedii*

The phenotypic characteristics of this species are generally consistent with *M. bovis*, with the exception that they fail to produce detectable amounts of MPB70 antigen. The organisms are acid-alcohol-fast, non–spore forming, and nonmotile bacilli with loose cord formation. Growth is generally enhanced by sodium pyruvate and usually occurs within 3–6 weeks of incubation on egg-based media at 36°–37°C. Colonies are dysgonic, rough, flat, and nonphotochromogenic. Isolates are negative for nitrate reduction and are generally negative for niacin accumulation, with some isolates demonstrating low to medium reactions for niacin. In addition, they are susceptible to PZA (50 μg/mL) and to TCH (1 μg/mL) (occasionally isolates have demonstrated resistance to 1 μg TCH/mL but are susceptible to 10 μg/mL).

Molecular Characterization of M. pinnipedii

Genetic properties indicate that the strains fall somewhat between *M. tuberculosis* and *M. bovis* genetically and are even more similar to *M. africanum* and *M. microti*. All isolates contain the sequences IS*6110*, IS*1081*, MPB70, and *mtp40*, yet fail to produce detectable MPB70 antigen. The *pncA* gene contains CAC (His) at codon

Table 26.3. Phenotypic properties of the seal bacillus compared with other members of the *M. tuberculosis* complex (from Cousins et al., 2003)

Species	Nitrate Reduction	Niacin Accumulation	Pyruvate Preference	Stimulated by Glycerol	MPB70 Antigen	TCH	PZA	Pathogenicity Guinea Pig	Rabbit
M. tuberculosis									
Classic	+	+	−	+	−	R	S	++	−
Asian	+	+	−	−	−	S	S	++	−
M. africanum									
Type I	−	V	−	−	−	S	S	++	±
Type II	+	V	−	−	−	R	S		
M. microti	−	−[a]	−	−	−	S[b]	S	−	
M. pinnipedii	−	−	+	−	−	S	S	++	+++
M. bovis	−	−	+	−	+	S	R	++	++
M. caprae	−	−	+	−	?	S[c]	S	NA	NA
M. bovis BCG	−	−	+	+	+	S	R	−	−

[a]Occasional strains, including the isolates from New Zealand, gave weak or positive reactions in the niacin accumulation test.
[b]New Zealand strains were resistant to 1 TCH/mL but were sensitive to 10 mg TCH/mL.
[c]Resistant to 1 and 2 mg TCH/mL, but sensitive to 5 and 10 mg TCH/mL.
Abbreviations: +, positive; −, negative; V, variable; S, sensitive; R, resistant.

57, and a G at nt 285 in the *oxyR* gene similar to *M. tuberculosis*, *M. microti*, and *M. africanum*. The isolates are susceptible to isoniazid, rifampicin, streptomycin, ethambutol, and paraminosalysilic acid. The type strain 6482^T has been lodged in the ATCC (BAA-688^T) and NCTC (13288^T) collections.

The seal spoligotypes form a unique cluster that is clearly different from all other members of the *M. tuberculosis* complex (Table 26.5) and that can be used as a method of identification, along with the genetic tests outlined in Table 26.4.

Pathogenicity and Zoonotic Risk

With the recent diagnosis of tuberculosis by histopathology in a New Zealand sea lion, disease has now been recorded in seven different species of pinniped global-ly, including three species of sea lion and four species of fur seal. Although pin-nipeds are clearly the natural host for *M. pinnipedii*, infection has spread from affected seals to a seal trainer working with them in a zoological park in Australia, from infected fur seals to Brazilian tapir, Chilean pudu and llama, and Western Lowland gorilla in a zoological park in the United Kingdom, and in a separate inci-dent, apparently from seals to cattle in New Zealand. The virulence of the organ-ism has been confirmed by experimental infection of guinea pigs and rabbits, and these findings indicate a potentially wide host range for the organism, similar to that of *M. bovis* (13). The range of hosts susceptible to *M. pinnipedii* has not been fully tested experimentally, but if the number of incidental infections to other species is any guide, it is likely to be more far ranging than *M. tuberculosis*, *M. africanum*, and *M. microti*. The finding of a bovine isolate in New Zealand with identical char-acteristics to those in New Zealand fur seals from this country confirms that this strain is capable of infecting cattle. However, tuberculosis in seals is considered to be of limited risk to cattle tuberculosis control programs, as there is generally lim-ited contact between these two species. At present, it is unknown whether *M. pin-nipedii* infection can be maintained in other hosts or whether they are merely spillover hosts. The organism is known to cause serious disease in these species, and in humans. The consulting physician of the human case was quoted as saying, "the organism seemed to be more pathogenic than *M. bovis*" (2). Because pinnipeds naturally inhabit a mostly a marine and coastal environment, there is more limited opportunity for infection of other animal species. It is not yet known whether this organism infects other marine mammals. Because of the proven zoonotic risk, and the fact that marine park workers, conservation or fisheries officers, and veterinar-ians may be required to handle potentially infected seals, it is important that they are aware of the risks of infection and take appropriate precautions when moving or handling such animals, or when collecting specimens from them (2,14)

Distribution of Pinniped Species Affected by *M. pinnipedii*

It is now well known that tuberculosis is endemic in sea lion and fur seal pop-ulations in the southern hemisphere. The population distributions of the different

Table 26.4. Genetic properties of the seal bacillus when compared with other members of the *M. tuberculosis* complex (from Cousins et al., 2003)

Species	IS6110	IS1081	Mtp40	PncA C57	KatG C463	OxyR n 285	GyrA C95	Spoligotyping: spacers 39–43
M. tuberculosis								
Classic	+	+	+[a]	CAC (His)	CTG (Leu), CGG (Arg)	G	AGC (Ser), ACC (Thr)	Present (1–5)
Asian	+	+	+	CAC	CTG/CGG	G	–	
M. africanum								
Type I	+	+	+[a]	CAC	CTG	G	ACC	Present (1–5)
Type II	+	+	+[a]	CAC	CTG	G	ACC	
M. microti	+	+	–[b]	CAC	CTG	G	ACC	Nil
M. pinnipedii	+	+	+	CAC	CTG	G	ACC	Nil
M. bovis	+	+	–	GAC (Asp)	CTG	A	ACC	Nil
M. caprae	+	+	–	CAC	CTG	A	ACC	Nil
M. bovis BCG	+	+	–	GAC	CTG	A	ACC	Nil

[a]Very occasionally, members of these species lack the genetic IS6110 or *mtp40* element (Liébana et al., 1996).
[b]7/7 isolates were negative for *mtp40* (Liébana et al., 1996), whereas one isolate tested by Bernardelli et al. (1996) was reported as positive.
Present (1–5) between 1 and 5 of the 3′ spacers (39–43) are present, Nil none of the five 3′ spacers (39–43) are present.

265

Table 26.5. Spoligotypes identified from *M. pinnipedii* isolates from Australia, Uruguay, Argentina, Great Britain, and New Zealand compared with reference strains of the *M. tuberculosis* complex (taken from Cousins et al., 2003)

Isolate/ strain/type	Spoligotype pattern observed with 43 spacers in DR locus	Number of isolates				
		Australia	Argentina/ Uruguay	Great Britain	New Zealand	Total
M. tuberculosis H37Rv	+++++++++++++++++++++−					
M. africanum TMC 03	+++++++++−−−++++++					
M. africanum TMC 12	+++++++++++++−−+++					
M. microti ATCC 0871	−−−−−−−−−−−−					
M. bovis BCG P3	−+−−−−++++++++−+++					
M. bovis Sp01	+++−+++++++++++−++					
M. pinnipedii SS-1	−−+++−−−−−−−+++++++	15	13			28
M. pinnipedii SS-2	−−+++−−−−−+++++		1			1
M. pinnipedii SS-3	−−+−−++−−−−+++			3		3
M. pinnipedii SS-4	++++++−−−−				3	3
Total		15	14	3	3	35

+ Hybridization with spacer, − no hybridization with spacer, TMC Trudeau Mycobacterium Collection, ATCC American Type Culture Collection.

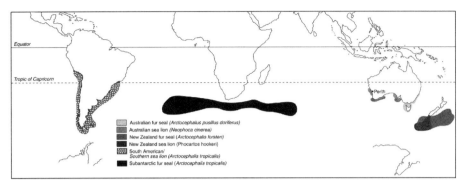

Figure 26.5. Geographical distribution of pinniped populations bacteriologically confirmed as *Mycobacterium pinnipedii* causing tuberculosis.

pinniped species known to be infected with *M. pinnipedii* are shown in Figure 26.5. There is some crossover between some of the populations (e.g., New Zealand fur seals and New Zealand sea lion and Australian sea lions), indicating that there is potential for spread between the various species. In fact, it is known that in some cases, different species of seals inhabit the same islands in Australia. The prevalence and incidence of disease in these populations remains unknown and extremely difficult to ascertain because of the difficulty of undertaking any form of survey using skin test or other methods such as gamma interferon. Opportunistic screening of seals using an ELISA developed for seal tuberculosis (15) has been of limited use in assessing the health status of wild-caught seals in Australia (Cousins, unpublished data).

Evolutionary Aspects

The finding of tuberculosis in these seven species of pinniped indicates that infection has been endemic in these animals for many thousands of years, if not hundreds of thousands. The population dynamics of the various species of pinniped affected by tuberculosis indicate possible routes of transmission for some of the seal populations; however, some of the affected species do not overlap and are likely to have been separated for centuries, if not thousands of years. Interestingly, the spoligotype patterns of the *M. pinnipedii* isolates from six different seal species isolated from five different countries (and four continents) over the 15-year period appear closely related, indicating either a very stable genotype or a relatively recent spread. Unless infection is found in another species known to have a wider migration route, it is unlikely that transmission has occurred in relatively recent times.

New DNA technologies that can detect large sequence polymorphisms or deletions (16,17) have been used to study the evolution of *M. tuberculosis* complex organisms. It has been shown that an increasing number of large sequence deletions in *M. bovis* Bacille Calmette-Güerin have occurred with its subculture and subsequent loss of virulence (16). It is now widely accepted that these large sequence deletions occur in a single direction and that such results can be used to define the taxonomic evolution of strains. Although *M. bovis* was once considered to be the precursor to human tuberculosis (18) (with the human pathogen evolving from *M. bovis* around the times when humans domesticated animals), this theory has now been discounted, and it has been shown that a rarely isolated member of the *M. tuberculosis* complex first isolated from a patient in Somalia and called *M. canettii* (11) is a precursor to *M. tuberculosis* and that *M. bovis* (and *M. bovis* Bacille Calmette-Güerin) is the youngest member of the complex (evolutionarily speaking). It has also been demonstrated that *M. bovis*–like organisms isolated from goats (19,20) and seals, which have been accepted as new members within the *M. tuberculosis* complex (*M. caprae* and *M. pinnipedii*), have evolved from *M. tuberculosis*, with *M. pinnipedii* and *M. africanum* evolving along a common side branch (Fig. 26.6).

Conclusion

Tuberculosis in pinnipeds is an endemic disease that affects at least seven species of seal in the southern hemisphere. Further studies may clarify whether this disease is confined to species in the southern hemisphere or whether it is a more global occurrence. Researchers, marine scientists, and conservationists are encouraged to examine sick or dying seals in coastal areas for evidence of tuberculosis to expand the host range and geographic spread of *M. pinnipedii*. Because of the known path-

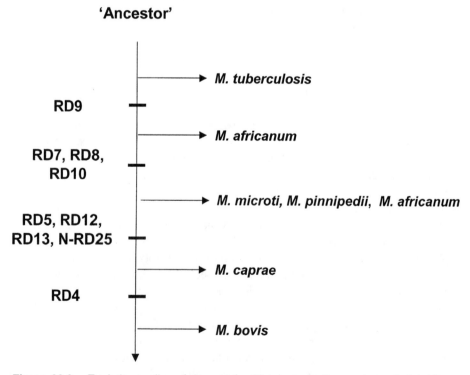

Figure 26.6. Evolutionary line of descent for *M. tuberculosis* organisms derived from large sequence polymorphisms and deletions (from Mostowy et al. 2004 [12]).

ogenicity of *M. pinnipedii* for humans, appropriate precautions should be taken by handlers of potentially affected seals.

Acknowledgments

I am grateful to Padraig Duignan from New Zealand, Miguel Castro and Helena Katz from Uruguay, and Sue Dow from the United Kingdom for providing updated statistics on seal cases for this chapter. I also thank Padraig Duignan for supplying photographs of the gross pathology and histopathology and David Forshaw, Department of Agriculture, Western Australia, for his comments on the pathology.

References

1. Forshaw, D. and G. R. Phelps (1991). "Tuberculosis in a captive colony of pinnipeds." *Journal of Wildlife Diseases* **27**: 288-295.
2. Thompson, P. J., D. V. Cousins, et al. (1993). "Seals, seal trainers and mycobacterial infection." *American Review of Respiratory Disease* **147**: 164-167.
3. Woods, R., D. V. Cousins, et al. (1995). "Diagnosis of tuberculosis in a free-ranging Australian fur seal (*Arctocephalus pusillus doriferus*) from Tasmania." *Journal of Wildlife Diseases* **31**(1): 83-86.
4. Castro Ramos, M., M. Ayala, et al. (1998). "Aislamiento de *Mycobacterium bovis* en Pinnipedos Otaria byronia (*Lobo marino comun*) en Uruguay." *Revista de Medicina Veterinaria* **79**(3): 197-200.
5. Bernardelli, A., R. Bastida, et al. (1996). "Tuberculosis in sea lions and fur seals from the south-western Atlantic coast." *Scientific and Technical Review Office International des Epizooties.* **15**(3): 985-1005.
6. Bastida, R., J. Loureiro, et al. (1999). "Tuberculosis in a wild subantarctic fur seal from Argentina." *Journal of Wildlife Diseases* **35**(4): 796-798.
7. Cousins, D. V., R. Bastida, et al. (2003). "Tuberculosis in seals caused by a novel member of the *Mycobacterium tuberculosis* complex: *Mycobacterium pinnipedii* sp. nov."
8. Hunter, J. E., P. J. Duignan, et al. (1998). "First report of potentially zoonotic tuberculosis in fur seals in New Zealand." *New Zealand Medical Journal* **111**: 130-131.
9. Cousins, D. V., B. R. Francis, et al. (1990). "Tuberculosis in captive seals: bacteriological studies on an isolate belonging to the *Mycobacterium tuberculosis* complex." *Research in Veterinary Science* **48**: 196-200.
10. Cousins, D. V., S. N. Williams, et al. (1993). "Tuberculosis in wild seals and characterisation of the seal bacillus." *Australian Veterinary Journal* **70**(3): 92-97.
11. Brosch, R., S. V. Gordon, et al. (2002). "A new evolutionary scenario for the *Mycobacterium tuberculosis* complex." PNAS **99**(6): 3684-3689.
12. Mostowy, S., D. Cousins, et al. (2002). "Genomic deletions suggest a phylogeny for the *Mycobacterium tuberculosis* complex." *Journal of infectious Diseases* **186**(1): 74-80.
13. O'Reilly, L. M. and C. J. Daborn (1995). "The epidemiology of *Mycobacterium bovis* infections in animals and man: a review." *Tubercle and Lung Disease* **76**(1): 1-46.
14. Bastida, R., J. Loureiro, et al. (1994). *Healths risks while handling eared seals.* 22nd International Marine Animal Trainers Association (IMATA) Conference, Tacoma, Seattle, USA, 1994.

15. Cousins, D. V. (1987). "ELISA for detection of tuberculosis in seals." *The Veterinary Record* **121**: 305. *International Journal of Systematic and Evolutionary Microbiology* **53**(Pt 5): 1305-1314.

16. Behr, M. A. and P. M. Small (1999). "A historical and molecular phylogeny of BCG strains." *Vaccine* **17**(7-8): 915-922.

17. Behr, M. A., M. A. Wilson, et al. (1999). "Comparative genomics of BCG vaccines by whole genome DNA-microarray." *Science* **284**(5419): 1520-1523.

18. Stead, W. W. (1997). "The origin and spread of tuberculosis. How the past explains the present and is the key to the future." *Tuberculosis* **18**(1): 65-77.

19. Aranaz, A., E. Liébana, et al. (1999). "*Mycobacterium tuberculosis* subsp *caprae* subsp. nov.: a taxonomic study of a new member of the *Mycobacterium tuberculosis* complex isolated from goats in Spain." *International Journal of Systematic Bacteriology* **49**(3): 1263-1273.

20. Aranaz, A., D. Cousins, et al. (2003). "Elevation of *Mycobacterium tuberculosis* subsp. *caprae* Aranaz et al. 1999 to species rank as *Mycobacterium caprae* comb. nov., sp. nov." *International Journal of Systematic and Evolutionary Microbiology* **53**(Pt 6): 1785-1789.

Chapter 27

Tuberculosis in Nonhuman Primates with and Emphasis on *Mycobacterium bovis*

P.A. Frost, DVM

Early Investigation and Natural History

Tuberculosis had been recognized clinically in animals, particularly in nonhuman primates (NHPs), before the identification of the bacillus. Initially, when Robert Koch discovered the tubercle bacillus, he believed that the same organism caused the disease in bovine and humans. This was to soon change when he noted small but consistent differences between the bacilli (1). Much of what is known about tuberculosis and its transmission, the route of infection, diagnosis, clinical course, progression of disease, and pathology, were discovered through evaluation of naturally occurring infection.

In 1884, Koch was the first to describe the course of tuberculosis in monkeys, stating that it was more rapid in these animals than in humans, and that lesions develop more widely throughout the organs of the body. In the beginning, there was tremendous discussion among the researchers as to the predominant route of infection. The two main schools of thought seemed to be divided as to whether the organisms enter through the lungs or the gastrointestinal tract. This yielded a flurry of experiments in NHPs as well as publications during this period. Early experiments reported feeding tubercle bacilli of both origins to delineate the clinical course, resulting in a primary focus of human strains resulting in pulmonary lesions and the bovine strain resulting in intestinal lesions. Meanwhile, alternate routes were noted when the animals were fed the organism that could pass without local lesions and spread systemically through the blood and lymph systems. Still other investigators would inoculate subcutaneously to see whether the organism could be spread through the blood and lymph system (2). As further experimentation proceeded, it quickly became apparent that both *M. bovis* and *M. tuberculosis* would have similar presentation, dependent on the route of exposure.

Acknowledging the incidence in captive animals was high, others sought to determine the source of the infection. Carpenter had suggested that the source of these infections in captive animals was most likely human contact because the numbers of wild primates under their study maintained their numbers, and early researchers could not find evidence of tuberculosis in that population. In newly captive *Macaca mulatta* held for export in India, few animals were noted as positive, whereas the incidence of the disease in this species held in captivity in the United States was found to be greater. The earliest means of transportation of these animals was by ship, and the animals were housed for variable periods of time with the animal dealer, providing an opportunity for transmission before their arrival in the United States. The prevalence of tuberculosis in captive colonies was widespread, with high morbidity and mortality (3).

In the natural course of disease investigation, after the etiologic agent is discovered, its routes of transmission and the recognition of high morbidity and mortality are identified. The next logical step is to develop diagnostic testing.

Early investigators showed that monkeys with tuberculosis would react similarly to man on the intradermal injection of a small amount of tuberculin. The method of injecting into the eyelid as a diagnostic method is historically credited to Schroeder (4). The reasoning behind the choice of the eyelid was the absence of hair and the looseness of the skin, which would allow for the greatest reaction.

The detection and elimination of positive animals was only part of the entire program of prevention and control. The recognition of the need for standards on husbandry and routine care to include improved shipping conditions, nutrition, and sanitation; better holding facilities; quarantine; and implementation of surveillance testing drastically decreased the incidence from a common occurrence to a sporadic event in captive NHPs.

Tuberculosis has occurred in prosimians, New World monkeys, Old World monkeys, and apes. There may be differences in susceptibility between the species, but all NHPs are susceptible to tubercle bacilli. Tuberculosis has been recognized most often in laboratory and zoological collections of Asian monkeys, particularly those of the genus *Macaca* (i.e., *M. mulatta, M. arctoides, M. nemestrina*, and *M. fasicularis*), and to a lesser extent in African cercopithecoids (i.e., Papio, Cercopithecus, erythrocebus), Cercocebus and pongids, (i.e., Pongo), Gorilla, and Pan. There are few reports of tuberculosis among New World monkeys, and these have been mainly in Saimiri, Aotus, and Ateles (5). Not all reports of tuberculosis have been diligent in reporting the exact mycobacteria involved. Estimates indicate that 10% of the tuberculosis outbreaks were caused by *M. bovis* (6).

Tuberculosis: Clinical Signs

Through the application of all that has been learned over the years regarding this disease came the development of industry standards that guide importation, husbandry, and medical management in association with regulatory oversight. As a result, the incidence of tuberculosis has been reduced precipitously, and many current, practicing veterinarians have never experienced an epizootic. For them, the introduction to tuberculosis in NHPs occurs through current literature, books, and review of recent epizootics in other facilities. Veterinary practice is based on a foundation of knowledge about disease and the probability of its occurrence. The fact that the incidence of tuberculosis is currently low, combined with a high morbidity and mortality, along with a significant zoonotic potential, make it a major threat to all colonies. For the clinician, there are no pathopneumonic signs, no clear hematologic presentation, nor a definitive diagnostic test. Although a diagnosis may be elusive even to the most skilled, one must keep this disease on one's list of differential diagnoses to exclude while determining a definitive diagnosis of a condition, to avoid overlooking it.

The clinical signs in NHPs are often nondescript and ill-defined. Tuberculosis can imitate a multitude of diseases such as pneumonia, neoplasm, and fungal infections. The clinical spectrum of symptoms can range from asymptomatic to multisymptomatic, being highly dependent on the route of exposure. Signs and symptoms can be related to generalized physiological systems and specific organ involvement, as well as pulmonary and neurological manifestations.

General clinical signs can include rough hair coat, anorexia, depression, lethargy, fever (low grade to intermittently persistent), weight loss, hepatomegaly, splenomegaly, and local or general lymphadenopathy (with or without draining tracts). A chronic or paroxysmal cough and dyspnea indicate pulmonary involvement, which mirrors influenza, acute bronchitis, or pneumonia. Neurological presentation with signs including anisocoria or ataxia may implicate meningitis (central nervous system involvement), and paresis to paralysis can indicate a peripheral neurological component that may be a result of spondylitis.

Species susceptibility and disease progression has long been suspected among NHPs. On the basis of disease progression, experimental studies have shown that *M. fasicularis* can be classified into three categories: rapidly progressive, acute/chronic infection, and latent (subclinical). This mirrors what is found in the human population. The mean survival time was dose dependent, and weight loss was observed in all groups; the weight loss was particularly remarkable, along with persistent temperature elevations in the high-dose group. (7)

Pathogenesis

The pathogenesis of tuberculosis in NHPs along with captive animals is well described in the literature (5,8–10). The site of introduction of the bacillus will depend on the route of exposure, with ingestion and inhalation being the most predominant methods. Transmission, however, has been documented through direct contact, and through contact with fomites such as a thermometer and a tattoo needle. Through sound medical practices such as the use of sterile disposables and effective sterilization procedures, one can minimize transmission.

At the site of entry, bacilli are processed by the regional macrophages by means of phagocytosis. The effectiveness of this process is macrophage dependent and is variable. Those organisms that survive the lysosomal enzymes and oxidative process within the cell continue to multiply and inevitably cause cell death, subsequently releasing their contents. The release of the cellular precuts and the secretion of cytokines stimulates recruitment of both T-lymphocytes and circulating monocytes to further phagocytize the bacilli. Macrophages transform into epitheloid cells that eventually become the center of the granuloma. Once the delayed hypersensitivity is activated, cytotoxic T-lymphocytes enhance the recruitment activation and destruction of these cells that form the central area of necrosis. Fusion of activated macrophages forms the multinucleated giant cell of Langhan's type. The proliferation of fibroblasts forms the encapsulation that surrounds the tubercle.

Calcification is rare in NHPs compared to what is observed in man. There is variation among the species of NHPs as to the degree of susceptibility. In *M. mulatta* the disease is progressive early in its course, followed by rapid dissemination and formation of caseous nodules.

Pathology

Gross and microscopic lesions in NHPs with tuberculosis can vary in duration and degree of the disease. Organs of predilection are the lung and adjacent hilar lymph nodes. Secondary dissemination occurs to the spleen, kidney, liver, and associated lymph nodes (Fig. 27.1). Additional sites reported but seen with decreased frequency include the omentum, ovary, cerebrum, spinal column, peripheral lymph nodes, skin, and mammary gland.

The extent of the lesions can range from no detectable lesions to wide dissemination of yellow-white-to-gray caseous granulomas, ranging from pinpoint to large coalescing lesions (Fig. 27.1). Distribution and appearance of the nodules in the lung can be focal, coalescing, and cavitary. The hilar lymph nodes that drain this region also are found to contain caseous nodules. The process of cavitation occurs when large granulomas in the lung expel their contents into adjacent airways. In areas where the affected lung is in association with the parietal pleura, adhesions can occur.

Tuberculous spondylitis and Pott's disease has been reported in the rhesus monkey (7,11). Early investigators suggested that it was attributable to the rupture of the pleural lesions and establishment of the local foci in the thoracic wall and along the vertebrae. Experimental findings indicate vertebral involvement from hematogenous seeding, as there was no evidence of rupture of the pleural lesions. Miliary

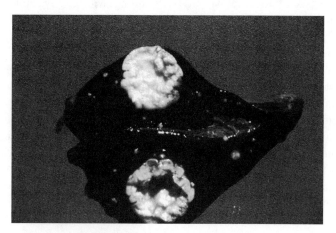

Figure 27.1.   Tuberculous lesion in liver of a rhesus monkey from which *Mycobacterium bovis* was isolated

spread to the eye has also been reported, with one of the animals having panophthalmitis as a result of a large granuloma that destroyed the eye. (7).

Histological Narrative

Histopathologic appearance is dependent on a multitude of factors, but most important, it is based on the duration and extent of the disease. The classic lesion is characterized by a central core of acellular necrotic debris surrounded by epitheloid macrophages with multinucleated Langhan's giant cells at the periphery (Fig. 27.2). The lung and intestines, being the site of early infections, may present with microscopic granulomas surrounded by a collection of epitheloid cells, with an occasional giant cell. These early lesions may have a collection of neutrophils in their center, making this a diagnostic challenge in distinguishing it from other granulomatous diseases. Use of acid-fast stains can help in the demonstration of acid-fast bacilli. In particular, *Nocardia* spp. represents the greatest test to the diagnostician, as clinically and diagnostically, the lesion distribution and dissemination are similar. Although this organism is partially acid-fast, most lesions have a predominant neutrophilic component and present as a pyogranuloma rather than what is seen in typical tubercles. *M. fasicularis* challenged with 10^4 and 10^5 colony-forming units presented with necrotic caseation with moderate numbers of epitheloid cells, few lymphocytes, and Langhan's giant cells. Lower dose ($\leq 10^3$) animals had a greater amount of infiltrates as a result of an enhanced immune response with a slower disease progression. The lesions seen in the lowest dose (10^1) are contained of dense cellular infiltrates (7).

Diagnostic Testing and Considerations

One of the major limitations for disease control appears to be detection of infected animals. The tuberculin skin test (TST) in primates has been the gold standard for

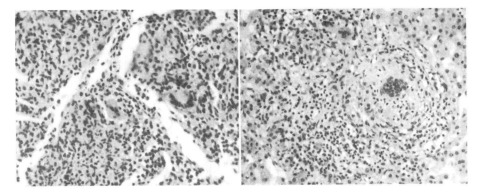

Figure 27.2.   Section of lung from a baboon from which *Mycobacterium bovis* was isolated. Granuloma of lymphocytes, epitheloid cells, and multinucleated giant cells with area of necrosis.

years for use in initial (quarantine) screening and surveillance for tuberculosis. In the development of TST, the concentration of antigen, site of administration, and product performance in the detection of disease were examined. In early studies comparing the *M. bovis* versus mammalian tuberculin, researchers (12) found that the latter was superior in the diagnosis of tuberculosis. The TST involves the intradermal administration of 0.1 mL Tuberculin Mammailian (*M. tuberculosis*), strains C, D^t, and P^n, into the eyelid (9). Alternate lids are recommended in sequential testing. The cell-mediated immunity measured by the TST is dependent on the production of cytokines by sensitized lymphocytes at the injection site in recognition of mycobacterial protein. The placement should be low enough on the lid so that swelling is easily visualized. Injection sites are observed at 24, 48, and 72 hours postadministration. The injection site is evaluated for edema and induration. The test is interpreted as positive when there is a swelling in conjunction with lid droop. The same trained individual or veterinarian should interpret these tests at each time point. Standard facility programs will dictate the length of time between tests and the number of tests applicable for quarantine and routine surveillance of the colony. This test is dependent on the animals' ability to elicit a cell-mediated response. Detection of positive animals is difficult early on and in advanced stages of the disease. A cell-mediated response in competent animals occurs approximately 4 weeks after exposure. This challenges the surveillance in possibly compromised individuals who are unable to mount a cell-mediated immunity such as postvaccination (measles), geriatrics, immunosuppressed (natural or experimental), and drug interference.

False-positive reactions have been seen in animals that have trauma as a result of administration, as a nonspecific reaction to the vehicle, and those that have been inoculated with complete Freund's adjuvant. Limitations in the past have revolved around availability of Tuberculin, limited shelf life, quality and purity of the product used, adequate volume used, skill in administration, thoroughness in recording bruise or lid trauma, visual access (group housed), accurate interpretation at all time periods, inadequate time interval between tests, or lack of documentation. All of these elements can jeopardize a surveillance program

Early and advanced stages of the disease frequently remain undetected using TST, mandating that clinicians seek supplemental testing to enhance their programs. Lymphoproliferative Assay (LPA) in comparison to the skin test appears to be a more sensitive indicator for the detection of disease. Under experimental conditions in *M. fasciularis,* Walsh (7) reported that all dose groups challenged displayed a positive response, including the high-dose animals (10^5). In the groups challenged with less than 10^4 colony-forming units, LPA responses were strongly positive. Peak responses tended to occur later and to be higher in those animals challenged with lower doses. LPA responses were highly dependent on the concentration of PPD, with responses to 10 and 1 ug/mL consistently greater than responses to 0.1 or 0.01 ug/mL (7). LPA assays have been also used in the *M. mulatta* to distinguish noninfected from infected animals.

In response to the bacilli, lymphocytes secrete cytokines including IFN-γ in an effort to stimulate macrophages. Through refinement of the LPA came the commercially available Primagam test that measures IFN-γ response to purified protein derivatives (PPDs) of *M. bovis* and *M. avium* (14). This test has been used to analyze the T-cell response to the antigens as a diagnostic aid in the detection of tuberculosis. Many species of NHPs have been tested using this system, including marmosets, squirrel monkeys, vervets, langurs, guenons, mandrills, gibbons, chimpanzees, orangutans, and gorillas. It has most recently been used in rhesus and cynomologus monkeys. During an outbreak of *M. bovis* in macaques (*M. mulatta* and *M. fasciularis*), it was shown that this test had good sensitivity (68%) and excellent specificity (97%) as compared to the animals' disease status based on pathologic findings. Comparative results for the TST were, respectively, 84% and 87%. Though both tests indicated intermittent positive and negative reactions on repeated testing, failure of determination of tuberculous animals by either test was not reported. The IFN-γ response to *M. bovis* PPD was low in *M. fasciularis*. In this species, parallel use of the TST and the Primagram test for maximal overall sensitivity in a tuberculosis screening program is recommended (15).

Other tests developed to survey for tuberculosis-infected animals involve detecting specific circulating antibodies (16). The problem with this type of test is in choosing a universal antigen as the test reagent. The difference in titers does not allow for a separation between infected and noninfected, but through repeated ELISA testing, it can categorize animals into negative, suspect, and positive animals when the TST is unsuccessful (17).

The culture and speciation of mycobacteria is difficult and time consuming. It can require valuable time to limit an outbreak, spending up to 6–8 weeks to grow, and speciation of the Mycobacterium may take up to 10–12 weeks following initial collection of the sample (18). Polymerase chain reaction for mycobacterial DNA may provide a more rapid alternative to other tests, but this test requires mycobacterial DNA.

There have been great inroads made in the understanding of this disease in NHPs and in the development of testing to augment the tuberculin skin test. Because each test has its inherent limitation to application, obtaining an accurate diagnosis of tuberculosis may require a battery of the tests available. In an effort to further our understanding, particularly of the early disease, effective detection will rely on the knowledge gained from further basic research to develop and refine additional diagnostics in cooperation, while applying these principles and tests to epizootic occurrences.

Radiographic

Clinical review of radiographs of the thorax may provide the clinician with an advantage in the diagnosis of tuberculosis (Fig. 27.3). Radiographically, *Nocardia* spp. cannot be distinguished from tuberculosis, offering a diagnostic challenge. However, radiograph examination of the chest in conjunction with additional diagnostic tests may facilitate detection. Walsh (7) suggests that examining radiographs of the chest is a highly sensitive tool for early detection of disease. In his investigation of *M. fasicularis*, he discovered had pulmonary infiltrates as early as two weeks after challenge. Radiographs were used to help monitor the progression, stabilization, and regression of disease.

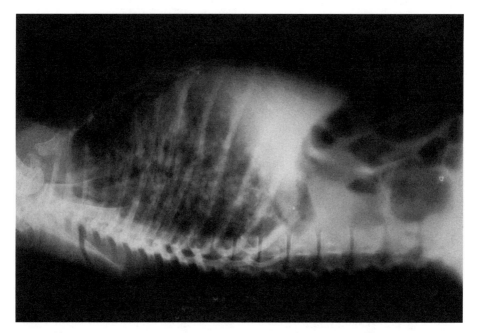

Figure 27.3. Lateral chest roentgenogram of a baboon with *Mycobacterium bovis* infection. Micronodular lesions up to 6 μm in diameter are observed.

Culture

Successful isolation of the organism depends on the quality of the specimen, the appropriate processing, and the culture techniques employed by the laboratory. Although *M. bovis* and *M. tuberculosis* are similar in clinical presentation, their culture requirements differ. In contrast to *M. tuberculosis*, poor or no growth in medium containing more than 1% glycerol is one of the distinguishing properties of *M. bovis*. Other distinguishing characteristics of *M. bovis* are that it does not reduce nitrate, and the niacin test is negative (1).

Samples should be carefully collected and handled by all involved, bearing in mind the potential of transmission. Cultures from animals early in the disease progression often show no growth. Every effort should be made to minimize contamination. Sputum (mucus or mucopurulent matter expectorated from the air passages), gastric lavage, bronchial lavages, and brushings are the most frequent submissions.

Staining

The cell wall contains mycolic acid, allowing this organism to stain with basic dyes, which contributes to the characteristic of acid-fast property that distinguishes mycobacteria from other bacteria. There are three types of staining procedures for rapid detection and confirmation of acid fast bacilli: fluorochrome, Ziel-Neelsen, and Kinyoun stain.

Hematologic

Chronic infectious inflammatory processes can decrease the red cell life and depress the bone marrow. In *M. mulatta*, a normocytic, normochromic anemia with an accompanying leukocytosis and a lymphopenia is found. Elevations in monocytes accompany bacterial and protozoal infections, chronic inflammatory conditions, and neoplasms. A recent outbreak of *M. bovis* in *M. mulatta* reported a hematologic picture presenting with a leukocytosis characterized by mature neutrophilia and a monocytosis; however, another presented only with a mild monocytosis (19).

Eryrthrocyte Sedimentation Rate (ESR)

A rise in ESR accompanies most inflammatory diseases and occurs when chronic inflammatory diseases exacerbate. Although considered a nonspecific test, ESR has three main functions: first as an aid in detection of the inflammatory process, second to monitor a disease course or activity, and finally as a screen for an inflammatory or neoplastic condition. ESR proved to be a useful parameter for monitoring the development of disease in the cynomologus monkey experimentally infected with *M. tuberculosis* (7). The ESR rose rapidly after infection, and the rapidity as well as the magnitude of the rise were highly dependent on the challenge dose.

The Great Apes: Special Diagnostic Challenge

The Great Apes, chimps (*Pan troglodytes*), orangutans (*Pongo pygaemus*), and gorillas (*Gorilla gorilla*), are all susceptible to infection by pathogenic mycobacteria (*M. tuberculosis, M. bovis,* and *M. avium*). As with all other primates, there is a concern for false negatives caused by immunocompetency, although a strong mitogen response will support immunocompetency. Separating the "false positives" and nonspecific responders from the true positives has always been a frustrating diagnostic challenge. Responders to the TST have been reported in chimps, gorillas, and the orangutan. There are no widely accepted universal standard protocols for the evaluation of NHPs that respond to tuberculin. One must consider a thorough understanding of an animal's clinical history to include all vaccines, particularly Bacille Calmette-Güerin immunizations. All animals should receive a complete physical examination, and although the signs, as in other primates, may appear as weight loss, lymphadenopathy, splenomegaly, hepatomegaly, ascites, pleural fluid, respiratory disease, and chronic draining wounds, tuberculosis should be in the differential. Diagnostically, orangutans appear to have a greater sensitivity to tuberculin than do gorillas or the chimpanzee (Fig. 27.4). It is thought that orangutans have a greater sensitivity than the other great apes to tuberculin, and they may be sensitized to mycobacterial antigens by exposure to nontuberculous mycobacteria (13). The palpebral TST is the most common primary site other than the arm, chest, or abdomen. Comparative testing involves the simultaneous administration of biologically balanced *M. bovis* PPD and *M. avium* PPD at separate sites on the abdomen to differentiate between *M. bovis* and infection and sensitization resulting from environmental mycobacteria. Nontuberculous mycobacteria have

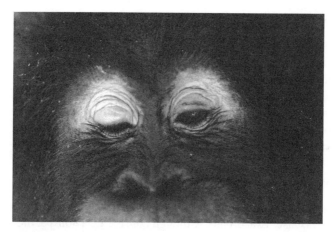

Figure 27.4.   Tuberculin skin test response in the eyelid of an orangutan (48 hours after injection of *Mycobacterium bovis* PPD).

been cultured from healthy orangutans and their environments (13). The challenges to this test are the interpretation and its reliability.

Repeated physical restraint of these animals to examine the site is often difficult because of its frequency. A complete diagnostic approach applies all other testing commonly applied to the other NHPs. A recent report of *M. bovis* was reported in a gorilla using the Primagam system. The combination of a positive TST and a strong Primagam result ruled out the possibility of a false positive or nonspecific responder. The response to bovine PPD was significantly greater than avian PPD, indicating infection with *M. bovis* or *M. tuberculosis*. The test incorporated two experimental antigens, ESAT-6 and CFP-10, to help eliminate a BCG reaction. Neither antigen is present in the BCG genome, so the strong response to these antigens strongly indicated that the animal was infected with *M. bovis* or *M. tuberculosis* (14).

Prevention and Control

The insidious nature of the disease and limits of current testing procedures continue to provide challenges for those who maintain NHPs. Prevention and control of the disease will always rely on a multipronged approach. Understanding all potential sources of infection will minimize the probability for exposure and transmission. Self-sustaining populations should limit the acquisitions of new additions whenever possible. Often, however, it is necessary to obtain animals with specific disease-free status, defined genetics, or protocol-required characteristics, or for adding to a zoological collection. Even among facilities fortunate to maintain a "closed colony," the risk of transmission through human contact will always exist. It is imperative to always know the source colony from which one is obtaining the animal, as well as that source's practices.

The choice of a shipping and transport company is most critical. This decision must be an informed one. It is necessary to apply the same level of scrutiny to a prospective transporter that is maintained at one's own facility. Several fundamental questions should be asked:

Do they have experience shipping NHPs?

For the species they are shipping, do they have knowledge of transmissible diseases, particularly tuberculosis?

Are their employees temporary hires, and do they have a surveillance program for tuberculosis? Are their employees trained in the use of personal protective equipment and clothing?

If they use metal crates, how are they disinfected (wooden crates must not be reused on the shipment)?

If animals from different sources are being shipped, are they physically separated, and do they have different air supplies?

Will the animals be held in a holding facility before they are transported to the destination?

Depending on the species and the time at which the exposure occurs, disease status may or may not be detected within the confines of the quarantine period. When new additions are acquired, a complete history should be transferred to the receiving institution before, or at the time of, shipment. The history should include pertinent health information and key information such as the original source of the animal, any holding facilities between the shipper and the recipient, and the name of the transporting organization. The stronghold of any institution is its animal data program. It is important to consider how one might obtain and track this data while still in the design phase. The historical information should be put in record for each animal for easy access, and the data system can then be searched by animal number (or its alias), location, and date, which will expedite the time it will take to build the epidemiologic pathway in the event of an outbreak. This will minimize the loss of valuable time identifying a potential source, contacts, number of personnel exposed, and the possibility that other institutions might be involved.

Quarantine is not just a facility or a repetitive exercise guided by a written program—it is a state of mind. It is the last barrier preventing introduction of disease into the colony and the first potential of exposure for personnel. Preparation for its operation begins before its occupation. Thoughtful planning as to the environmental support to the unit such as HVAC systems, electrical services such as lights/timers that include back-up generators, drainage maintenance, pest control, and cage operation will minimize the number of ancillary individuals involved in the quarantine process. It is important to confine the number of individuals involved in the process to a small number of highly qualified, trained individuals capable of identifying the subtle subjective and objective clinical and behavioral changes in primates that precede overt onset of disease. Quite often these individuals have been through the process innumerable times. However, it remains vital to ensure that these personnel have reviewed and maintain a clear understanding of the report structure, sampling handling, waste removal, potential diseases, clinical signs, and transmission and surveillance testing that includes tuberculin administration and, more important, its interpretation.

Space is a limiting factor for most institutions when it comes to management decisions. Every effort should be made to maintain the fundamental recommendation not to comingle animals of different species. In addition, when it is possible to keep new arrivals collectively isolated, particularly if the objective is for short-term holding, this will prevent contact with the stock colony. Movements between holding areas should be kept to a minimum and documented conscientiously even if it is only on a temporary basis for facility maintenance. Animals that are maintained for public display should be held behind a solid barrier because of the number and frequency of contacts with humans. All facilities should have areas for general housing, swing space for maintenance, clinical support space, and quarantine and isolation. Space should be available to allow for separation for further testing and surveillance.

To meet the challenge of primate social requirements, more facilities are choosing to house them in large groups. Because social contact is not only frequent in such an environment but also inherently extremely proximate, with transmission probable, some managers have chosen to incorporate a disinfectant that has tuberculocidal properties in their wash-down routines in an effort to drop the environmental load and to minimize aerosolization of tubercle bacilli.

The potential for transmission of multiple diseases, including tuberculosis, between humans and NHPs exists; therefore, all facilities should develop, implement, and maintain a comprehensive personnel health program with continuous review of its effectiveness. A formal program should include standard operating procedures, a clear understanding of the disease and its transmission, and the importance of the personnel protection equipment. An excellent resource pertaining to NHPs is the 2003 NRC publication "Occupational Health and Safety in the Care and Use of Nonhuman Primates." The oversight of such a program should include an occupational health professional. Depending on the background of this individual, additional information from consulting physicians and veterinarians knowledgeable in nonhuman primates may be warranted. The majority of institutions' programs are comprehensive and delineates those who are employees, investigators, postdoctoral fellows, and maintenance workers, however, short-term students, volunteers, and those employees who "moonlight" supporting other primate-holding facilities may not be given the attention that they should. Requiring the same education and training that the entire staff receives can reduce concern for the latter. Lapses or exemptions in the enforcement of such a program may create an opportunity for the source of a future outbreak of tuberculosis. Sanctuaries—free-ranging colonies that allow direct contact with humans without personal protective equipment—are of greatest risk of introducing sources into their colonies.

Institutions frequently face the request to assume responsibility for accepting NHPs as pets. Often they have lived a number of years in direct contact with humans and innumerable visitors. The institution must consider the financial, space, and behavioral effects when making a decision but must also determine the risk to, liability for, and effect on the existing population. There must be adequate isolation space to test, separate, and monitor any positives that are identified. This is particularly important among group-housed animals.

Consideration of treatment of tuberculosis in NHPs should be a well-thought-out process (20,21). Current treatment modalities should be sought to maximize efficacy, particularly as there is a rise in drug-resistant strains of the disease in the human population. Application of fundamental principles and standards are the key to maintaining a healthy colony. There must be diligent surveillance of the two primary sources of the disease: man and animal. The cost of surveillance is minimal when one considers the effect on primate holdings, breeding colonies, and research, or the potential devastation of an endangered species. Tuberculosis still remains a major diagnostic challenge, and the threat to primate colonies should not be underestimated.

Acknowledgment

I acknowledge the University of Louisiana at Lafayette's Library Resources, and in particular the Interlibrary Loan Department, in their searches for the historical background articles. Also thanks to Mr. Al Lamperez of the Division of Research Resources at New Iberia Research Center for his advice, support, and technical expertise in the preparation of this chapter.

References

1. Thoen, C. O. and B. R. Bloom. 1995. *Mycobacterium bovis* Infection in Animals and Humans, 1st ed. Ames: Iowa State University Press.
2. Kennard, M. 1941. Tuberculosis and tuberculin tests in subhuman primates. *Yale J Biol Med* 13:795-812.
3. Carpenter, C. R. 1940. Rhesus monkeys (*Macaca mulatto*) for American laboratories. *Science* 92:284-86.
4. Schroeder, C. R. 1938. A diagnostic test for the recognition of tuberculosis in nonhuman primates: a preliminary report. *Zoologica* 23:469-75.
5. King Jr, N. W. 1993. Monographs on Pathology of Laboratory Animals Sponsored by the International Life Sciences Institute, "Nonhuman Primates I," 141-148.
6. Kaufmann, A. F. 1975. A perspective of simian tuberculosis in the United States— 1972. *J Med Primatol* 4:278-86.
7. Walsh, G. P. 1996. The Philippine cynomologus monkey (*Macaca fasciularis*) provides a new human primate model of tuberculosis that resembles human disease. *Nat Med* 2:430-36.
8. Thoen, C. O. 1994. Tuberculosis in wild and domestic mammals. *In* B. R. Bloom (ed.), Tuberculosis: Pathogenesis, Protection and Control. Washington, DC: ASM Press, Washington, 157-162.
9. Gibson, S. 1998. Nonhuman Primates in Biomedical Research Diseases. Washington, DC: Academic Press, 59-102.
10. Thoen, C. O. and R. G. Barletta. 2004. Mycobacterium. *In* C. L. Gyler, J. F. Prescott, J. G. Songer, and C. O. Thoen (ed.), Pathogenesis of Bacterial Infections in Animals, 3rd ed. Ames, IA: Blackwell Publishing, 69-76.
11. Fox, J. G. 1974. Tuberculosis spondylitis and Pott's paraplegia in a rhesus monkey. *Lab Anim Sci* 24:335-39

12. McLaughlin, R. M. and G. E. Marrs. 1978. Tuberculin testing in nonhuman primates: OT vs. PPD. *In* R. J. Montali (ed.), Mycobacterial Infections in Zoo Animals. Washington, DC: Smithsonian Press, 123-27.

13. Calle, P. and C. O. Thoen. 1989. Tuberculin skin test response, mycobacteriologic examinations of gastric lavage, and serum enzyme-linked immunosorbent assays in Orangutans (*Pongo pygmaeus*). *J Zoo Wildl Med* 20:307-14.

14. McCracken, H. 2002. Gamma interferon enzyme immunoassays and their use in the investigation of tuberculosis in a western lowland gorilla. Proc Am Assoc Zoo Vet, pp. 352-358.

15. Garcia, M. A. 2004. Diagnosis of tuberculosis in macques, using whole-blood in vitro interferon-gamma (PRIMAGAM). *Testing Comperative Med* 54:86-92.

16. Thoen, C. O., K. Mills, and M. P. Hopkins. 1980. Enzyme-linked protein A: An enzyme-linked immunosorbent assay reagent for detecting antibodies in tuberculous exotic animals. *Am J Vet Res* 40:833-37.

17. Corcoran, K. and C. O. Thoen. 1991. Application of an enzyme immunoassay for detecting antibodies in sera of *Macaca fasicularis* naturally exposed to *Mycobacterium tuberculosis*. *J Med Primatol* 20:404-408.

18. Kaneene, J. B. andC. O. Thoen. 2004. Tuberculosis. *J Am Vet Med Assoc* 224:685-91.

19. Garcia M. A., D. M. Bouley, M. J. Larson, B. Lifland, R. Moorhead, M. D. Simkins, D. C. Borie, R. Tolwani, and G. Otto. 2004. Outbreak of *Mycobacterium bovis* in a conditioned colony of rhesus (*Macaca fascicularis*) macaques. *Comp Med* 54:578-84.

20. Wolf, R. H., S. V. Gibson, and E. A. Watson. 1988. Multidrug chemotherapy of tuberculosis in rhesus monkeys. *Lab Anim Sci* 38:25-30.

21. Thoen, C. O. Tuberculosis and other mycobacterial diseases in captive wild animals. *In* M. E. Fowler (ed.), Zoo and Wild Animal Medicine. Denver, CO: W.B. Sanders, Denver, 45-49.

Chapter 28
DNA Vaccines Against Tuberculosis

O. Chacon, MD, PhD, and J.P. Bannantine, PhD

Introduction

Since its early development more than 200 years ago, vaccination has become one of the most effective measures to prevent infectious diseases. The use of vaccines is responsible for global eradication of smallpox and also for saving millions of human lives that otherwise would have been lost or severely impaired because of diseases such as polio, tetanus, and measles, among others (54,58).

An ideal vaccine should elicit long-lasting protective immunity, preferably soon after its administration, without causing disease in the recipient or subsequent contacts; allow detection of infected versus immunized individuals without interfering with available diagnostic tests; be cost effective and easy to produce in large quantities; be easy to store and transport, preserving its immunobiological properties under different environmental conditions; be easy to administer to large populations, ideally in a single dose, without causing side effects; be safe enough to be used in immunocompromised hosts; have therapeutic potential; and be compatible with other vaccines so that they can be administered simultaneously without interfering with each other's effectiveness and safety. In addition, consideration should be given to the different environments and societies in which the vaccine must be administered, as those factors will directly affect individual's compliance with any proposed immunization regimen (4,13).

Vaccine Implementation against Tuberculosis

Vaccine implementation is particularly useful in preventing diseases caused by intracellular pathogens such as viruses, certain bacteria, and parasitic protozoa. These microorganisms are etiologic agents of endemic, epidemic, or emerging infectious diseases worldwide. For example, mycobacteria cause a number of diseases, including tuberculosis (TB), in humans and animals. This disease is the leading cause of human death in the world caused by a single infectious agent (7). *Mycobacterium tuberculosis* is the principal cause of TB in humans and other primates—it is estimated that it infects one-third of the world human population (57). This mycobacterial species is also occasionally seen in dogs, pigs, and cattle (53). In contrast, *Mycobacterium bovis*, the etiologic agent of bovine TB, has a wide host range and infects ruminants, carnivores, and primates, including humans. It has been calculated that *M. bovis* infects more than 50 million cattle worldwide, resulting in an economic loss of about $3 billion annually (63). Although *M. tuberculosis* is responsible for 80%–90% of all TB cases in humans, the number of cases attributed to *M. bovis* is increasing (56) (http://www.who.int/vaccines-documents/PP-WER/wer7904.pdf). For *M. bovis* and *M. tuberculosis* in both humans and animals, contaminated aerosols are the most common routes of transmission (12). *M. tuberculosis* and *M. bovis* are members of the *M. tuberculosis* complex. This complex also includes the human pathogens *Mycobacterium africanum* and *Mycobacterium canettii*. Another member of the complex is *Mycobacterium microti*, the etiologic agent of TB in wild voles (27,74,77).

TB is a chronic, granulomatous, devastating disease. The only licensed vaccine for TB is the attenuated strain Bacillus Calmette-Güerin (BCG). This vaccine has been rated as one of the safest vaccines ever developed. BCG is inexpensive to produce and can be safely administered to young children (3). Regarding its effectiveness, BCG is considered to have moderate efficacy in humans (62). This situation is paralleled in cattle, in that BCG confers only partial protection against *M. bovis* (10). Although BCG has been able to reduce the risk of infection by 50% and deaths by 70% (14), there are variations among the repertoire of BCG substrains used for vaccination that may affect vaccination efficiency (39). Furthermore, BCG does interfere with TB diagnosis, as it converts vaccines to a positive skin test. For this reason, routine use of this vaccine has been deterred in the United States. It is evident that, although BCG is still widely administered in several countries around the world, it is not an ideal vaccine against TB. This highlights the need to develop more effective vaccines that might prove compatible with diagnostic tests. New vaccines to prevent TB in humans and animals would be very useful in improving their health. Potential applications of animal vaccination against tuberculosis, including prevention of disease transmission to humans and other animals, have been reviewed (60). Excellent reviews on new approaches to TB vaccinations are also available (9,37,47).

DNA Vaccines Encoding Protective Antigens

In addition, new live attenuated vaccines based on genetically modified mycobacteria and alternate approaches to generate novel antimycobacterial vaccines include subunit vaccines based on mycobacterial proteins or DNA sequences. DNA vaccination is based on observations that administration of recombinant plasmid DNA resulted in expression of the exogenous protein encoded by the plasmid (24,79,80). RNA-based subunit vaccines might become a new alternative for antimycobacterial vaccination. In this context, recent studies in mice indicate that RNA vaccination has the potential to provide effective short-term protection against TB without the potential side effects of DNA vaccines (81). At present, ample use of DNA vaccination is very appealing, as production of pure DNA is less expensive and demanding than isolation and manipulation of pure proteins or RNA. However, in addition to the immunological aspects of protection, there are many other factors that should be considered before attempting production of a DNA vaccine practical for general use. For example, the DNA vaccine vehicle must be amenable to transfer and maintain stable recombinant DNA. Expression of antigens encoded by the vaccine should be in the proper conformation and in the proper location to allow induction of the preferred immune response. It is also necessary that the final vaccine does not carry antibiotic resistance markers to prevent the possibility of transfer of these resistance markers to other pathogenic organisms in the environment. Finally, to prevent secondary effects such as tumor formation resulting from inactivation of tumor repressor genes, any possibility of foreign DNA insertion in the host chromosome must be ruled out before any candidate DNA vaccine may be considered for practical use in humans or animals.

DNA vaccination against TB has been attempted using naked DNA or various vectors encoding a broad selection of mycobacterial antigens. Several proteins and lipoproteins secreted by mycobacteria may be recognized by the immune system early during infection. Thus, they may be used to modulate the initial immune response, and their genes become candidates for DNA vaccines (1). Several of these antigens, including secreted *M. bovis* (MPB) and *M. tuberculosis* (MPT) proteins, antigen Ag85, ESAT-6, Apa, and PstS-3, as well as several nonsecreted mycobacterial heat shock proteins have been used, among others, as candidates for DNA vaccination against tuberculosis (3,17,38,48,59,67,69,75,76,78). Recently, the two sequences, Ag85A and PstS-3, were combined in a double-gene DNA vaccine that appears capable of protecting against reactivation of TB as well as reinfection (29). Somatic mycobacterial antigens are also processed in macrophages and elicit a cell-mediated immune response. Nevertheless, the issue of whether somatic antigens could be protective against TB is controversial, although substantial evidence exists in favor of a protective role for secreted antigens (3,4,31). Because cell-mediated immunity, including interferon-gamma (IFNγ)–secreting T-lymphocytes, plays a key role in protection against TB, it is important to select as vaccine sources mycobacterial antigens that preferentially induce that type of immune response. In antimycobacterial vaccines, DNA has been administered alone or in the presence of a variety of adjuvants and carriers. Routes of administration include classical intramuscular injection, electroporation, aerosol application, and gene gun bombardment (64,73). Furthermore, the immune response generated by DNA vaccination against TB has been boosted by the subsequent administration of mycobacterial proteins or attenuated strains, including BCG (60,61,66,75,76).

Selection of Suitable DNA Vaccines

When selecting new candidates for antimycobacterial DNA vaccines, consideration must be given to possible variations in the immune response and in the protection conferred by different antigens. Even closely related sequences exhibiting high DNA homology may confer different protection levels. For example, intramuscular immunization of mice with PstS-1, PstS-2, and PstS-3 DNA, encoding *M. tuberculosis* highly homologous putative phosphate binding proteins, indicated that only PstS-3 DNA conferred significant protection against parenteral challenge with virulent *M. tuberculosis* (67). In the same context, a mouse model used to compare immunogenicity of injected Hsp65 and Hsp70 DNA vaccines showed that the intensity of immune response generated, measured among others by serum IFNγ levels and nitric oxide in intraperitoneal macrophages, was higher after Hsp65 DNA vaccination immunization (18). Vaccination of mice with injected plasmid DNA encoding Hsp65 conferred a level of protection to *M. tuberculosis* challenge similar to the one conferred by BCG (69). Vaccines based on Hsp65 DNA may also have a potential therapeutic effect, as evidenced in *M. tuberculosis*–infected mice treated with *Mycobacterium leprae* Hsp65 DNA. This effect is probably a result of CD8+ lung cell activation, with recovery of IFNγ levels and resulting reduction in lung injury (8).

Using similar cattle vaccination protocols for the inoculation of DNA vaccines encoding *M. leprae* Hsp65 or the serodominant antigens MPB70 or MPB83 indicated that the former DNA vaccine appears to be more effective than the latter in inducing protective immune responses. In both cases (vaccination with Hsp65 and vaccination with MPB70 or MPB83), immunization with DNA did not cause a delayed-type hypersensitivity response, indicating a potential advantage of DNA vaccines regarding their lack of interference with diagnostic tests (75,78). These studies highlight the importance of selecting adequate antigens for vaccination, as lung lesions were larger in animals vaccinated with MPB70 or MPB83 compared to in the BCG-vaccinated group. Moreover, boosting MPB70 DNA-primed animals with MPB70 protein was accompanied by increased production of specific IgG. This increase might even have contributed to an increase in lung pathology of *M. bovis*–challenged animals (78). In the same context, recent studies indicate that humoral responses characterized by an increase in MPB83-specific IgG1 correlate with an increased severity of lesions and bacterial loads (46).

In some cases, it might be useful to consider more than one antigen or epitope to be present in the same DNA formulation (52). For example, mice and guinea pigs vaccinated by inoculation with MTB72F DNA (a tandem sequence of immunogenic MTB32 and MTB39 DNA) were protected from an aerosol challenge with virulent *M. tuberculosis*. This vaccine is currently in a phase I clinical trial (59). Other divalent vaccines, including both the Ag85B gene and either MTB64 or Hsp60, confer better protection than BCG in *M. tuberculosis* murine models of infection (45,71). However, caution must be taken with the use of this and other DNA vaccine formulations, including those with the gene encoding for the *M. leprae* Hsp60 protein, as they may actually induce severe necrosis in animals previously exposed to *M. tuberculosis* (70). Noteworthy, vaccination of mice with a DNA divalent vaccine encoding Ag85A and ESAT-6, followed by priming with live attenuated *M. bovis* strains, did not increase the protective efficacy of the monovalent vaccines, although there was a significant increase in the number of IFNγ-secreting cells (61). Hence, combining antigens does not necessarily result in DNA vaccine improvement, even when there are indicators of an adequate immune response. Nevertheless, this strategy has the potential to be used in immunocompromised individuals, as suggested by the protection of CD4−/− mice against aerogenic infection with *M. tuberculosis* after inoculation with a DNA vaccine cocktail containing antigens Ag85B, ESAT-6, KatG, MPT84, MPT12, MPT63, MPT64, and MPT83 DNA. Activation of antigen-presenting cells in these CD4−/− mice might be related to Toll-like receptors capable of binding to all or some of the cocktail antigens. Furthermore, recognition of DNA CpG motifs by Toll-like receptor 9 might act as an adjuvant in these and other DNA vaccines (22,30). A cocktail vaccine including 10 different DNA antigens was either fused to a Tissue Plasminogen Activator signal sequence to increase the expression level of secreted proteins, to significantly induce humoral and cell mediated immunity, or conjugated to ubiquitin to increase intracellular protein degradation and elicit cytokine responses in the absence of specific antibody production. Intramuscular injection of mice with these two vaccines conferred protection to aerogenic infection with virulent *M. tuberculosis* similar to that conferred by BCG (21). Ubiquitin as well as spacer sequences have been used to modulate murine cellular immune responses to DNA vaccines on the basis of MPT64 and 38KDa protein epitopes (76).

Boosting DNA Vaccines

The efficacy of DNA vaccines has been improved by boosting with microorganisms or proteins. In this context, subcutaneous BCG boosting in cattle after vaccination with Hsp65, Hsp70, and Apa DNA resulted in enhanced protection against intratracheal challenge with virulent *M. bovis* (60). Similarly, levels of antigen-specific T-cells were increased in cattle vaccinated with Ag85A DNA and boosted with intradermal inoculation of a modified vaccinia virus Ankara expressing the same antigen. The increase in antigen-specific T-cells was more evident when the animals were primed intradermally with Ag85A DNA, probably because of a higher number of antigen-presenting cells in skin than in muscle (68). The improved protective efficacy of an Ag85A DNA vaccine was also observed in guinea pigs after two doses of the monovalent Ag85A DNA vaccine were administered by gene gun bombardment before subcutaneous boosting with an Ag85A synthetic peptide (64). Subcutaneous protein boosting with ESAT-6 also resulted in improved immunogenicity of an injected ESAT-6 DNA vaccine in mice (76). Protection conferred by some antigens may only be evident when a protein boost accompanies the corresponding DNA vaccination protocol. This effect may be evident regardless of the antigen's immunogenicity. For example, although intradermal immunization with Apa (a rare glycosylated mycobacterial protein with potential T-cell epitopes) is able to stimulate IFNγ-secreting T-cells, guinea pigs immunized intradermally with *M. tuberculosis* Apa DNA vaccine were not protected against parenteral challenge with virulent *M. tuberculosis*. However, protection was achieved by boosting with a recombinant poxvirus expressing the same Apa antigen. Protection levels were similar to those conferred by BCG vaccination. It is not clear whether the degree of protection could be different after challenge by aerosolization (38).

DNA Vaccine Enhancement

Particulate and nonparticulate adjuvants play an important role in DNA vaccination (16,42). These molecules may be selected because of their immunogenic properties. Trehalose dimicolate, for example, is a glycolipid of the mycobacterial cell wall characterized by its ability to elicit secretion of Th1-type cytokines. This type of immune response is usually, although not always, protective against TB (32,43). In this context, a single administration of coencapsulated Hsp65 DNA and trehalose dimicolate into biodegradable poly-glycolide-co-dl-lactide microspheres resulted in an immune response and protection levels similar to those achieved with three doses of naked DNA administration. In this case, it is possible that the results were caused by a combination of the adjuvant trehalose dimicolate's immunogenic capacity and the sustained presentation of the antigen by the poly-glycolide-co-dl-lactide microspheres (42,44). Adjuvant properties have been attributed to DNA sequences, such as bacterial CpG motifs (36). Experiments in other microbial systems such as *Mycoplasma hyopneumoniae* and human papillomavirus E7 indicate that mycobacterial sequences similar to those encoding ESAT-6 and Hsp70 may have the potential to increase protective immunity and act as adjuvants in DNA vaccination (35,50,73). Thus, it might be worthy to explore whether the same effect is to be observed when those sequences are added to antimycobacterial DNA vaccines.

Coinjection of immunomodulator genes may also be used to manipulate the qualitative and quantitative characteristics of the immune response generated by DNA vaccines. For example, a potent increase in IFNγ levels has been observed in mice spleens after coinjection of *M. tuberculosis* Hsp65 DNA and murine IL-12 or GM-CSF DNA (2). DNA vaccines may also be improved by the correct selection of carriers. In this context, promising results have been reported using cationic submicron emulsions to deliver DNA vaccines to the pulmonary tissue. Those emulsions are able to transfect epithelial cells in the lung, probably inducing cross priming of antigen-presenting cells and stimulation of antigen-specific T-cells (6). Cationic poly-DL-lactide-co-glycolide particles were used as carrier in a DNA vaccine encoding Ag85A. The amount of DNA required to confer protection in mice challenged by aerosolization was significantly lower in the presence of poly-DL-lactide-co-glycolide, compared to the corresponding naked DNA vaccine (51). Cationic and neutral colipid formulations have been also used to improve the immunogenicity and protection levels conferred by intramuscularly or intranasally administered Ag85A, Ag85B, and PstS-3 DNA (23). Similar results have been observed when dimethyl dioctyldecyl ammonium bromide was added to Ag85B, MPT83, and ESAT-6 DNA vaccines (11).

Recombinant intracellular microorganisms have the potential to act as biological carriers in intracellular targeting strategies for DNA vaccines. For example, a self-destructing attenuated strain of *Lysteria monocytogenes* carrying expression vectors for *M. bovis* Ag85 or MPB/MPT51 was successfully used to induce protective immunity against *M. tuberculosis* in mice (48). Routes of vaccination may also have a potential effect on protection levels conferred by DNA vaccination. In this context, as shown in small-animal models, improved T-cell responses were observed in cattle when intramuscular injection of plasmid DNA encoding *M. leprae* Hsp65 was followed by electroporation (72). Interestingly, although immunization of mice with Hsp65 DNA by gene gun bombardment requires a smaller amount of DNA to be immunogenic, the immune response generated by a gene gun was less protective than the one obtained by intramuscular injection (41). Similarly, gene gun immunization of mice with Ag85A DNA vaccine did not protect them against *M. tuberculosis* challenge (65).

Genomic Approaches to Obtain Ideal DNA Vaccine Candidates

With the availability of the complete genome sequences of *M. bovis* (28) and two strains of *M. tuberculosis* (15,26), there is the opportunity to take a step back and reevaluate protective DNA sequences in an unbiased manner. This can be accomplished through the expression library immunization method described by Johnston and Barry (34). Furthermore, instead of a random expression library, the genome sequence allows investigators to generate a directed expression library, which limits the number of clones necessary to be screened for protective effects. There are currently 3951 open reading frames defined for the *M. bovis* genome (28), and each one of those genes must be cloned into a DNA vaccine vector in the directed expression library approach. These 3951 genes are arrayed and used to immunize mice, with each group of mice receiving a subset of the cloned genes (clone pools). Protective pools identified in the initial round are further subdivided and moved forward for a second round of screening in mice, and this process continues until a very limited number of solidly protective clones remains. This method has recently been proven successful in identifying a protective sequence against *Coccidioides* spp. infections in mice (33).

It may be possible to trim down the list of clones even before screening begins, but this approach may exclude genes contributing to protection. Another caveat to this approach is that by selectively excluding genes to screen or test, human bias is introduced. Nonetheless, there are many genes that should theoretically have a limited effect on protective responses. Housekeeping genes that perform routine functions including DNA metabolism and amino acid biosynthesis are often conserved across many microbial species and are examples of sequences that can be "safely" excluded. In contrast, proteins that are pathogen-specific are more relevant for vaccine development, as they are potentially involved in colonizing or damaging the host. The genomic differences in the form of single nucleotide polymorphisms and insertions or deletions have been well characterized between pathogenic *M. tuberculosis* H37Rv and the *M. bovis* vaccine strain BCG (5,55). A thorough comparison of the genomes of *M. tuberculosis* and BCG, followed by selection of TB-specific sequences/epitopes, is another logical approach to TB vaccine development (20).

Conclusions

In summary, although lack of a consensus in immunization and challenge protocols makes it difficult to compare the results obtained with DNA vaccination against TB, the following common themes can be recognized. First, several conserved antigens, such as Hsp65 DNA, have been identified as potential candidates for effective vaccines. Second, there has been improved protection conferred by DNA vaccines after boosting with proteins or live attenuated vectors, where in some cases the same antigen was expressed. Third, there has also been better protection after intramuscular immunization, despite a need for larger amounts of DNA to be inoculated. Fourth, there is a potential use of a variety of adjuvants to improve immunogenicity and protection, and possibly to reduce the amount of vaccine DNA required for protection. Finally, regarding other subunit vaccines, there is a possibility of eliminating the delayed-type hypersensitivity response by selecting appropriate antigens, and hence eliminating interference with current diagnostic tests. A comprehensive summary of DNA vaccines against tuberculosis is provided (Table 28.1).

It is noteworthy that the ability of an antigen to trigger potentially protective immune responses *in vitro* does not necessarily correlate with its effectiveness *in vivo,* making it necessary to test the corresponding DNA vaccine under different protocols and conditions. Care should be taken to follow immunization protocols that are the least invasive as possible. Furthermore, it would be advisable to follow bona fide challenge protocols resembling natural routes of infection, such as aerosolization. Aspects for future research on DNA vaccination against TB include the selection of the best antigens or combination of antigens, adjuvants, and administration routes. Because peptide epitope recognition by T-cells is MHC restricted (19,40), it is likely that more than a single gene will be necessary for protection to be achieved using a DNA subunit vaccine in a population. Emphasis should be given to the evaluation of the potential side effects of long-term persistence of DNA in the host. Problems common to DNA vaccination approaches include chromosomal integration that leads to mutagenesis or an autoimmune response (25). Ethical aspects to be considered are the introduction of foreign genetic material and its potential effect on the host's genome and transcription machinery. However, this could be overcome by the use of appropriate vectors, including the pVAX plasmids, designed not to include the mammalian DNA sequences that could be responsible for homologous recombination between the DNA vaccine vector and the host's chromosome (49). In conclusion, by selecting the correct antigens that are able to induce adequate and lasting CMI, and possibly humoral, response, plus the appropriate combination of vectors, adjuvants, and route of administration, a protective DNA vaccine against tuberculosis in humans and animals is presently feasible.

Acknowledgments

Thanks to Drs. A. Restrepo and C. Thoen for critical review of the manuscript, and to Ms. D. Zinniel for technical assistance.

Table 28.1. DNA vaccines against tuberculosis.

Antigen DNA	Model	Vehicle Adjuvant	Route and immunization protocol	Challenge	Conclusions	Reference
M. leprae Hsp65	Cattle	Plasmid	IM–1 mg plasmid– wk 0, 3 and 6 IM–1 mg plasmid wk 0 SC recombinant protein in IFA wk 3 (1 mg) and wk 6 (0.5 mg) SC–BCG 1×10^6 CFU–wk 0 and 6 Responses evaluated 3 wks after final vaccination.	N/A	No interference with tuberculin test. DNA-prime boosting resulted in improved cell and humoral immunogenicity.	75
	Murine BALB/c	Plasmid DNA/TDM	IM–100 g naked plasmid–wk 0, 1 and 2 IM–30 g Plasmid/ TDM–single dose	IT–*M. tuberculosis* H37Rv 1×10^5 CFU–approximately 2 wk after last immunization. Cytokine examination in splenocytes from mice killed 2 wk (naked DNA) or 4 wk (DNA/TDM). Antibody evaluation in sera collected after completion of vaccination. Mice killed 5 or 30 days after challenge.	TDM use allowed 10 times dose reduction to achieve protection. It also induced high levels of IFN in lungs and specific IgG2.	44

Continues

Table 28.1. Continued

Antigen DNA	Model	Vehicle Adjuvant	Route and immunization protocol	Challenge	Conclusions	Reference
M. tuberculosis Hsp65	Murine C57BL/6	Plasmid	IM–200 g Hsp65 DNA plasmid and 200 g cytokine plasmid–wk 0, 2 and 4 BCG 1×10^5 CFU–wk 3 and 6	Aerosol–*M. tuberculosis* H37Rv–4 wk after final immunization. Mice euthanized 20 wks after challenge. Sera collected at first immunization and 2 wk after every immunization. Splenocytes collected from mice sacrificed 3 wk after last immunization.	Immune response was not the same with all cytokines. Co-injection of IL-12 expressing plasmid induced a significant increase in cell and humoral immunity.	2
M. tuberculosis Hsp65, Apa and Hsp70	Cattle	Plasmid	ID (0.1 mg) and IM (0.9 mg) plasmid–wk 0 ID (0.05 mg) and IM (0.45 mg) plasmid–wk 3 SC–BCG and BCG boost 1×10^6 CFU–wk 6	IT–*M. bovis* strain 83/6235 1.5×10^3 CFU–13 wk after initial immunization. Cattle necropsy approximately 16 wk after challenge. Cytokine levels measured from wk 10 after initial vaccination. PPD at wk 10 after initial vaccination.	Increase in protection parameters was higher after DNA/BCG boost vaccination. Also lowest PPD response. Strong INF response did not correlate with protection.	60
M. tuberculosis Apa	Guinea pigs	Plasmid	ID–200 g plasmid (wk 0, 4, 8 and 12)	IM–*M. tuberculosis* NTI64719 2×10^5	Significant level of protection	38

	Poxvirus to boost	and poxvirus 1 × 10^7 PFU (4 wk after last injection) BCG 1 × 10^6 CFU–wk 0	CFU–approximately 4 wk after last immunization.	conferred by Apa DNA + APAMVA boost.	
M. tuberculosis Ag85A	Murine Balb/c	Plasmid PLG	IM. 100 g plasmid or 50 g, 10 g or 1 g PLG-DNA–wk 0 and approximately wk 4 IV–BCG 1 × 10^5 CFU–wk 0	Aerosol–*M. tuberculosis* H37Rv 200 CFU/lung or 5 × 10^5 CFU IV. INF secreting cells analyzed 5 d after last vaccination.	Ag8A DNA/PLG induced Th1 type cell response and protection similar to BCG and significantly higher than naked DNA.	51
	Guinea pigs	Plasmid	Gene gun–50 g plasmid DNA– wk 0 and 3 SC–peptide boost 0.5 mg in IFA BCG 10 g BCG Tokyo	Aerosol–*M. tuberculosis* Kurono strain 1 × 10^6 CFU. Calculated uptake–400 CFU/animal. Guinea pigs sacrificed 7 wk after infection OR followed for up to 7 mo.	Long lasting protective efficacy improved significantly by peptide boosting. Similar to BCG.	64
	Catte	Plasmid Fowlpox virus (FP) and Vaccinia virus (MVA)	Plasmid DNA–ID (2 mg) and IM (2 mg)–wk 0. Boosted with MVA-85A 5 × 10^8 PFU (IV or ID–wk 4), 1 × 10^9 PFU (IV or ID–wk 24) and 1 × 10^9 PFU (IV or ID–wk 72)	N/A	T cell responses enhanced by MVA-85A boosting. Intradermal priming more effective than intramuscular priming. Overall bias towards CD4+ T cell responses.	68

Continues

Table 28.1. Continued

Antigen DNA	Model	Vehicle Adjuvant	Route and immunization protocol	Challenge	Conclusions	Reference
			Plasmid DNA–4 mg ID or IM–wk 0 and 4. Boosted with MVA-85A 1 × 10^9 PFU (ID–wk 8 and 12) FP-85A 2x10^8 PFU (ID). Boosted with MVA-85A 1 × 10^9 PFU (ID–wk 4 and 8)			
M. tuberculosis Ag85A and ESAT-6 fusion	Murine Balb/c and C57BL/6	Plasmid	IM–100 g plasmid DNA–wk 0 and 4 SC–boost with plasmid DNA or *M. bovis* BCG or Wag520 1x10^6 CFU wk 8	Aerosol–virulent *M. bovis*. Calculated inhalation and retention of approximately 10 CFU/mouse. 14 or 24 wk after initial vaccination. Mice killed 5 wk after challenge.	Vaccination with DNA alone induced strongest humoral immune response. DNA priming with avirulent *M. bovis* boosting increased cellular immune response. Not better than BCG.	61
BCG Ag85A, Ag85B and MPB51	Murine Balb/c and C57BL/6	*Listeria monocytogenes*	IV (Balb/c) approximately 1 × 10^6 CFU or IP (C57BL/6) approximately 1 × 10^7 CFU recombinant *L. monocytogenes*– wk 0, 2 and 6	IV–balb/c 5 × 10^5 CFU *M. tuberculosis* H37Rv– approximately 8 wk after last immunization.	Protection similar to BCG	48

296

M. tuberculosis 85B and MPT64	Murine C57BL/6	Plasmid	SC–BCG 1×10^6 CFU twice at 2 wk interval (Balb/c) or IP–BCG 1×10^7 CFU once (C57BL/6) IM–100 g plasmid DNA–wk 0, 3 and 6 SC–BCG 5×10^6 CFU–wk 0	Mice sacrificed 10 wks later. IV–M. tuberculosis H37Rv, 1×10^6 CFU–8 wk after final immunization. Mice sacrificed 8 wk later.	Increased cell and humoral immunity induced by divalent vaccine. Increased protection. Survival rate higher than BCG.	71
M. tuberculosis 32$_C$-Mtb39-Mtb32$_N$	Murine C57BL/6 and Guinea pigs	Plasmid	IM (Mice)–100 g plasmid DNA or 8 g recombinant protein with adjuvant–wk 0, 3 and 6 IV–BCG in base of tail vein 5×10^4 CFU once Mice sacrificed 3 weeks after last boost for immunogenic studies. IM (Guinea pigs)–200 g plasmid DNA or 20 g recombinant protein with adjuvant–wk 0, 3 and 6 ID–BCG 1×10^3 CFU once	Mice–aerosol–M. tuberculosis H37Rv. Calculated dose of 50–100 CFU. 30 d after last immunization. Mice euthanized 4 wk later. Guinea pigs –aerosol. M. tuberculosis H37Rv. Calculated dose 20–50 CFU. 13 wk after last immunization. Guinea pigs followed up to 70 wk.	Protection similar to BCG.	59

Table 28.1. Continued

Antigen DNA	Model	Vehicle Adjuvant	Route and immunization protocol	Challenge	Conclusions	Reference
M. tuberculosis MPB70 and MPB83	Cattle	Plasmid	IM–1 mg plasmid -wk 0, 3 and 6 1 mg plasmid (IM)–wk 0 and 1 mg recombinant protein in IFA (SC) wk 3 and 6 SC–BCG 4 × 10⁵ CFU wk 0 and 6 Immune responses evaluated at 0, 3, 6, 9 and 13 wk after initial vaccination. Responses evaluated 3 wk after final vaccination.	IT–virulent *M. bovis* 5 × 10³ CFU. 13 wk after initial vaccination. Immune responses evaluated at 0, 2, 5, 10 and 17 wk after challenge. Animals sacrificed 17 wk after challenge.	Immune responses not significant in animals vaccinated with DNA alone. Protein boost increased immune responses (mainly humoral) and increased lung pathology. No interference with tuberculin test. No protection.	78
M. tuberculosis PstS-1, PstS-2, PstS3 and Ag85A	Murine C57BL-6	Plasmid	IM–100 g plasmid DNA–wk 0, 3 and 6 IV–BCG 1 × 10⁶ CFU–wk 0	IV–*M. tuberculosis* H37Rv 1 × 10⁶ CFU. Approximately 8 wk after last plasmid DNA injection or 14 wk after BCG. Mice sacrificed at different time points after challenge.	Significant levels of highly Ag-specific Abs, IL-2 and INF after all vaccinations. PstS3 DNA vaccination induced highest IL-2 and INF production and significant protection for 3 mo after challenge.	67

APAMVA: Poxvirus expressing Apa, D: days, IM: intramuscular, IV: intravenous, ID: intradermal, IT: intratracheal, IFA: incomplete Freund's adjuvant, Mo: months, N/A: not applicable, PLG: poly (DL–lactide-co-glycolide), SC: subcutaneous, TDM: trehalose dimicolate, Wk: weeks.

References

1. Andersen, P. 1994. Effective vaccination of mice against *Mycobacterium tuberculosis* infection with a soluble mixture of secreted mycobacterial proteins. *Infect Immun* 62:2536-44.
2. Baek, K. M., S. Y. Ko, M. Lee, J. S. Lee, J. O. Kim, H. J. Ko, J. W. Lee, S. H. Lee, S. N. Cho, and C. Y. Kang. 2003. Comparative analysis of effects of cytokine gene adjuvants on DNA vaccination against *Mycobacterium tuberculosis* heat shock protein 65. *Vaccine* 21:3684-9.
3. Baldwin, S. L., C. D'Souza, A. D. Roberts, B. P. Kelly, A. A. Frank, M. A. Lui, J. B. Ulmer, K. Huygen, D. M. McMurray, and I. M. Orme. 1998. Evaluation of new vaccines in the mouse and guinea pig model of tuberculosis. *Infect Immun* 66:2951-9.
4. Barletta, R. G., R. O. Donis, O. Chacon, H. Shams, and J. D. Cirillo. 2000. Vaccines against intracellular pathogens. *Subcell Biochem* 33:559-99.
5. Behr, M. A., M. A. Wilson, W. P. Gill, H. Salamon, G. K. Schoolnik, S. Rane, and P. M. Small. 1999. Comparative genomics of BCG vaccines by whole-genome DNA microarray. *Science* 284:1520-3.
6. Bivas-Benita, M., M. Oudshoorn, S. Romeijn, K. van Meijgaarden, H. Koerten, H. van der Meulen, G. Lambert, T. Ottenhoff, S. Benita, H. Junginger, and G. Borchard. 2004. Cationic submicron emulsions for pulmonary DNA immunization. *J Control Release* 100:145-55.
7. Bloom, B. R., and C. J. Murray. 1992. Tuberculosis: commentary on a reemergent killer. *Science* 257:1055-64.
8. Bonato, V. L., E. D. Goncalves, E. G. Soares, R. R. Santos Junior, A. Sartori, A. A. Coelho-Castelo, and C. L. Silva. 2004. Immune regulatory effect of pHSP65 DNA therapy in pulmonary tuberculosis: activation of CD8+ cells, interferon-gamma recovery and reduction of lung injury. *Immunology* 113:130-8.
9. Britton, W. J., and U. Palendira. 2003. Improving vaccines against tuberculosis. *Immunol Cell Biol* 81:34-45.
10. Buddle, B. M., G. W. de Lisle, A. Pfeffer, and F. E. Aldwell. 1995. Immunological responses and protection against *Mycobacterium bovis* in calves vaccinated with a low dose of BCG. *Vaccine* 13:1123-30.
11. Cai, H., X. Tian, X. D. Hu, Y. H. Zhuang, and Y. X. Zhu. 2004. Combined DNA vaccines formulated in DDA enhance protective immunity against tuberculosis. *DNA Cell Biol* 23:450-6.
12. Carleton, P. 1993. Respiratory tuberculosis, p. 493-502. *In* K. V. F. Jubb (ed.), Pathology of Domestic Animals. Orlando, FL: Academic Press.
13. Clements, C. J., G. Larsen, and L. Jodar. 2004. Technologies that make administration of vaccines safer. *Vaccine* 22:2054-8.
14. Colditz, G. A., T. F. Brewer, C. S. Berkey, M. E. Wilson, E. Burdick, H. V. Fineberg, and F. Mosteller. 1994. Efficacy of BCG vaccine in the prevention of tuberculosis. Meta-analysis of the published literature. *JAMA* 271:698-702.
15. Cole, S. T., R. Brosch, J. Parkhill, T. Garnier, C. Churcher, D. Harris, S. V. Gordon, K. Eiglmeier, S. Gas, C. E. Barry, 3rd, F. Tekaia, K. Badcock, D. Basham, D. Brown, T. Chillingworth, R. Connor, R. Davies, K. Devlin, T. Feltwell, S. Gentles, N. Hamlin, S. Holroyd, T. Hornsby, K. Jagels, B. G. Barrell, et al. 1998. Deciphering the biology of *Mycobacterium tuberculosis* from the complete genome sequence. *Nature* 393:537-44.
16. Cui, Z., and R. J. Mumper. 2003. Microparticles and nanoparticles as delivery systems for DNA vaccines. *Crit Rev Ther Drug Carrier Syst* 20:103-37.

17. Dai, W., H. Huang, Y. Yuan, J. Hu, and Y. Huangfu. 2001. Comparative study on the immunogenicity between Hsp70 DNA vaccine and Hsp65 DNA vaccine in human *Mycobacterium tuberculosis*. *J Tongji Med Univ* 21:181-3.

18. Dai, W., L. Liang, H. Gao, H. Huang, Z. Chen, J. Cheng, and Y. Huangfu. 2004. Construction, expression and identification of a recombinant BCG vaccine encoding human *Mycobacterium tuberculosis* heat shock protein 65. *J Huazhong Univ Sci Technolog Med Sci* 24:107-11, 123.

19. Daugelat, S., C. H. Ladel, and S. H. Kaufmann. 1995. Influence of mouse strain and vaccine viability on T-cell responses induced by *Mycobacterium bovis* bacillus Calmette-Guerin. *Infect Immun* 63:2033-40.

20. De Groot, A. S., A. Bosma, N. Chinai, J. Frost, B. M. Jesdale, M. A. Gonzalez, W. Martin, and C. Saint-Aubin. 2001. From genome to vaccine: in silico predictions, ex vivo verification. *Vaccine* 19:4385-95.

21. Delogu, G., A. Li, C. Repique, F. Collins, and S. L. Morris. 2002. DNA vaccine combinations expressing either tissue plasminogen activator signal sequence fusion proteins or ubiquitin-conjugated antigens induce sustained protective immunity in a mouse model of pulmonary tuberculosis. *Infect Immun* 70:292-302.

22. Derrick, S. C., C. Repique, P. Snoy, A. L. Yang, and S. Morris. 2004. Immunization with a DNA vaccine cocktail protects mice lacking CD4 cells against an aerogenic infection with Mycobacterium tuberculosis. *Infect Immun* 72:1685-92.

23. D'Souza, S., V. Rosseels, O. Denis, A. Tanghe, N. De Smet, F. Jurion, K. Palfliet, N. Castiglioni, A. Vanonckelen, C. Wheeler, and K. Huygen. 2002. Improved tuberculosis DNA vaccines by formulation in cationic lipids. *Infect Immun* 70:3681-8.

24. Dubensky, T. W., B. A. Campbell, and L. P. Villarreal. 1984. Direct transfection of viral and plasmid DNA into the liver or spleen of mice. *Proc Natl Acad Sci USA* 81:7529-33.

25. Elanschezhiyan, M., K. L. Karem, and B. T. Rouse. 1997. DNA vaccines—a modern gimmick or a boon to vaccinology? *Crit Rev Immunol* 17:139-154.

26. Fleischmann, R. D., D. Alland, J. A. Eisen, L. Carpenter, O. White, J. Peterson, R. DeBoy, R. Dodson, M. Gwinn, D. Haft, E. Hickey, J. F. Kolonay, W. C. Nelson, L. A. Umayam, M. Ermolaeva, S. L. Salzberg, A. Delcher, T. Utterback, J. Weidman, H. Khouri, J. Gill, A. Mikula, W. Bishai, W. R. Jacobs Jr., J. C. Venter, and C. M. Fraser. 2002. Whole-genome comparison of *Mycobacterium tuberculosis* clinical and laboratory strains. *J Bacteriol* 184:5479-90.

27. Garcia-Pelayo, M. C., K. C. Caimi, J. K. Inwald, J. Hinds, F. Bigi, M. I. Romano, D. van Soolingen, R. G. Hewinson, A. Cataldi, and S. V. Gordon. 2004. Microarray analysis of *Mycobacterium microti* reveals deletion of genes encoding PE-PPE proteins and ESAT-6 family antigens. *Tuberculosis (Edinb)* 84:159-66.

28. Garnier, T., K. Eiglmeier, J. C. Camus, N. Medina, H. Mansoor, M. Pryor, S. Duthoy, S. Grondin, C. Lacroix, C. Monsempe, S. Simon, B. Harris, R. Atkin, J. Doggett, R. Mayes, L. Keating, P. R. Wheeler, J. Parkhill, B. G. Barrell, S. T. Cole, S. V. Gordon, and R. G. Hewinson. 2003. The complete genome sequence of *Mycobacterium bovis*. *Proc Natl Acad Sci USA* 100:7877-82.

29. Ha, S. J., B. Y. Jeon, J. I. Youn, S. C. Kim, S. N. Cho, and Y. C. Sung. 2005. Protective effect of DNA vaccine during chemotherapy on reactivation and reinfection of *Mycobacterium tuberculosis*. *Gene Ther.* 12:634-8

30. Hemmi, H., O. Takeuchi, T. Kawai, T. Kaisho, S. Sato, H. Sanjo, M. Matsumoto, K. Hoshino, H. Wagner, K. Takeda, and S. Akira. 2000. A Toll-like receptor recognizes bacterial DNA. *Nature* 408:740-5.

31. Horwitz, M. A., B. W. Lee, B. J. Dillon, and G. Harth. 1995. Protective immunity against tuberculosis induced by vaccination with major extracellular proteins of *Mycobacterium tuberculosis*. *Proc Natl Acad Sci USA* 92:1530-4.

32. Hovav, A. H., J. Mullerad, L. Davidovitch, Y. Fishman, F. Bigi, A. Cataldi, and H. Bercovier. 2003. The *Mycobacterium tuberculosis* recombinant 27-kilodalton lipoprotein induces a strong Th1-type immune response deleterious to protection. *Infect Immun* 71:3146-54.

33. Ivey, F. D., D. M. Magee, M. D. Woitaske, S. A. Johnston, and R. A. Cox. 2003. Identification of a protective antigen of Coccidioides immitis by expression library immunization. *Vaccine* 21:4359-67.

34. Johnston, S. A., and M. A. Barry. 1997. Genetic to genomic vaccination. *Vaccine* 15: 808-9.

35. Kim, T. W., C. F. Hung, D. Boyd, J. Juang, L. He, J. W. Kim, J. M. Hardwick, and T. C. Wu. 2003. Enhancing DNA vaccine potency by combining a strategy to prolong dendritic cell life with intracellular targeting strategies. *J Immunol* 171:2970-6.

36. Krieg, A. M., A. K. Yi, S. Matson, T. J. Waldschmidt, G. A. Bishop, R. Teasdale, G. A. Koretzky, and D. M. Klinman. 1995. CpG motifs in bacterial DNA trigger direct B-cell activation. *Nature* 374:546-9.

37. Kumar, H., D. Malhotra, S. Goswami, and R. N. Bamezai. 2003. How far have we reached in tuberculosis vaccine development? *Crit Rev Microbiol* 29:297-312.

38. Kumar, P., R. R. Amara, V. K. Challu, V. K. Chadda, and V. Satchidanandam. 2003. The Apa protein of *Mycobacterium tuberculosis* stimulates gamma interferon-secreting CD4+ and CD8+ T cells from purified protein derivative-positive individuals and affords protection in a guinea pig model. *Infect Immun* 71:1929-37.

39. Lagranderie, M. R., A. M. Balazuc, E. Deriaud, C. D. Leclerc, and M. Gheorghiu. 1996. Comparison of immune responses of mice immunized with five different *Mycobacterium bovis* BCG vaccine strains. *Infect Immun* 64:1-9.

40. Launois, P., R. DeLeys, M. N. Niang, A. Drowart, M. Andrien, P. Dierckx, J. L. Cartel, J. L. Sarthou, J. P. Van Vooren, and K. Huygen. 1994. T-cell-epitope mapping of the major secreted mycobacterial antigen Ag85A in tuberculosis and leprosy. *Infect Immun* 62:3679-87.

41. Lima, K. M., V. L. Bonato, L. H. Faccioli, I. T. Brandao, S. A. dos Santos, A. A. Coelho-Castelo, S. C. Leao, and C. L. Silva. 2001. Comparison of different delivery systems of vaccination for the induction of protection against tuberculosis in mice. *Vaccine* 19:3518-25.

42. Lima, K. M., S. A. dos Santos, J. M. Rodrigues, Jr., and C. L. Silva. 2004. Vaccine adjuvant: it makes the difference. *Vaccine* 22:2374-9.

43. Lima, K. M., S. A. dos Santos, R. R. Santos, I. T. Brandao, J. M. Rodrigues, Jr., and C. L. Silva. 2003. Efficacy of DNA-hsp65 vaccination for tuberculosis varies with method of DNA introduction in vivo. *Vaccine* 22:49-56.

44. Lima, K. M., S. A. Santos, V. M. Lima, A. A. Coelho-Castelo, J. M. Rodrigues, Jr., and C. L. Silva. 2003. Single dose of a vaccine based on DNA encoding mycobacterial hsp65 protein plus TDM-loaded PLGA microspheres protects mice against a virulent strain of *Mycobacterium tuberculosis*. *Gene Ther* 10:678-85.

45. Luo, X. D., D. Y. Zhu, Q. Chen, Y. Jiang, S. Jiang, and C. Yang. 2004. [A study of the protective effect of the DNA vaccine encoding tubercle antigen 85B with MPT64 in mice challenged with *Mycobacterium tuberculosis*]. *Zhonghua Jie He He Hu Xi Za Zhi* 27:611-6.

46. Lyashchenko, K., A. O. Whelan, R. Greenwald, J. M. Pollock, P. Andersen, R. G. Hewinson, and H. M. Vordermeier. 2004. Association of tuberculin-boosted antibody responses with pathology and cell-mediated immunity in cattle vaccinated with *Mycobacterium bovis* BCG and infected with *M. bovis*. *Infect Immun* 72:2462-7.

47. McMurray, D. N. 2003. Recent progress in the development and testing of vaccines against human tuberculosis. *Int J Parasitol* 33:547-54.

48. Miki, K., T. Nagata, T. Tanaka, Y. H. Kim, M. Uchijima, N. Ohara, S. Nakamura, M. Okada, and Y. Koide. 2004. Induction of protective cellular immunity against *Mycobacterium tuberculosis* by recombinant attenuated self-destructing *Listeria monocytogenes* strains harboring eukaryotic expression plasmids for antigen 85 complex and MPB/MPT51. *Infect Immun* 72:2014-21.
49. Milan, R., R. Alois, C. Josef, B. Jana, and W. Evzen. 2004. Recombinant protein and DNA vaccines derived from hsp60 *Trichophyton mentagrophytes* control the clinical course of trichophytosis in bovine species and guinea-pigs. *Mycoses* 47:407-17.
50. Minion, F. C., S. A. Menon, G. G. Mahairas, and M. J. Wannemuehler. 2003. Enhanced murine antigen-specific gamma interferon and immunoglobulin G2a responses by using mycobacterial ESAT-6 sequences in DNA vaccines. *Infect Immun* 71:2239-43.
51. Mollenkopf, H. J., G. Dietrich, J. Fensterle, L. Grode, K. D. Diehl, B. Knapp, M. Singh, D. T. O'Hagan, J. B. Ulmer, and S. H. Kaufmann. 2004. Enhanced protective efficacy of a tuberculosis DNA vaccine by adsorption onto cationic PLG microparticles. *Vaccine* 22:2690-5.
52. Morris, S., C. Kelley, A. Howard, Z. Li, and F. Collins. 2000. The immunogenicity of single and combination DNA vaccines against tuberculosis. *Vaccine* 18:2155-63.
53. O'Reilly, L. M., and C. J. Daborn. 1995. The epidemiology of *Mycobacterium bovis* infections in animals and man: a review. *Tuber Lung Dis* 76 Suppl 1:1-46.
54. Orenstein, W. A., M. Wharton, K. J. Bart, and A. R. Hinman. 2005. Immunization, p. 3557-3589. *In* G. L. Mandel, J. E. Bennett, and R. Dolin (ed.), Principles and Practice of Infectious Diseases. Philadelphia, PA: Churchill Livingstone.
55. Philipp, W. J., S. Nair, G. Guglielmi, M. Lagranderie, B. Gicquel, and S. T. Cole. 1996. Physical mapping of Mycobacterium bovis BCG pasteur reveals differences from the genome map of *Mycobacterium tuberculosis* H37Rv and from *M. bovis*. *Microbiology* 142(Pt 11):3135-45.
56. Pritchard, D. G. 1988. A century of bovine tuberculosis 1888-1988: conquest and controversy. *J Comp Pathol* 99:357-99.
57. Raviglione, M. C. 2003. The TB epidemic from 1992 to 2002. *Tuberculosis (Edinb)* 83:4-14.
58. Rojas, W., and L. E. Cano. 2004. Inmunizacion, p. 451-464. *In* Corporacion para Investigaciones Biologicas (ed.), Inmunologia, 13th ed. Medellin: Corporacion para Investigaciones Biologicas.
59. Skeiky, Y. A., M. R. Alderson, P. J. Ovendale, J. A. Guderian, L. Brandt, D. C. Dillon, A. Campos-Neto, Y. Lobet, W. Dalemans, I. M. Orme, and S. G. Reed. 2004. Differential immune responses and protective efficacy induced by components of a tuberculosis polyprotein vaccine, Mtb72F, delivered as naked DNA or recombinant protein. *J Immunol* 172:7618-28.
60. Skinner, M. A., B. M. Buddle, D. N. Wedlock, D. Keen, G. W. de Lisle, R. E. Tascon, J. C. Ferraz, D. B. Lowrie, P. J. Cockle, H. M. Vordermeier, and R. G. Hewinson. 2003. A DNA prime—*Mycobacterium bovis* BCG boost vaccination strategy for cattle induces protection against bovine tuberculosis. *Infect Immun* 71:4901-7.
61. Skinner, M. A., A. J. Ramsay, G. S. Buchan, D. L. Keen, C. Ranasinghe, L. Slobbe, D. M. Collins, G. W. de Lisle, and B. M. Buddle. 2003. A DNA prime-live vaccine boost strategy in mice can augment IFN-gamma responses to mycobacterial antigens but does not increase the protective efficacy of two attenuated strains of *Mycobacterium bovis* against bovine tuberculosis. *Immunology* 108:548-55.
62. Snider, D. E., Jr., and J. R. La Montagne. 1994. The neglected global tuberculosis problem: a report of the 1992 World Congress on Tuberculosis. *J Infect Dis* 169:1189-96.

63. Steele, J. H. 1995. Introduction (Part 2 Regional and Country Status Reports), p. 169-172. *In* C. O. Thoen and J. H. Steele (ed.), *Mycobacterium bovis* Infection in Animals and Humans. Ames: Iowa State University Press.

64. Sugawara, I., H. Yamada, T. Udagawa, and K. Huygen. 2003. Vaccination of guinea pigs with DNA encoding Ag85A by gene gun bombardment. *Tuberculosis* (Edinb) 83:331-7.

65. Tanghe, A., O. Denis, B. Lambrecht, V. Motte, T. van den Berg, and K. Huygen. 2000. Tuberculosis DNA vaccine encoding Ag85A is immunogenic and protective when administered by intramuscular needle injection but not by epidermal gene gun bombardment. *Infect Immun* 68:3854-60.

66. Tanghe, A., S. D'Souza, V. Rosseels, O. Denis, T. H. Ottenhoff, W. Dalemans, C. Wheeler, and K. Huygen. 2001. Improved immunogenicity and protective efficacy of a tuberculosis DNA vaccine encoding Ag85 by protein boosting. *Infect Immun* 69:3041-7.

67. Tanghe, A., P. Lefevre, O. Denis, S. D'Souza, M. Braibant, E. Lozes, M. Singh, D. Montgomery, J. Content, and K. Huygen. 1999. Immunogenicity and protective efficacy of tuberculosis DNA vaccines encoding putative phosphate transport receptors. *J Immunol* 162:1113-9.

68. Taracha, E. L., R. Bishop, A. J. Musoke, A. V. Hill, and S. C. Gilbert. 2003. Heterologous priming-boosting immunization of cattle with *Mycobacterium tuberculosis* 85A induces antigen-specific T-cell responses. *Infect Immun* 71:6906-14.

69. Tascon, R. E., M. J. Colston, S. Ragno, E. Stavropoulos, D. Gregory, and D. B. Lowrie. 1996. Vaccination against tuberculosis by DNA injection. *Nat Med* 2:888-92.

70. Taylor, J. L., O. C. Turner, R. J. Basaraba, J. T. Belisle, K. Huygen, and I. M. Orme. 2003. Pulmonary necrosis resulting from DNA vaccination against tuberculosis. *Infect Immun* 71:2192-8.

71. Tian, X., H. Cai, and Y. X. Zhu. 2004. Protection of mice with a divalent tuberculosis DNA vaccine encoding antigens Ag85B and MPT64. *Acta Biochim Biophys Sin (Shanghai)* 36:269-76.

72. Tollefsen, S., M. Vordermeier, I. Olsen, A. K. Storset, L. J. Reitan, D. Clifford, D. B. Lowrie, H. G. Wiker, K. Huygen, G. Hewinson, I. Mathiesen, and T. E. Tjelle. 2003. DNA injection in combination with electroporation: a novel method for vaccination of farmed ruminants. *Scand J Immunol* 57:229-38.

73. Trimble, C., C. T. Lin, C. F. Hung, S. Pai, J. Juang, L. He, M. Gillison, D. Pardoll, L. Wu, and T. C. Wu. 2003. Comparison of the CD8+ T cell responses and antitumor effects generated by DNA vaccine administered through gene gun, biojector, and syringe. *Vaccine* 21:4036-42.

74. van Soolingen, D., T. Hoogenboezem, P. E. de Haas, P. W. Hermans, M. A. Koedam, K. S. Teppema, P. J. Brennan, G. S. Besra, F. Portaels, J. Top, L. M. Schouls, and J. D. van Embden. 1997. A novel pathogenic taxon of the *Mycobacterium tuberculosis* complex, Canetti: characterization of an exceptional isolate from Africa. *Int J Syst Bacteriol* 47:1236-45.

75. Vordermeier, H. M., D. B. Lowrie, and R. G. Hewinson. 2003. Improved immunogenicity of DNA vaccination with mycobacterial HSP65 against bovine tuberculosis by protein boosting. *Vet Microbiol* 93:349-59.

76. Wang, Q. M., S. H. Sun, Z. L. Hu, M. Yin, C. J. Xiao, and J. C. Zhang. 2004. Improved immunogenicity of a tuberculosis DNA vaccine encoding ESAT6 by DNA priming and protein boosting. *Vaccine* 22:3622-7.

77. Wayne, L. G., and G. P. Kubica. 1986. The Mycobacteria, p. 1435-1457. *In* P. H. A. Sneath and J. G. Holt (ed.), Bergey's Manual of Systematic Bacteriology, vol. 2. Baltimore, MD: Williams & Wilkins.

78. Wedlock, D. N., M. A. Skinner, N. A. Parlane, H. M. Vordermeier, R. G. Hewinson, G. W. de Lisle, and B. M. Buddle. 2003. Vaccination with DNA vaccines encoding MPB70 or MPB83 or a MPB70 DNA prime-protein boost does not protect cattle against bovine tuberculosis. *Tuberculosis (Edinb)* 83:339-49.
79. Will, H., R. Cattaneo, H. G. Koch, G. Darai, H. Schaller, H. Schellekens, P. M. van Eerd, and F. Deinhardt. 1982. Cloned HBV DNA causes hepatitis in chimpanzees. *Nature* 299:740-2.
80. Wolff, J. A., R. W. Malone, P. Williams, W. Chong, G. Acsadi, A. Jani, and P. L. Felgner. 1990. Direct gene transfer into mouse muscle in vivo. *Science* 247:1465-8.
81. Xue, T., E. Stavropoulos, M. Yang, S. Ragno, M. Vordermeier, M. Chambers, G. Hewinson, D. B. Lowrie, M. J. Colston, and R. E. Tascon. 2004. RNA encoding the MPT83 antigen induces protective immune responses against Mycobacterium tuberculosis infection. *Infect Immun* 72:6324-9.

Chapter 29

Bovine Tuberculosis: Environmental Public Health Preparedness Considerations for the Future

D.A. Ashford, DVM, MPH, DSc, L. Voelker DVM, MPH, and J.H. Steele, DVM

In the United Kingdom, the incidence of bovine tuberculosis increased 10-fold between 1979 and 2000, and because "scientific analysis [had] recently identified significant TB threats that could lead to the spread of the disease in the United States and compromise international and domestic trade in U.S. animals and animal product," the Secretary of the U.S. Department of Agriculture declared an emergency funding allocation for *Mycobacterium bovis* surveillance and control programs in October 2000. Increases in autogenous incidence, decreases in pre-mortem testing of cattle, increased importation to the United States of human cases with increased travel, and globalization in general present public health with new preparedness challenges. We review the science surrounding transmission of this organism and general concerns for public health preparedness.

Bovine tuberculosis is primarily caused by *Mycobacterium bovis*. *M. bovis* is a member of the *Mycobacterium tuberculosis* complex of mycobacteria. The complex includes *M. tuberculosis*, *M. bovis*, *Mycobacterium africanum*, *Mycobacterium microti*, and *Mycobacterium canetti*. These are slowly growing, nonphotochromogenic, acid-fast bacilli. Infection of humans with any one these five mycobacteria can result in the disease termed tuberculosis. Regardless of which species in this complex is the cause of disease in humans, the resulting disease is indistinguishable clinically, radiologically, and pathologically. However, before bovine tuberculosis control programs, and in areas of the world where milk is still the primary vector for this *Mycobacterium*, *M. bovis* was and is more commonly associated with primary tuberculosis outside of the lung (extrapulmonary disease) (1,2). Before the control of bovine tuberculosis and pasteurization programs in Northern Europe, the majority of cases of *M. bovis* infection among humans were extrapulmonary, with the following organ systems being affected in decreasing order of frequency: lymph nodes, skin, skeletal, genitourinary, and central nervous (meningitis) (3–5).

Following exposure, development of disease in humans depends on the ability of the *Mycobacterium* to establish infection and grow within host cells, and there is some evidence that *M. bovis* does not establish itself in human beings as readily as *M. tuberculosis* (6). Following infection, *M. bovis* is phagocytized by macrophages and is carried to lymph nodes, parenchyma of the lung, and other sites. In the macrophage, the bacilli resist being killed through escaping the phagolysosome, blocking maturation and fusion of phagosomal compartments, limiting their differentiation into active vacuoles, and natural resistance to the oxidative burst (5). Thus, the bacilli are able to multiply, destroy phagocytes, and escape into intracellular spaces. This, in turn, stimulates the accumulation of other phagocytes creating the typical histopathological lesion of tuberculosis—the granuloma. These granulomas can continue to expand with new phagocytic cell infiltration, giant cell formation, and fibrosis, and eventually macroscopic lesions, known as tubercles, are formed. The resulting disease is known as tuberculosis. The incubation period can be weeks to decades.

Although the diagnosis of tuberculosis in humans is usually suspected on the basis of radiographic findings and microscopic examination of smears of sputum (or other secretions or tissues), using acid-fast or other stains, the identification of the specific etiological agent (as *M. bovis* or another mycobacteria) depends on the ability to culture the organism and identify any *Mycobacteria* that are isolated (7). Both culture and identification of these mycobacterial species are complicated, potentially dangerous, and require expertise that is uncommon in the developed world and is extremely rare in the developing world. Because identification of the infecting species has a minimal effect on management of the tuberculosis patient, there is little incentive from health care providers to identify the mycobacterial species associated with tuberculosis. In the United States, the current molecular probe diagnostic assay, which is routinely used for confirmation of suspected tuberculosis cases, does not distinguish among the species in the *M. tuberculosis* complex.

Because identification of the species of infecting mycobacteria among tuberculosis cases is difficult and not routine in most of the world, and because no specific serological or skin test exists, the precise incidence and prevalence of human disease caused by *M. bovis* is unknown. However, it is possible to estimate the burden of *M. bovis* infections among humans from existing data for tuberculosis incidence and some data regarding the proportion of tuberculosis caused by *M. bovis* in various parts of the world (8). In Europe and North America, it is estimated that *M. bovis* now makes up about 0.5%–1.0% of human tuberculosis cases (9–12). This is a reduction from before the 1960s, when *M. bovis* caused 5%–20% of tuberculosis cases (before intensification of bovine tuberculosis control programs; 6). In countries where bovine tuberculosis is still common and pasteurization of milk rare, it is estimated that 10%–15% of human cases of tuberculosis are caused by *M. bovis* infection. In South American countries such as Argentina, where the prevalence of infection in cattle may be higher than in North America or Northern Europe, but where milk is routinely pasteurized or boiled before consumption, *M. bovis* infection makes up 1%–6% of human tuberculosis cases (13,14).

In the last decade, worldwide, an estimated 9 million cases of tuberculosis occurred each year (approximately 10% among human immunodeficiency virus [HIV]–infected individuals), and an estimated 1.9 million people die each year of tuberculosis (15,16). From worldwide country and regional data indicating that 1%–15% of those cases may be caused by *M. bovis*, we can estimate an annual world incidence of between 90,000 and 1,350,000 cases of *M. bovis*–associated tuberculosis. The prevalence of bovine tuberculosis in the world has been recently reviewed (17).

Subpopulations at risk for *M. bovis* infection include any population consuming unpasteurized contaminated milk, abattoir workers, veterinarians, hunters, and HIV-infected or other immunologically compromised populations (6,18–22). Given that both HIV and *M. bovis* transmission are high in Africa, with 90% of the African population living in areas where neither pasteurization nor bovine tuberculosis programs occur and up to 1 in 10 adults are infected with HIV, the association between these two diseases is of particular concern for much of the African continent (20).

M. bovis is the cause of tuberculosis in a broad range of mammalian hosts including cattle and other ruminants, felids, canids, lagomorphs, porcids, camilids, cervids, and primates including humans (23–31). Maintenance of *M. bovis* is believed to be primarily related to ruminants; however, other species of animals have been shown to maintain infection from generation to generation (24–30). Unpasteurized contaminated milk (32) and other secretions or tissues from any of these species (but primarily from cattle) can serve as the source of infection for humans (6). Although *M. bovis* may survive in soil, on fomites, and in feces for days to months, depending on local environmental conditions and sunlight, soil is not considered an important source of infection for humans (but may be for cattle; 33).

M. bovis can enter human hosts through ingestion, inhalation, or direct contact with mucous membranes or broken skin. Milk is still regarded as the principal vehicle for transmission to humans in countries in which bovine tuberculosis is not controlled, and ingestion of contaminated milk or other dairy products is more often associated with scrofula, abdominal tuberculosis, and other extrapulmonary forms of the disease (34,35). Among cattle, *M. bovis* is spread primarily by the respiratory route, and humans can also be infected by this route (21,22,35,36). Though considered uncommon, contact of broken skin with contaminated animal products can lead to cutaneous tuberculosis, also known as Butcher's or Prosector's wart (37). By any route, the infectious dose for humans is unknown but is estimated to be in the tens to hundreds of bacilli by the respiratory route, and in the millions by gastrointestinal route (2). On the basis of animal models and outbreak investigations, it is known that the infectious dose is influenced by the species of host (potentially higher for humans than cattle), other host factors (immune status, etc.), route of infection (higher for ingestion), and strain of bacteria (38).

Human-to-human transmission of *M. bovis* infection has been reported, but it is considered unlikely (3). One report of human-to-human transmission occurred among HIV-infected individuals in a hospital setting (39), and the HIV epidemic might increase the potential for human-to-human spread of *M. bovis*.

Changing Epidemiology

In the late 20th and early 21st centuries, in developed countries, bovine tuberculosis has reemerged among humans as an urban disease associated with immigration, as well as among relaxed cattle of bovine tuberculosis control programs (40). As trends in globalization continue, the importation of human cases of bovine tuberculosis from areas where the disease remains endemic in livestock and where milk pasteurization or heating may not be universally implemented may become an expanding risk. A similar reemergence of bovine-related tuberculosis has been observed for the southwestern United States (41,42). The incidence and prevalence of *M. bovis* infection in developing countries has been recently reviewed, and the infection remains common throughout the developing world (43). Surveillance information from developing countries is complicated by a lack of veterinary public health infrastructure, inability to distinguish *M. bovis* from other species using microscopy, limited availability of diagnostic reference laboratories for culture, and incomplete surveillance systems in general. Nonetheless, according to Cosivi et al., "Approximately 85% of cattle and 82% of the human population are in areas where bovine TB is either partly controlled or not controlled at all" (43). In Asia, 94% of the human population lives in countries where livestock tuberculosis is under no control or under limited control programs. In Latin America, country prevalence estimates range from 0.1% to 67% of total cattle populations, and 60% of the human population is estimated to live in areas in which cattle undergo no or limited control of bovine TB. High potential rates of contaminated animal products do not translate into a high risk alone if pasteurization, sanitation, and proper handling and cooking of meat are followed. Many developed countries still allow sales of unpasteurized milk. In most developing countries, consumption of raw milk remains common. In one study in Ethiopia, only 3% of the heads of households responded that they did not consume raw milk and milk products, and consumption of raw milk was associated with lower education (44). However, consumption of raw meat was found to be present among 9% of the respondents and did not differ significantly with education level. Forty-three percent of cattle in the same area were found to react to skin testing, and 25% of households reported having had tuberculosis among the family members. This is an example of a situation where closer study revealed a critical combination for the potential for high transmission of *M. bovis* to humans, but the degree to which *M. bovis* was contributing to the local human disease remained unknown.

In addition to this potential emerging threat of importation of human cases with increased global migration into areas of more intensive control of the bovine TB problem, such as North America and Europe, autogenous transmission continues on those continents as well. The increases in incidence among cattle in some of those countries may represent an increased risk in autogenous cases as well. In 1995, France estimated its incidence of *M. bovis* infection as 0.07/100,000, constituting about 0.5% of tuberculosis cases (45). In 1994, estimates for Australia were that *M. bovis* constituted 1.5% of annual TB cases (46). In some developed countries, there has been a resurgence of the disease in cattle. In the United Kingdom, for example, there were 1031 herds and 9000 livestock cases in 2000, compared with 89 herds and 600 cases in 1979. In the United Kingdom, this resurgence has resulted in locally acquired human infection from cattle as late as 2004, when a family was infected with *M. bovis*, and infected cattle were known to have been present on the farm tended by the family. Similar to underdeveloped parts of the world, developed countries also suffer from a lack of centralized capacity to distinguish the infecting mycobacterial species of human cases, and therefore, the true burden of *M. bovis* in the developed world also remains unclear. In 2004, almost 15,000 cases of human TB were reported to the Centers for Disease Control and Prevention. The number of those cases that were caused by *M. bovis* is unknown. Among cattle, the TB eradication program of the U.S. Department of Agriculture has nearly eliminated bovine TB from the United States; however, a few infected herds of cattle are reported each year in the United States, most often in the Texas, New Mexico, and Michigan milksheds, but in 2002 an infected herd was reported in California. The role of wildlife is incompletely studied and was accelerated in 1984 with the discovery of infected bison in 10 states, and one study of prevalence (by Lasher) indicates that the prevalence of TB among wild *cervidae* in the United States is much greater than expected (47). In 2004, there were 12 outbreaks of bovine TB among livestock, 52 cases reported to the OIE from the United States, compared to nine outbreaks and 26 cases in 1996. The numbers of outbreaks and cases among cattle vary from year to year in the United States for that period, with a high of 13 outbreaks in 2001 and 500 cases in 1998 (http://www.oie.int).

Is Meat a Threat?

With the resurgence in interest in bovine tuberculosis that has coincided with increasing incidence among livestock in the United Kingdom, the issue of transmission in meat has resurfaced. Tuberculosis lesions in bovine skeletal muscle of infected animals are rare. The lymph node, liver, spleen, and kidney may be positive on culture without lesions present. As an intracellular pathogen associated with the reticuloendothelial systems, it is possible for the organism to be present throughout the host at different times in acute and chronic infection. In general, the literature indicates that skeletal muscle is an infrequent source of *M. bovis*, when infected animals are examined postmortem by gross pathology and culture (48).

Environmental Considerations

M. bovis can survive for months in the open environment, particularly in cold, moist environments out of direct sunlight. *M. bovis* has been isolated for up to 8 weeks from various feeds kept at 75°F and 14 weeks from feeds kept at 32°F. One study in Australia for soil survival showed that survival in artificial environments mimicking the natural environment for Queensland was 4–8 weeks. *M. bovis* was not reisolated from any substrates held in sunlight or from fecal material at 4 weeks (the first sampling time after inoculation) (49).

In the infected carcasses of various mammalian species, *M. bovis* can survive for many weeks. Little et al. showed that *M. bovis* could survive for 2 weeks in the carcass of a tuberculous badger lying in a pasture in ambient conditions in the United Kingdom, and the organism survived for 6 weeks in an infected buffalo carcass in South African ambient conditions. (50,51)

Terrorism Planning

M. bovis could be considered a potential terrorist agent because of its potential for aerosol transmission and stability in the environment. Such a use could result in prejudicing livestock products of the affected country. Although it is unclear what the actual morbidity or mortality of such an attack on animals or human might be, it is critical to keep in mind that the anthrax attacks of 2001 demonstrated that the effect on society and government are to a large part independent of actual morbidity and mortality. In that case, 22 people were affected by the organism, among at least 10,000 exposed, and four people died. No animal cases of anthrax were discovered. All levels of government were involved in a multimillion dollar—if not billion dollar—response as a result. Scientists and public health practitioners should, at least in part, separate themselves from arguments of the effectiveness of an agent in causing morbidity and mortality if used in an attack and should consider the many other potential effects of the use of any particular agent. Outcomes such as the loss of trust and the disruption of local or national economies are not solely based on the "efficacy" of a pathogen chosen by the terrorist to cause harm. Those outcomes are equally rooted in the public's perceptions of the act itself as a terrorist act and in perceptions of risk following such an attack.

The effect of the disposal of carcasses on environmental contamination and as risks for human health should be considered in planning against the potential use of *M. bovis* by terrorists. According to the Pan American Health Organization, most zoonotic diseases do not survive in dead animals (52). Most carcass disposal methods will attenuate or eliminate the infectivity of most pathogens. However, because a terrorist pathogen may not behave in expected ways, the ecology of the specific organism of concern in relation to the conditions created by body decomposition and carcass disposal should be considered in each situation. The environmental health risk assessment is complicated by the fact that some pathogens can survive on body surfaces, in feces, and in the environment surrounding a dead carcass. In the case of agroterrorism, the resulting dead animals may represent a risk to human health. As such, public health practitioners should be familiar with zoonotic diseases present in their area. The terrorist agent that caused the death of the animals may not be the primary zoonosis of concern. Foot and mouth disease, for example, has limited transmission to and pathogenicity for humans but caused the culling of millions of animals in the United Kingdom.

During the 2001 Foot and Mouth Disease outbreak in the United Kingdom, no human cases of Foot and Mouth Disease were reported, but four animal workers contracted *Coxiella burnetti* infection (Q fever) from infected sheep (53). Zoonotic tuberculosis could be a concern for those handling animal carcasses, and it is very resistant to adverse environmental conditions, desiccation, and many disinfectants. Funeral directors, who are exposed to bodies but are not involved in opening cavities, have an increased risk of human tuberculosis (54). This indicates that tuberculosis transmission from intact bodies occurs, and the knowledge of the existing prevalence of *M. bovis* in potentially affected domestic and wild animal species would be of use in estimating the risk to first responders managing the carcasses following a terrorism attack.

In 2000, the Centers for Disease Control and Prevention categorized possible bioterrorist agents/biological toxins into categories A, B, and C on the basis of their threat to public health and national security. Category A agents were considered the highest risk. Though most category A, B, and C pathogens are zoonotic or cause disease in both man and animals, tuberculosis is not listed among them (http://www.cdc.gov/mmrr/preview/mmwrhtml/rr4904a1.html). The U.S. Department of Agriculture list, "High Consequence Livestock and Plant Pathogens and Toxins," can be found at http://www.aphis.usda.gov/programs/ag_selectagent/ag_bioterr_toxinslist.html.

The length of time of survival and infectiousness of *M. bovis* in animal tissue is not precisely known, but it is at least up to several weeks, and scavengers are susceptible to infection from infected carcasses (51,52,53). Infected carcasses should be considered potentially infectious if left on the surface or buried in landfills. Incineration and alkaline hydrolysis, an alternative method for treatment and disposal of infectious animal waste, have been shown to effectively eliminate *M. bovis* from contaminated carcasses (55,56).

It is of interest that approximately 2% of the U.S. feedlots produce 75% of the beef consumed in the United States (57). Although *M. bovis* is not seen as a high threat, its purposeful introduction into the livestock population in areas relatively free of the pathogen could cause a loss of confidence in animal products. Following such an attack, the risk analysis for livestock and humans would be complicated by several variables including a long incubation period, the difficulty of diagnosis, the gaps in data on consumption of unpasteurized milk products in the United States, the gaps in data on the risk from meat contaminated with the organism, and the potential roles of wildlife in spread or maintenance of new foci.

Effect on Control

Because the organism can infect nearly all warm-blooded animals, control strategies are complicated, as they must be for any such multihost zoonotic disease. Wild animals in nearly all affected nations may be infected and play another critical role in the local ecologies of disease. However, the role of wild animals is not clearly understood in most situations, and where the issue of the influence of one host on another is investigated, they are often found to be victims of cattle infection. In some countries, such as New Zealand, the host range may be limited enough (in that case, ferrets and brush tailed possums) for successful containment and control. However, empirical estimates of the individual contributions of these species to livestock infection are needed before any such control strategies could even be suggested.

In general, diseases such as bovine tuberculosis know no borders, and the problems of one country can quickly become the problems of the world. Improvement in international surveillance activities will depend on adequate international investment in improved testing and veterinary services for cattle in all countries. As this disease is primarily transmitted from cattle to humans in milk, human infection can be reduced with control of bovine tuberculosis and pasteurization. Testing of cattle with an intradermal tuberculosis test (or by inspection at slaughter), combined with removal or quarantine of infected herds and pasteurization of milk, has proven very effective in reducing the incidence of *M. bovis* infection in humans (23,24). It is important to keep in mind that humans have served as sources of infection for cattle on more than one occasion, and special consideration should be given to the potential role of human cases introducing new strains to nonendemic or controlled areas in which animals may be particularly susceptible, genetically, to them. Elimination is complicated by the several wild animal reservoirs of *M. bovis* present in most of the world, but practical elimination of human infection can be achieved with control programs targeting only domestic animals. Such control programs may seem simple, but they require political commitment, public agreement regarding the benefit, adequate public funding for what can be a very expensive disease control program, an extensive public or private veterinary infrastructure, organized meat inspection for identification and tracing of infected herds, availability and maintenance of skin-test antigen for identification of infected animals, and a centralized dairy industry that employs pasteurization or public education regarding the risks of unpasteurized dairy products. Without these requirements, as seen in much of the developing world, *M. bovis* will continue to be a common public health problem. Further study is needed regarding the role of meat and offal in local transmission in countries where raw or inadequately cooked meat and offal from infected herds are consumed.

References

1. Griffith, A. S. 1937. Bovine tuberculosis. *Vet Rec* 49, 982.
2. Mollers, B. 1928. Der M. tuberklbazillus. *In* Handbook of Pathogenesis Mikroorgznismen. Berlin: Kolle & Waserman, 827.
3. Francis, J. 1950. Control of infection with the bovine tubercle bacillus. *Lancet* 258:34-39.
4. Griffith, A. S. 1937. Bovine tuberculosis in man. *Tubercle* 18:529-543.
5. Schmiedel, A. 1968. Rapid decline in human tuberculosis and persistence of widespread tuberculosis of cattle. An unusual epidemiological situation and its consequences. *Bull Int Union Tuberc* 41:297-300.
6. Grange, J. M. 1995. Human aspects of *Mycobacterium bovis* infection. *In* C. O. Thoen & J. H. Steele (eds.), *Mycobacterium bovis* Infection in Animals and Humans. Ames: Iowa State University Press, 29-46.
7. Collins, C. H., J. M. Grange, and M. D. Yates. 1985. Organization and practice in tuberculosis bacteriology. London: Butterworths.
8. Kleeberg, H. H. 1984. Human tuberculosis of bovine origin in relation to public health. *Rev Sci Tech Off Int Epiz* 3:11-32.
9. Hardie, R. M. and J. M. Watson. 1992. *Mycobacterium bovis* in England and Wales: past, present and future. *Epidemiol Infect* 109:23-33.
10. Salfelder, T., T. Schliesser, and H. Jungbluth. 1983. Folgerungen aus dem derzeitigen Vorkommen von *Mycobacterium bovis* bei Mensch und Tier. *Fortschr Vet Med* 37:141-45.
11. Schliesser, T. 1986. Prevalence of *M. bovis* in man 20 years after eradication of bovine tuberculosis in cattle. *Bull Int Union Tubercul* 61:58-59.

12. Wigle W.D., Ashley M.J., Killough E.M., Cosens M. (1972). Bovine tuberculosis in humans in Ontario. *Am. Rev. Respir. Dis.*, 106:528-534.

13. De Kantor, I. N. and V. Ritacco. 1994. Bovine tuberculosis in Latin America and the Caribbean: current status, control, and eradication programs. *Vet Microbiol* 40:137-51.

14. Latini, M. S., O. A. Latini, M. L. Lopez, and J. O. Cecconi. 1990. Tuberculosis bovina en seres humanos. *Rev Argent Torax* 51:13-16.

15. Meslin, F.-X. and O. Cosivi. 1995. Introduction—World Health Organization. *In* C. O. Thoen and J. H. Steele (ed.). *Mycobacterium bovis* Infection in Animals and Humans. Iowa State University Press, Ames, Iowa, 3-14.

16. Navin, T. R., S. J. N. McNabb, and J. T. Crawford. 2002. The continued threat of tuberculosis. *Emerg Infect Dis* 8:1187.

17. Cosivi, O., J. M. Grange, C. J. Daborn, M. C. Raviglione, T. Fujikura, D. Cousins, R. A. Robinson, H. F. Huchzermeyer, I. de Kantor, and F.-X. 1998. Zoonotic tuberculosis due to *Mycobacterium bovis* in developing countries. *Emerg Infect Dis* 4:1-17.

18. Danker, W. M., N. J. Waecker, M. A. Essey, K. Moser, M. Thompson, and C. E. Davis. 1993. *Mycobacterium bovis* infections in San Diego: a clinico-epidemiologic study of 73 patients and a historical review of a forgotten pathogen. *Medicine* 72:11-37.

19. Dankner, W. M. and C. E. Davis. 2000. *Mycobacterium bovis* as a significant cause of tuberculosis in children residing along the United States–Mexico border in the Baja California region. *Pediatrics* 105:E79.

20. Grange, J. M., D. Daborn, and O. Cosivi. 1994. HIV-related tuberculosis due to *Mycobacterium bovis*. *Eur Respir J* 7:1564-6.

21. Liss, G. M., L. Wong, D. C. Kittle, A. Simor, M. Naus, P. Martiquet, and C. R. Misener. 1994. Occupational exposure to *Mycobacterium bovis* infection in deer and elk in Ontario. *R Can J Publ Hlth* 85:326-29.

22. Robinson, P., D. Morris, and R. Antic. 1988. *Mycobacterium bovis* as an occupational hazard in abattoir workers. *Aust NZ J Med* 18:701-3.

23. Barlow, A. M., K. A. Mitchell, and K. H. Visram. 1999. Bovine tuberculosis in Llama (*Lama glama*) in the UK. *Vet Rec* 145:639-40.

24. Bolske, G., L. Englund, H. Wahlstrom, G. W. de Lisle, D. M. Collins, and P. S. Croston. 1995. Bovine tuberculosis in Swedish deer farms: epidemiological investigations and tracing using restriction fragment analysis. *Vet Rec* 136:414-17.

25. Cheeseman, C. L., J. W. Wilsmith, and F. A. Stuart. 1989. Tuberculosis: the disease and epidemiology in the badger, a review. *Epidemiol Infect* 103:113-25.

26. Collins C. H. and J. M. Grange. 1987. Zoonotic implications of *Mycobacterium bovis* infection. *Irish Vet J* 41:363-66.

27. Cordes, D. O., J. A. Bullians, D. E. Lake, and M. E. Carter. 1981. Observations on tuberculosis caused by *Mycobacterium bovis* in sheep. *NZ Vet J* 29:60-62.

28. De Lisle G. W., K. Crews, J. de Zwart, et al. 1993. *Mycobacterium bovis* infections in wild ferrets. *NZ Vet J* 41:148-49.

29. Monies, R. J., M. P. Cranwell, N. Palmer, J. Inwald, and R. G. Hewinson. 2000. Bovine tuberculosis in domestic cats. *Vet Rec* 146:407-8.

30. Morris, R. S., D. U. Pfeiffer, and R. Jackson. 1994. The epidemiology of *Mycobacterium bovis* infections. *Vet Microbiol* 40:153-77.

31. Stumpf, C. D., M. A. Essey, D. H. Person, et al. 1984. Epidemiologic study of *M. bovis* in American bison. *Proc US Anim Health Assoc* 88:1.

32. Stahl, S. 1939. A tuberculosis epidemic caused by milk-borne infection. *Brit J Child Dis* 36:83-89.

33. Duffield, B. J. and D. A. Young. 1985. Survival of *Mycobacterium bovis* in defined environmental conditions. *Vet Microbiol* 10:193-97.

34. Ashford, D. A., E. S. Whitney, P. Raghunathan, and O. Cosivi. 2001. epidemiology of selected mycobacteria that infect humans and other animals. *Rev Sci Tech Off Int Epiz* 20:325-37.

35. Sigurdson, J. 1945. Studies on the risk of infection with bovine tuberculosis to the rural population. With special reference to pulmonary tuberculosis. *Acta Tuberc Scand* Suppl. XV:1-250.

36. Dalovisio, J. R., M. Stetter, and W. Mikoto-Wells. 1992. Rhinoceros, rhinorrhea: cause of an outbreak of infection due to airborne *Mycobacterium bovis* in zookeepers. *Clin Infect Dis* 15:598-600.

37. Grange, J. M., M. D. Yates, and C. H. Collins. 1988 inoculation mycobacterioris. *Clin Exp Dermatol* 13:211-20.

38. Skinner, M. A., D. N. Wedlock, and B. M. Buddle. 2001. Vaccination of animals against *Mycobacterium bovis*. *Rev Sci Tech Off Int Epiz* 20:112-32.

39. Guerrero, A., J. Cobo, J. Fortun, E. Navas, C. Quereda, A. Asensio, J. Canon, J. Blazquez, and E. Gomez-Mampaso. 1997. Nosocomial transmission of *Mycobacterium bovis* resistant to 11 drugs in people with advanced HIV-1 infection. *Lancet* 350:1738-42.

40. European Commision (2003). The Health Status of the European Union—Narrowing the Health Gap. Luxemburg: Office of Official Publications of the European Communitites, 58.

41. Dankner, W. and C. Davis. 2000. *Mycobacterium bovis* as a significant cause of tuberculosis in children residing along the United States–Mexico border in the Baja California region. *Pediatrics* 105:E79.

42. Dankner, W. M., N. J. Waecker, M. A. Essey, K. Moser, M. Thompson, and C. E. Davis. 1993. *Mycobacterium bovis* infections in San Diego: a clinicoepidemiologic study of 73 patients and a historical review of a forgotten pathogen. *Medicine* 72:11-37.

43. Cosivi, O., J. M. Grange, C. J. Daborn, M. C. Raviglione, T. Fujikura, D. Cousins, R. A. Robinson, H. F. Huchzermeyer, I. de Kantor, and F. X. Meslin. 1998. Zoonotic tuberculosis due to *Mycobacterium bovis* in developing countries. *Emerg Infect Dis* 4:59-70.

44. Ameni, G., K. Amenu, and M. Tibbo. 2003. Bovine tuberculosis: prevalence and risk factor assessment in cattle and cattle owners in Wuchale-Jida District, Central Ethiopia. *Int J Appl Res Vet Med* 1,

45. Robert, J., F. Boulahbal, D. Trystam, et al. A national survey of human *Mycobacterium bovis* infection in France. *Int J Tuberc Lung Dis* 3:711-14.

46. Cousins, D. V. and D. J. Dawson. 1999. Tuberculosis due to *Mycobacterium bovis* in the Australian population: cases recorded during 1970-1994. *Int J Tuberc Lung Dis* 3:715-21.

47. Lasher, G. 2002. Department of community health confirms human case of bovine TB. Available at: http://www.bovinetb.com.

48. Drieux, H. 1984. Post-mortem inspection and judgement of tuberculosis carcasses. *In* Meat Hygiene. Food and Agricultural Organisation of the United Nations. Geneva: Switzerland, 195-215.

49. Buffield B. J. and D. A. Young. 1985. *Mycobacterium bovis* in defined environmental conditions. *Vet Microbiol* 10:193-97.

50. Little, T. W. A., P. F. Naylor, and J. W. Wilesmith. 1982. Laboratory study of *Mycobacterium bovis* infection in badgers and calves. *Vet Rec* 111:550-57.

51. Tweddle, N. E. and P. Livingstone. 1994. Bovine tuberculosis control and eradiation programs in Australia and New Zealand. *Vet Microbiol* 40:23-29.

52. Pan American Health Organization. 2004. Management of dead bodies in disaster situations. Washington, DC: Pan American Health Organization.

53. UK Public Health Laboratory Service. (2001). Foot and mouth disease: disposal of carcasses. Third report on results of monitoring public health. Available at: http://www.hpa.org.uk/infections/topics_az/footmouth/FMD-Results%20of%20Monitoring3.pdf.

54. Centers for Disease Control and Prevention. 2004. Medical examiners, coroners, and biologic terrorism. *Morb Mortal Wkly Rep* 53:1-27.

55. Wisconsin Department of Natural Resources. 2002. An analysis of risks associated with disposal of deer from Wisconsin in municipal solid waste landfills. Available at: http://www.whitetailsunlimited.com/pages/cwd/risk_analysis.pdf.

56. Kaye, G. I., P. B. Weber, A. Evans, and R. A. Venezia. Efficacy of alkaline hydrolysis as an alternative method for treatment and disposal of infectious animal waste. *Contemporary Topics Lab Anim Sci* 37:43-46.

57. Breeze, R. 2004. Agroterrorism: betting far more than the farm. *Biosecurity Bioterrorism Biodefense Strategy Pract Sci* 2:1-14.

Index